PREGNANCY,
BIRTH
AND ABORTION

PREGNANCY, BIRTH AND ABORTION

PAUL H. GEBHARD

WARDELL B. POMEROY

CLYDE E. MARTIN

CORNELIA V. CHRISTENSON

of the
Institute for Sex Research, Inc.
Founded by Alfred C. Kinsey
Indiana University
Bloomington, Indiana

GREENWOOD PRESS, PUBLISHERS
WESTPORT, CONNECTICUT

Library of Congress Cataloging in Publication Data

Indiana. University. Institute for Sex Research.
   Pregnancy, birth, and abortion.

   Reprint of the ed. published by Harper, New York.
   Bibliography: p.
   Includes index.
   1. Pregnancy. 2. Abortion--United States.
3. Sex research. I. Gebhard, Paul H. II. Title.
[DNLM: 1. Abortion, Induced. 2. Illegitimacy.
3. Sex behavior. HQ18.U5 I39p 1958a]
[HQ767.5.U5I54 1976]   301   75-37383
ISBN 0-8371-8663-3

Originally published in 1958 by Harper & Brothers, Publishers
and Paul B. Hoeber, Inc., Medical Books, New York

Reprinted with the permission of Harper & Row, Publishers, Inc.

Reprinted in 1976 by Greenwood Press, Inc.
51 Riverside Avenue, Westport, Connecticut 06880

Library of Congress catalog card number 75-37383
ISBN 0-8371-8663-3

Printed in the United States of America

10 9 8 7 6 5 4 3 2

To

ALFRED CHARLES KINSEY
1894–1956

Scientist and Teacher
Pioneer in studies of human sexual behavior
Founder of the Institute for Sex Research

CONTENTS

Tables and Figures are listed under the appropriate headings in the Index.

INTRODUCTION

The Institute for Sex Research, founded by the late Dr. Alfred C. Kinsey and located at Indiana University, Bloomington, Indiana, is a nonprofit scientific research organization devoted to the study of human sexual behavior. The primary purpose of the Institute is to secure data on all aspects of human sexual behavior that lend themselves to scientific investigation, to analyze the data, and to make the findings available for others to use.

The research began in 1938, and a corporate organization to carry it on was formed in 1947. During the history of the research it has been continuously supported in part by Indiana University and, for various periods, by the Medical Division of the Rockefeller Foundation, the National Research Council, and the United States Public Health Service. In addition, all book royalties and lecture fees have been used to continue the research program. The Institute is particularly indebted to Indiana University, its Board of Trustees, and its president, Dr. Herman B Wells, for the continuous support and encouragement given us.

The Institute has produced two major publications, *Sexual Behavior in the Human Male* (1948) and *Sexual Behavior in the Human Female* (1953). Both volumes dealt with sexual behavior per se; the reproductive consequences of a part of such behavior were scarcely touched upon since the Institute planned to publish on that subject at some future date as part of a projected series of studies. This omission may seem strange to those of purposivistic thought to whom sex and reproduction are essentially synonymous, but actually only one type of sexual behavior—that is, heterosexual coitus—can end in reproduction and only a small percentage of that type does so.

As a result of correspondence with Dr. Mary Steichen Calderone, the medical director of the Planned Parenthood Federation of America, which began in 1953, Dr. Kinsey took part in the Arden House Abortion Conference sponsored by the Planned Parenthood Federation and held at Harriman, New York, in 1955. There he was made keenly aware that the data he presented concerning conception and the outcome of conception were of primary and immediate importance to the participants of the conference and to many other persons. Consequently, it was decided to publish those particular data in the proceedings of the meeting, and that the Institute for Sex Research would prepare a more comprehensive study to be issued as a separate volume. It was realized that such a volume would contain information of unique social and scientific value.

This project, which has been financially supported by the Institute itself and by the National Research Council's Committee for Research in Problems of Sex, proved to be far more complex and time-consuming than had been anticipated. Numerous statistical problems arose, necessitating additional analyses and revisions, and for his guidance in preparing these we owe a great deal to Dr. Christopher Tietze. In the midst of this preliminary work the Institute lost its founder, which indirectly caused further delay.

At this point it is appropriate to add that the staff members of the Institute have always functioned as a team, jointly devoting their attention to the studies in hand. Consequently, a number of staff members who do not appear as authors of this volume deserve recognition for the important part they play in the research as a whole and, to varying degrees, in this particular study:

William Dellenback, Research Assistant, Photographic Studies
Alice Field, Trustee
Dorothea Funk, Secretary
Mary Louise Hare, Research Assistant, Library
Hedwig Leser, Research Assistant, Translator
Werner Manheim, Research Assistant, Translator
Henry Remak, Research Assistant, Translator
Theodore Torrey, Trustee
Mary Winther, Research Assistant

In connection with this book we are keenly aware of the limitations of our data necessarily resulting from the fact that sample size is a product of available time, personnel, and money, and that an interview must be kept within a reasonable time limit. With equal keenness we feel we have something of value to present. In the presentation we have tried to be forthright and to make available all relevant data, so that our findings may be evaluated and properly used. But human behavior is not simple, and any scientific description and analysis of it must be buttressed with detail and qualifications.

The specialized nature and restricted scope of this volume place it in sharp contrast to our two earlier books, but this break with precedent was not unplanned. We have always thought of the Institute as having a continuing research program, periodically publishing large volumes, small volumes, journal articles, and monographs, the form depending upon the phenomena being studied and the available data.

Our major contribution in this book concerns phenomena ordinarily concealed from, or not investigated by, persons collecting data on human reproductive behavior. Much is known about live birth within marriage; live birth outside marriage is difficult to conceal and a moderate amount is known of its prevalence. Spontaneous abortion has been studied, usually through clinic and hospital patients, and some knowledge exists of the prevalence of spontaneous abortion of pregnancies sufficiently advanced to require medical attention. However, despite much writing, estimating, and guessing, there have been very few factual data on conceptions among unmarried females and the prevalence of induced illegal abortion among both married and unmarried females in this country. It is precisely on these subjects that we can provide much needed, factual information.

While this and subsequent volumes cannot represent writing and analyses done directly by Dr. Kinsey, it should be obvious that they owe their existence to him. Our future publications will stem from a research organization that he founded, and for years many of the data utilized will be those that he personally accumulated. As the Institute for Sex Research continues to produce work of value, the debt science and society in general owe to Dr. Kinsey will continue to increase.

PREGNANCY,
BIRTH
AND ABORTION

Chapter 1

TERMS AND METHODS

The worth of any scientific endeavor depends largely upon the clarity of the terms used and the soundness of the methods. In this first chapter we shall be primarily concerned with definition and less concerned with justification; it is unprofitable to devote much space to arguments why one particular term or method was chosen over another. The reasons for our choices are in many cases self-evident, or become so later in the volume.

TERMS

TERMS RELATING TO REPRODUCTION

Here one must differentiate between capacity and performance and, unfortunately, no standard and universally accepted terminology exists. In general we have followed demographic practice and used the following terms:

Fecundity, fecund: capacity to conceive.

Sterility, sterile: incapacity to conceive.

Fertility, fertile: having conceived, having demonstrated fecundity.

Infertility, infertile: not having conceived.

Thus a female who had not had coitus or who had always employed contraceptives during her coitus would be termed infertile but probably fecund.

Conception: the fertilization of the egg (ovum) by the spermatozoa.

Pregnancy: the condition of having an embryo, at any stage of development, within the body.

Embryo: we use this term to describe the product of conception from the moment of conception throughout its intrauterine development. The old distinction between embryo and fetus serves no useful purpose.

Live birth: an embryo sufficiently developed to live outside the uterus and alive when separated from the mother even though it may die shortly thereafter. While a few five- or six-month-old embryos are born and survive, the vast majority of live births is of embryos aged seven months or older.

Spontaneous abortion: death of the embryo not preceded by (and presumably not the result of) any intentional act by the mother or another person. For example, if a woman were forced to climb a long flight of stairs to go to and from her apartment, and aborted presumably because of the exertion, this would be considered a spontaneous abortion. On the other hand, if this woman deliberately climbed stairs repeatedly with the hope of causing an abortion, this would be considered an induced abortion. Actually, however, this fine discrimination seldom arises: most spontaneous abortions are the result of some defect in the embryo or in its environment and are not the result of physical exertion by the mother. The woman in the example above who reported that she induced an abortion by stair climbing would probably have spontaneously aborted even if she had never climbed one step. A normal embryo in a reasonably healthy woman is extremely difficult to dislodge. *Contrary to general usage, we include under spontaneous abortion not only what are commonly called miscarriages (embryos that perish before they are developed enough to live outside the uterus) but also stillbirths (embryos developed enough to live outside the uterus but born dead).* Stillbirths constitute only a small proportion of total births, roughly 2 to 3 per cent; hence our spontaneous abortion figures are not seriously altered by their inclusion. To attempt to differentiate stillbirths from late miscarriages would be most difficult since our data were derived from interviews with women rather than with their physicians. It should be noted that our definitions of live birth and spontaneous abortion differ slightly from those of the World Health Organization.

Induced abortion: expulsion or removal of the embryo preceded by (and presumably the result of) some intentional act by the mother or another person before it had developed to a point where it could survive. In a few questionable cases, as where abortion follows the taking of some substance of dubious efficacy, we have felt justified in agreeing with the woman and considering the event an induced abortion: the intent was present, the substance may have played some part in the abortion, and had the abortion not occurred, the woman would probably have resorted to more effective means. The vast majority of induced abortions do not entail such problems of definition. We have not ordinarily differentiated between illegal and legal (therapeutic) abortions except in Chapter 8, since legal abortions are numerically so few and medical practices in the matter vary so widely.

Outcome: the ultimate result of conception in live birth, spontaneous abortion, or induced abortion. The term "outcome" is used synonymously with the word "termination." Neither of these words is entirely satisfactory; the one is too easily punned on, the other carries the implication that the pregnancy was intentionally ended.

Coital years: a coital year is ordinarily a twelve-month period during which coitus has been experienced at least once. For the unmarried we have considered as coital years the period of time between the age at which the post-pubescent individual first had coitus and the age at which she married or, if she never married, the age at which she was interviewed. The assumption that pre-marital coitus, once begun, continues at a rate of at least once a year was made necessary by practical considerations involved in calculations. Actually this assumption proves true in such a high proportion of cases that the error involved is not particularly significant. For the married, we considered coital years as synonymous with marital years, including periods of temporary physical separation. We excluded periods of time between a final formal or informal separation and subsequent divorce, and also periods of time following an alienation and separation that gave indications of becoming permanent.

Post-adolescent: we are concerned in this study only with females physiologically mature enough to be fecund, and in this connection we have used the term "post-adolescent" to denote a female who has developed pubic hair and begun menstruation. The adjective "post-pubescent" is more accurate, but we have retained the term "post-adolescent" in order to conform to the usage in our previous publications, where we always spoke of pre-adolescence rather than pre-pubescence.

TERMS RELATING TO SOCIAL PHENOMENA

Since this study of reproductive behavior is set in its social context, definition of the social terminology is necessary.

Single: neither married at the age concerned nor ever previously married. The term "unmarried" is used synonymously.

Pre-marital: the period before the first marriage, or the period before the interview if the person was single at the time of interview.

Married: persons were considered married if they were living with their spouses either in a legal marriage or in a common-law relationship that had existed continuously for at least one year. In the latter instance, both spouses had to consider themselves married, and live together openly as man and wife. If a legally married couple had been separated for several months or more, and one or both stated that he or she did not intend to resume their marriage, we considered the marriage ended even though a formal divorce had not been obtained.

Marital: that period during a marriage. Thus marital coitus is coitus with a spouse during marriage.

Ever-married: a term applied to people who have ever been married, regardless of their marital status at the time they were interviewed.

Previously married: not married at the time but having been married.

Post-marital: that period following the end of a marriage and before the contraction of another marriage, if any.

Extra-marital: this term is used to distinguish sexual behavior and its reproductive result, if any, between a married woman and a man not her husband.

S.D.W. or ever-S.D.W.: an abbreviation distinguishing persons who have ever been separated, divorced, or widowed, regardless of their marital status at interview. This group is usually compared with a group of women who had married once and were still married at the time of the interview.

Age at marriage: in our usage, this refers solely to the woman's age at the beginning of her first marriage.

Grade school (0-8): this term is applied to persons who did not go beyond the eighth grade (or its equivalent if their education was not formal). Girls still in grade school and who therefore may go beyond the eighth grade are excluded from this category unless we specifically state otherwise.

High school (9-12): this term is applied to women who completed the eighth grade (or its equivalent) and went into, but not beyond, high school (Grades 9-12). Again, girls still in high school are excluded from this category unless otherwise stipulated.

College (13-16): this term is applied to those who completed the twelfth grade (or its equivalent) and entered college but did not complete more than four years of college work (regardless of the actual number of years spent as a college student). Persons still in college at interview are kept in this category despite the fact that a few may go into postgraduate work.

Postgraduate (17+): this term is applied to those who completed four years of college work (or its equivalent), received an appropriate degree, and at least began postgraduate work.

Note regarding educational level: we have classified individuals on the basis of the highest grade that they entered, whereas the U.S. Census classifies on the basis of the highest grade completed. This difference in procedure does not, however, seriously affect comparisons of our data and census data.

Decade of birth: the ten-year period during which the subject was born. We have made the following categories: 1880-1889, 1890-1899, 1900-1909, 1910-1919, 1920-1929, although in some instances we have been forced to combine the two earliest decades.

Devout: this term is applied to persons who, at the time they were interviewed, appeared to be deeply religious. By this we mean that they accepted the tenets of the faith or denomination to which they belonged and were seriously attempting to govern their behavior accordingly. As primary criteria for arriving at this judgment we used regularity of attendance at church or synagogue and degree of active participation in activities sponsored by such institutions. With Roman Catholics we inquired about frequency of confession, and with Jews we inquired about the observance of holy days and dietary restrictions.

Inactive: this term is applied to those who, at the time they were interviewed, appeared to be relatively indifferent or even opposed to religion, and who never or rarely attended church or synagogue, and who never or rarely participated in religious activities sponsored by these institutions. The term "inactive" includes all atheists and most agnostics, but the bulk of the inactive consists of persons who hold some religious beliefs.

Moderately devout: this term is applied to those who came in between devout and inactive. This category unfortunately but inescapably includes a sizable proportion of persons who were emotionally and intellectually non-devout but who did participate to some degree in church or synagogue services and/or activities for social reasons or because of pressure exerted by a spouse or relatives.

Note regarding religious classification: this classification suffers from several defects, the first of which is the error introduced by forcing humans into only three degrees of devoutness. Also we realize that even within one of our categories there is a difference between the members of the different religions in the intensity of their devotion. This precludes combining into three categories, regardless of religious affiliation, all the devout, all the moderately devout, and all the religiously inactive. A more serious defect is that the woman was classified on the basis of her practice at the time of interview. Despite these defects, degree of devoutness as we have measured it has shown itself to be a potent factor in the present study.

Prison: in this volume we consider as a prison any public building for the confinement or safe custody of misdemeanants or felons or others committed by law to such an institution. Mental hospitals are excluded. When we refer to prison females or our prison sample, we refer solely to women who were in prison at the time they were interviewed.

Non-prison: this adjective denotes women who were not in prison at the time they were interviewed.

White: we are concerned with the social rather than the genetic aspects of race. Our use of the term "white" corresponds with that of the U.S. Census.

Negro: we have classed as Negro any female who considers herself gro and/or who is considered a Negro by the people with whom ~.. lives and associates. Again the definition is social rather than genetic.

METHODS

Our methods were to a large degree determined by the quantity and form of our raw data. It must be remembered that this particular piece of research is post facto: we did not set out to gather data specifically for a study of pregnancy and its outcome, we set out to gather data on sexual behavior; its reproductive results were accorded less attention. Consequently this particular piece of research might be described as a study of data peripheral to our main interests.

Of many possible statistical treatments only a few are feasible in view of the size of our sample. At many points it would be desirable to subdivide the sample simultaneously according to numerous criteria but this is frequently impossible. Since our subsamples are often small, we have thought it wise to make our presentation as simple statistically as possible. However, what at first glance seems simple is in actuality most complex. A reader must bear in mind not only the various limitations as defined for any particular table of statistics but also the qualifications we append. He must continually be aware, too, that some variables are interdependent and that many statistics are influenced by hidden variables which, because of sample size, we cannot isolate or hold constant. For example, our data on the use of contraceptives are not sufficiently detailed to permit us to make allowance for the factor of contraception; hence our study is one of reproductive behavior rather than reproductive capacity.

While we have sought for simplicity we also realize that simplification can be distortion. Therefore we have not smoothed out fluctuations and inconsistencies. Measures of statistical significance and expected variation have not been employed. The nature of our data makes such measures meaningless, since they are appropriate only to a probability sample, which ours is not.

We feel that our results are useful. Our only fear is that some readers will, in spite of reiterated warnings and qualifications, misinterpret what we present.

In a study of this sort we are, basically, concerned with discovering how often a particular phenomenon occurs among a particular group of individuals, and with drawing inferences about the group from that discovery. We want to find out what happens, how often it happens, to whom it happens, and in what circumstances it happens. To answer these questions we have used several types of statistical measurement, which are described below.

Whatever our measurements, they must ordinarily take into account the age of the females involved. To say that a certain percentage of females has induced abortions is meaningless unless we know whether the percentage refers to teen-age girls, to women in their twenties, or to the experience of a lifetime. Thus in addition to being concerned with what happens we must be concerned with when it happens. In dealing with age or any other expression of time, we have taken one year as the minimal unit. The beginning rather than the mid-point of the year has been used: for example, we treat a female who married at the age of twenty-one as having been married on her twenty-first birthday. Our next largest unit for expressing time and age is a five-year period. Whereas U.S. Census and various studies use a quinquennial year as the initial year for their five-year periods (e.g., 20-24, 25-29), we have always used the quinquennial year as the terminal year for the five-year periods (e.g., 21-25, 26-30). Since our interviewing methods and all our statistics have followed this usage, it is impractical at this stage to change.

We have four basic measurements that we have applied in this study, each of which measures our data in a different way. However, we did not use all four measurements in every instance; in certain instances it was impossible or inappropriate to employ one or another of them.

1. **Accumulative experience.** This measurement shows what percentage of post-adolescent females in our sample has had a particular type of experience by a given age. This is the question most commonly asked by the public, usually phrased as, "How many married women *ever* have an abortion?" or "How many girls get pregnant before they marry?" While the concept of accumulative experience is simple enough, some explanation of how we arrived at the measurement is in order. Let us assume we are interested in determining the percentage of females who have experienced a pre-marital pregnancy by age twenty. Obviously we can use only females who have completed their twentieth year of life. We take the number of women aged twenty-one and over who experienced a pre-marital pregnancy before age twenty-one; dividing this number by the total number of women who had reached age twenty-one, the percentage is obtained. Repeating this process, calculating for successive ages, one would logically expect the percentages to show a continued increase. However, one finds that they sometimes decrease, especially at age forty and older. This decrease simply means that the people on whom we calculated our percentage for age forty, for example, had had experience different from that of the people on whom we calculated our percentages for younger ages. An example can make this clearer: let us assume

we are calculating what percentage of women has ever voted before marriage. Our percentages, starting with the youngest voting age, twenty-one, would successively increase until perhaps age fifty; then we would find the percentages dropping and finally by around age seventy reaching nearly zero. The reason for this decline is obvious: the women around age seventy and older had nearly all married before women were allowed to vote; the women in their fifties and sixties were, during their marriageable years, still in an era when relatively few women did vote. This illustration is not precisely comparable to our material, since one may assume that pre-marital coitus and its consequences have existed always, but it does show how variation in the sample by age-periods can influence accumulative experience percentages. Lastly, of course, small subsamples can also cause variations.

In our tables any figure derived from a sample of fewer than 50 females is italicized, and the number constituting the sample (the N) is also italicized. Where the number of females involved is considerably fewer than 50 a figure is ordinarily not given. This same procedure also applies to accumulative rate.

2. **Accumulative rate.** While the preceding measurement tells us what percentage of women in our sample had a particular type of experience up to a given age, we need to know how *often* they had that experience. Accumulative rate is expressed in terms of per hundred post-adolescent females; thus, for example, a pre-marital accumulative conception rate of 15 by age thirty would mean that every hundred women completing age thirty had experienced 15 pre-marital pregnancies. This accumulative rate does not tell us when these pregnanies took place—only that they occurred before age thirty-one. Like accumulated experience, and for the same reasons, accumulative rates can be less at older ages than at younger ages.

3. **Age-specific rate.** This is the rate at which post-adolescent females had a particular experience within given age-periods, for instance 16-20, 21-25, and so on. The rate is variously expressed in terms of rate per hundred pre-marital years lived, or per hundred pre-marital coital years (years in each of which coitus presumably occurred at least once), or per hundred marital years (presumed to be coital years), or per hundred post-adolescent years lived. Thus, for instance, a marital pregnancy rate of 24 per hundred marital years would mean that for every hundred years of marriage, 24 marital pregnancies resulted. This calculation can also tell us approximately the number of women involved. For example, within age-period 21-25 the marital conception rate of 24 also means that in any single year of the age-

period an average of 24 per cent of the married women conceived. This inference can be drawn by assuming, legitimately, that an insignificant number of women conceive twice within one year—in brief, we assume that in any single year one female had only one pregnancy. Although our age-periods are five-year periods, one must not multiply by five the percentage of women who conceived in any one year with the expectation of obtaining the percentage who conceived within the five-year period. This cannot be done because a considerable number of married women have more than one conception within a five-year period. In a few instances where figures for five-year age-periods could not be computed because of smallness of sample, we have used what may be considered an age-limited rate. Such a rate is expressed in terms of per hundred years for females ranging in age from adolescence to forty-five.

For married women, this measurement is based solely upon first marriages. The reason for this is the complexities involved in attempting to take into account multiple marriages.

While in the foregoing descriptions and discussions of experience and rate we have referred only to conception, it should be understood that we have also similarly calculated experience and rate of live birth, spontaneous abortion, and induced abortion.

In our tables any figure derived from less than 250 coital or marital years is italicized. Ordinarily no figure derived from less than 200 coital or marital years is expressed.

4. **Outcome ratios.** This measurement is concerned with the relative proportions of each of the three possible terminations of pregnancy: live birth, spontaneous abortion, and induced abortion. We excluded from this statistic the few pregnancies among females who were pregnant when interviewed. In certain instances, as when studying outcome among the unmarried, we added a fourth outcome that has sociological implications—outcome in subsequent marriage. From a social point of view, the interest is in what the pregnant unmarried female does—does she bear an illegitimate child, or does she abort, or does she get married?

Two types of outcome ratios have been employed:

a. The outcome ratio regardless of age at the time of the outcome. This is an over-all measurement useful in formulating generalizations and in cases where sample size precludes age-specific outcome ratio.

b. Age-specific outcome ratios. These represent the proportions of live birth, spontaneous abortion, and induced abortion within a given five-year age-period such as 16-20, 21-25, and so on. In our tables any figure derived from fewer than 50 conceptions or terminations is italicized. If there were considerably fewer than 50 conceptions or terminations, ordinarily no figure is expressed.

Note regarding tables. If data are inapplicable, this is shown by three dots. If a quantity is nil, this is expressed by 0. A quantity more than zero but less than 0.05 is indicated by 0.0. All percentages and rates have been rounded to one decimal place.

Chapter 2

THE SAMPLE

The data presented in the main body of this study represent a portion of the information secured from 5,293 white non-prison females who contributed their case histories to our study of human sexual behavior.[1] In addition, and described separately in Chapter 6, are data derived from 572 Negro non-prison females plus 309 Negro women interviewed in prison, and 900 white women interviewed in prison. These data on women with prison experience seem to have no precedent in the literature.

All of these females provided information on coitus, conception, and the termination of conception during their life spans and in various marital statuses. Those who had experienced induced abortion provided data as to method, agent, cost, and sequelae.

This study of reproduction is greatly enhanced by being a part of a study of total sexual behavior: we have at our disposal many relevant data concerning pre-marital coitus, marital coitus, extra-marital coitus, post-marital coitus, coital frequency, common-law marriages, informal separations, and many other items not incorporated in other demographic studies. On the other hand, we do not have systematically gathered data on attitudes and motives concerning conception and type of outcome. However, attitudes and motives may be inferred to a considerable extent from overt behavior.

This study also has the advantage of being based upon personal and confidential interviews. We have described our interview in our previous volumes (1948:35-70; 1953:58-64), but some salient features should be repeated here. The data were recorded, in code, during the interview. Thus any confusion about the point of the question or any ambiguity in the answer could be corrected as it arose. Furthermore, our reputation for keeping personal information confidential, our training in establishing rapport, and the hard-won ability to obtain the truth in those few instances where deception was attempted, all combined to result in our obtaining factual material that could not have been

---

[1] Females interviewed as patients in sterility clinics and interviewed in homes for unmarried mothers and detention homes are excluded from all groups considered in this volume.

11

obtained through the use of questionnaires. Nor could it have been obtained by interviewers who limited themselves solely to questions of reproductive behavior. One other technique has facilitated our gathering of information: we do not pass judgment upon an individual's behavior nor do we attempt to modify it. This true objectivity is sensed by the person interviewed and makes much easier the admission of socially disapproved behavior. For many the interview provided an opportunity to put into words experiences that they had previously been unable to discuss with others; this could not occur in a questionnaire study—one cannot establish rapport with a piece of paper.

In discussing interviewing the question soon arises: How valid are the reported data? While we dealt with reliability and validity in our previous volumes, we have devised a test of validity specifically for this study.

COMPARISON OF DATA FROM PAIRED SPOUSES

One test of the validity of data on the number and type of outcome of pregnancies is the analysis of reports from 586 white, paired spouses.

Table 1. Comparison of Data: Number of Spouses Reporting on Occurrence of Spontaneous and Induced Abortions in Marriage

For 586 Paired Spouses

Number reported by husband	NUMBER OF SPOUSES REPORTING ON SPONTANEOUS ABORTION							NUMBER OF SPOUSES REPORTING ON INDUCED ABORTION						
	Number reported by wife						Total husbands reporting	Number reported by wife						Total husbands reporting
	0	1	2	3	4	5+		0	1	2	3	4	5+	
0	483	5	2	0	0	0	490	518	8	0	0	0	1*	527
1	7	48	8	2	0	0	65	7	33	2	0	0	0	42
2	3	5	11	1	0	0	20	1	1	6	3	0	0	11
3	0	0	2	4	0	0	6	0	1	1	1	1	1	5
4	0	0	0	0	1	0	1	0	0	0	0	0	0	0
5+	0	0	0	0	0	4	4	0	0	1†	0	0	0	1
Total wives reporting	493	58	23	7	1	4	586	526	43	10	4	1	2	586

Bold face figures indicate agreement as to number and type of termination reported by husband and wife.

*One husband reported no induced abortions whereas his wife reported 8.

†One husband reported 6 induced abortions whereas his wife reported 2.

Concerning live birth, 99.8 per cent of the reports of the spouses were in agreement; for spontaneous abortion, 94.0 per cent; and for induced abortion, 95.2 per cent. In summary, 90.3 per cent were in complete agreement about the number of pregnancies and their outcome. One woman reported a birth that was not her husband's child although he believed it to be. Sixteen wives reported 24 induced abortions and 18 wives reported 22 spontaneous abortions that their husbands did not report, whereas 12 husbands reported 17 induced abortions and 17 husbands reported 20 spontaneous abortions that their wives did not report. In several cases the wife reported the termination as an induced abortion, whereas the husband had been led to believe the abortion was spontaneous. The greater number of induced abortions reported by the husbands may be interpreted to mean some evasion by their wives. Hence, the induced abortion figures reported by the females may be assumed to be somewhat too low.

Because of the very considerable agreement between spouses in their reporting on these items we believe that the validity of the histories in our total sample concerning marital pregnancy and its outcome is of a high degree.

We have other indications of validity that will be presented later in the book. Comparisons have been made, usually in the form of footnotes, with the findings of other studies, and census data have been similarly utilized (see Tables 4 to 7). Lastly, the internal consistency of our material suggests a high degree of validity.

Obviously our data are based upon recall. In the case of live birth and induced abortion this presents no problem: it is unlikely that a woman would forget either event. In the case of spontaneous abortion, memory is more fallible, but this defect is minor compared with the more serious problem of whether females correctly identify early spontaneous abortions.

In summary, we feel that our data and findings are sound enough to permit their use, within the limitations imposed by our sample, by anyone concerned with the study of human reproduction.

SOURCES OF THE SAMPLE

In our previous publications there are detailed discussions of our method of collecting data (1948:11-16, 102-104; 1953:22-38), and consequently a brief description must suffice here. We obtained our case histories primarily through working with groups; some were formally organized, such as Parent-Teacher Association groups, while others were informal, such as groups of business associates and friends. Our aim was to choose a definable group and obtain interviews from all or a high proportion of its members, thereby avoiding selective bias within the group. Over 85 per cent of our sample was derived from such groups. In choosing groups we tried to diversify our sample in order to reach individuals in many walks of life. While this method cannot substitute for random sampling, and while we necessarily took the opportunities that arose, we have accumulated a large body of case histories, the analyses of which permit one to draw inferences about larger segments of the population, even though the sample as a whole is not representative of any particular universe. Comparison of our sample data and census data will be made later in this chapter.

The majority of the groups was, almost necessarily, made up of persons who had some interest in, and comprehended the value of, sex research: teachers, students, P.T.A. members, women's clubs, civic organizations, social workers, and the staffs of hospitals and clinics. We were also able to secure case histories from church groups, groups of friends, individual housewives, unions, business offices, and so forth, but these groups constitute a numerical minority.

A detailed listing of the numerous groups with which we have worked would be difficult to compile, especially since some were informal (such as groups of neighbors or friends). Also, the title of a group might mislead the reader about the nature of its members. For example, included under the term "staffs of clinics and institutions," a term suggesting professional personnel, we have case histories of some of the typists and cleaning women who were employed there. The important thing is the characteristics of the females of our sample rather than the description of the source through which we met them, and these characteristics are given in our descriptive sample tables.

However, it is desirable to describe in at least a rough way the sources of our sample. Taking these in order of numerical size, the largest source of case histories consists of college students; there are 2,228 college females of whom 279 had married. The second largest source consists of small groups of friends or neighborhood groups and individual women. These provide 806 women of whom 524 had married. The third largest source consists of professional personnel or those associated with organizations that are professional: the staffs of clinics and institutions, teachers, nurses, and so forth. These total 681 females of whom 376 had married. We should point out, here, that not all these individuals were employed in professions: for example, if through having met a male physician employed in a clinic we obtained the case history of his mother, this history is listed as having been derived from the clinic. The fourth largest source of female case histories comprises classes in adult education: 335 females of whom 186 had married. Parent-Teacher Association groups are the fifth largest source, accounting for 323 females of whom 296 had married. The sixth largest source consists of church memberships and religious interest groups, comprising 311 females of whom 229 had married. The seventh largest source consists of women's clubs and civic organizations: 260 females of whom 175 had married.

The remaining sources are diverse in nature and none consists of as many as 200 females: union groups, personnel of business offices, groups of medical patients, persons in the fine arts, high school students, and so forth.

It is clear that many of these sources provide numerous employed women; consequently the proportion of employed women in our sample exceeds that of the general population. Census data for 1950 show that the birth rate for wives employed outside the home is markedly less than that for wives not so employed, and this in part explains the lower live birth rates of our married sample, which will be discussed later.

CONSTITUTION OF THE SAMPLE

The 5,293 white non-prison women, the subjects of the main body of this study, were interviewed in the years 1938 to 1955. About 97 per cent of the interviews occurred during 1940-1949, with January, 1946, being the median date of interview.

The women were almost exclusively in urban settings and from urban backgrounds; 96 per cent had lived as urban residents most of their adult years.

The geographic distribution of the women by primary region of adult residence is given below:

Table 2. Sample Description: Geographic Distribution of
Females in Sample Compared to 1950 U.S. Census

| REGION | FEMALES IN SAMPLE | | | | 1950 CENSUS URBAN WHITE FEMALES |
| | Total | | Ever married | | |
	Number	Per cent	Number	Per cent	Per cent
North East	2,462	46.5	973	43.8	34.0
North Central	1,825	34.5	694	31.2	30.3
South	447	8.4	261	11.8	20.9
West	514	9.7	279	12.6	14.8
Unclassified	45	0.9	14	0.6	...
Total	5,293	100.0	2,221	100.0	100.0

The comparison with census indicates that our sample suffers from an overrepresentation of women from the northeastern states and an underrepresentation of women from the South.

The composition of our sample of white non-prison women is given in Tables 8 to 13 in terms of age at reporting, marital status, educational achievement, age at marriage, decade of birth, and religious affiliation and degree of devoutness. From these tables it will be seen that, in terms of age at reporting, about four fifths of the sample consist of women aged 16-30. As to marital status, the sample is largely unmarried (58 per cent), and of those who did marry, a relatively large number were subsequently separated, divorced, or widowed. Included are 12 common-law marriages contracted by women

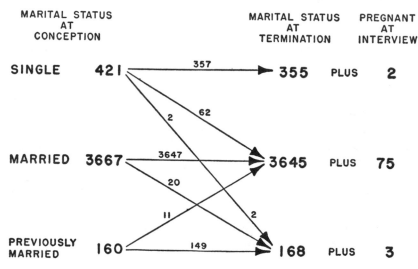

Figure 1. Pregnancies Experienced by White Non-Prison Females by Marital Status at Conception and at Termination.

Data from Table 13.

who married once and were still married at interview, and 80 common-law marriages contracted by 59 women who were ever separated, divorced, or widowed. The median age at reporting for females who had not married was 20.8 years; for those who had married once and were still married, 32.5; and for the separated, divorced, or widowed, 39.9. Roughly four fifths of the sample had had some college education: 90 per cent of the never-married, and 72 per cent of the ever-married. The sample is less out of balance when age at marriage is considered: most of the women married between the ages of twenty-one and twenty-five. As to the various decades of birth, the sample is heavily weighted by those born in 1920 and later (54 per cent). Turning to religious affiliation, one can see that our sample consists almost wholly of Protestants, Catholics, and Jews; the Protestants comprising 62 per cent, the Catholics 11 per cent, and the Jews 28 per cent.[2] Taken as a whole, 40 per cent of the Protestants, Catholics, and Jews of our sample were religiously inactive.

While the sample, taken as a whole, can be used as a basis for inferences only for the educationally upper 20 per cent of the U.S. population, it should be said that as the sample is subdivided, some of its categories (e.g., the high school educated) provide findings applicable to larger segments of the urban white population. In other instances in which several categories are compared, one may make inferences from the trends even though the absolute figures for some categories are subject to question. For example, one can infer that pre-marital conception is less often encountered among the religiously devout even though one may question the exact percentage.

For additional information concerning the material at our disposal the reader should refer to the N's of the subsequent tables. It will be seen that the N's of our analytical tables are as informative as the N's of our sample description tables. For example, sample description Table 8 indicates that 34 females were between the ages of eleven and fifteen when interviewed, but analytical Table 15 shows that our knowledge of what occurred at this young age is based upon not a mere 34 females but upon 5,258 who had reached or passed age fifteen who reported upon that early period of their lives as well as upon later periods.

The number of females who experienced conception and various types of outcome is given in the table below.

Table 3. Sample Description: Number of Females with
Experience in Conception, Birth, and Abortion*

For White Non-Prison Females

By Marital Status at Event

MARITAL STATUS AT EVENT	NUMBER OF WHITE NON-PRISON FEMALES					
	Type of experience					
	Conception	Any type termination	Live birth	Spontaneous abortion	Illegal abortion	Therapeutic abortion
Single	327	268	19	19	230	5
Married	1,408	1,372	1,192	390	304	43
Previously married	105	108	20	15	81	3
All statuses	1,609	1,568	1,219	418	531	51

*Figures in this table cannot be added horizontally or vertically since some females change marital status following conception and since one female may appear more than once in the vertical columns.

[2] In view of the relatively high educational attainment of our sample, these proportions are not unreasonable. See recent Current Population Survey data.

For a description of the number of conceptions and terminations experienced by the females of our sample, classified by marital status at the time of the event, see Table 13, Figure 1.

CENSUS COMPARISON

A comparison of our sample with U. S. Census data is made below by Dr. Christopher Tietze. Dr. Tietze is the author of "Introduction to the Statistics of Abortion," presented at the Pregnancy Wastage Conference (1953) and of the 1954 study, *Statistics on Abortion,* prepared for the Population Division of the United Nations.

COMPARISON WITH THE URBAN WHITE POPULATION

The methods employed by the Institute for Sex Research in the collection of sexual histories were not designed to produce a representative sample of the population of the United States. In a statistical sense the histories represent only themselves. It is possible, nevertheless, to compare the sample with the general population and to draw useful conclusions from this comparison about the nature and validity of the data collected.

Major differences between the group of respondents and the general population relate to race, urban-rural residence, age, and educational level. First, the histories discussed in this chapter were all obtained from white non-prison women. Histories contributed by Negro women are not included in Chapters 2 to 5 of the present report.[3] Second, the

Table 4. Census Comparison: Age Distribution

For White Non-Prison Females in Sample Compared with Estimate for Urban White Females, 15 Years of Age and Over, in 1945

AGE	WHITE NON-PRISON FEMALES IN SAMPLE		ESTIMATE FOR URBAN WHITE FEMALES
	Number	*Per cent*	*Per cent*
−14	22	*	*
15–19	1,203	22.8	9.6
20–24	1,507	28.6	11.1
25–29	645	12.2	11.3
30–34	480	9.1	10.6
35–39	478	9.1	10.0
40–44	375	7.1	9.2
45–49	261	5.0	8.4
50–54	150	2.8	7.5
55+	172	3.3	22.3
All ages	5,293	100.0	100.0

* Not included in computation of percentages.

[3] Information on pregnancies and their outcome among Negro females is contained in Chapter 6.

great majority of histories collected are those of women raised and residing in an urban environment. Only 167 among the 5,293 women in the sample (3.2 per cent) had lived on a farm most of their lives after age eighteen. The most appropriate standard for comparison would, therefore, seem to be the urban white population of the United States.

Age distribution. Table 4, arranged in conventional five-year age groups rather than in those used elsewhere in this volume, compares the age distribution of our sample with an estimated distribution of urban white females, fifteen years of age and over, in 1945, as approximated by the average of distribution reported in the population censuses of 1940 and 1950. The year 1945 was chosen for the estimate because it corresponds to the midpoint of the period during which the histories were obtained. The differences between our sample and the general population are immediately apparent. More than half the females in the sample were in the two age groups 15-19 years and 20-24 years, compared with only one fifth of the urban white females. Conversely, only 3 per cent of the females in our sample were fifty-five years old and over when their histories were recorded, while 22 per cent of the urban white females fell into that age group. The age structure of the sample clearly reflects the large number of histories obtained from college students.

Table 5. Census Comparison: Educational Level

For White Non-Prison Females in Sample Compared with Estimate for Urban White Females in 1945, Adjusted to Age Distribution of Sample

EDUCATIONAL LEVEL	WHITE NON-PRISON FEMALES IN SAMPLE		ESTIMATE FOR URBAN WHITE FEMALES
	Number	*Per cent*	*Per cent*
0–8	124*	2.3	27.1
9–12	809*	15.3	59.7
13–16	3,217	60.8	8.8†
17+	1,143	21.6	4.4†
All levels	5,293	100.0	100.0

*Girls still in school classified by current attendance (see page 4).
†13–15 and 16+ years.

Educational level. A fourth important difference between our sample and the general population concerns educational attainment. The proportion of women with better than average education is much higher in our group than in the urban white population and even further removed from the educational level of the total population of the United States. Table 5 shows the distribution of the sample by four educational levels, identified by the numbers of school years reported: 0 to 8 years, elementary school; 9 to 12 years, high school; 13 to 16 years, college; and 17 + years, postgraduate education. For comparison, the table also shows an estimated percentage distribution, by educational attainment, of the urban white female population in 1945. This estimated distribution is adjusted to the age structure of the sample, i.e., it applies to a group of females with the same age distribution as the sample, but with an educational attainment, in each age group, equal to that of the urban white population.

The educational categories of our sample and of the census's urban white population are only approximately comparable since our categories are defined in terms of attendance, while the census data are in terms of highest grade completed. Thus, according to the rules followed by the Institute, a woman who left college after attending for one semester is assigned to the educational level 13-16 years; according to census rules, the same woman is assigned to the group with 9-12 years of schooling. The category with the highest educational attainment in the sample (17 +) comprises only women who have at least begun studies beyond the level of the baccalaureate, while the highest census category (16 +) includes all college graduates, with and without postgraduate experience.

These variations in definition are, however, of minor importance compared with the real differences in educational attainment between the sample and the urban white population. More than four fifths of the women in the sample (82 per cent) had attended or were still attending college, compared with 13 per cent of the urban white females. Conversely, the sample's share of women with only elementary education was less than one tenth of the corresponding figure in the third column of Table 5. In rough approximation it can be said that the educational level of the women who contributed histories, taken as a group, equals the attainment of the highest 16 to 20 per cent of the urban white population of the United States.

Marital status. In terms of marital status, the sample includes 3,072 single females, 1,467 women married once, living with husband, and 754 in other categories. The last group comprises those ever-married women who had experienced at least one dissolution of marriage, i.e., those who were separated, divorced, or widowed, or were remarried at the time their histories were recorded. For convenience in reference they are designated the "ever-S.D.W." women. The high proportion of never-married females in the sample is obviously related to the low average age of the respondents.

Table 6 presents a cross tabulation by marital status and age at

Table 6. Census Comparison: Marital Status and Age at Interview

For White Non-Prison Females in Sample Compared with Estimate for Urban White Females in 1945, Adjusted to Educational Level Distribution of Sample

AGE AT INTERVIEW	WHITE NON-PRISON FEMALES IN SAMPLE		ESTIMATE FOR URBAN WHITE FEMALES
	Never Married		
	Number	*Per cent*	*Per cent*
−14	22		
15–19	1,150	95.6	93.9
20–24	1,174	77.9	62.7
25–29	254	39.4	29.0
30–34	139	29.0	19.9
35–39	137	28.7	18.9
40–44	66	17.6	19.3
45–49	54	20.7	20.7
50–54	36	24.0	20.9
55+	40	23.3	20.9
	Married Once, Living with Husband		
15–19	37	3.1	4.9
20–24	289	19.2	32.5
25–29	303	47.0	59.8
30–34	231	48.1	64.7
35–39	219	45.8	62.9
40–44	184	49.1	59.6
45–49	99	37.9	55.7
50–54	63	42.0	51.1
55+	42	24.4	37.1
	Ever Separated, Divorced, Widowed		
15–19	16	1.3	1.2
20–24	44	2.9	4.8
25–29	88	13.6	11.2
30–34	110	22.9	15.4
35–39	122	25.5	18.2
40–44	125	33.3	21.1
45–49	108	41.4	23.6
50–54	51	34.0	28.0
55+	90	52.3	42.0

interview of the sample and comparable estimates for urban white females in 1945, based on the censuses of 1940 and 1950.[4]

These estimates are adjusted to the distribution of the sample data by level of education. While the general patterns of the two distributions are similar, each age group of the sample comprises a smaller proportion of women married once, living with husband, than the corresponding age group in the adjusted urban white population. Conversely, with

Table 7. Census Comparison: Age at Interview, Number of
Live Births, and Accumulative Live Birth Rate

For Ever-Married White Non-Prison Females in Sample
Compared with Estimate for Urban White Females in
1945, Adjusted to the Distribution of the Sample
by Educational Level and Marital Status (Married
Once, Living with Husband; or Ever Separated,
Divorced, Widowed)

AGE AT INTERVIEW	EVER-MARRIED WHITE NON-PRISON FEMALES IN SAMPLE			ESTIMATE FOR URBAN WHITE FEMALES
	Number of females	Number of live births	Live births per female	Live births per female
15–19	53	6	0.11	0.40
20–24	333	63	0.19	0.56
25–29	391	279	0.71	1.02
30–34	341	426	1.25	1.39
35–39	341	474	1.39	1.58
40–44	309	442	1.43	1.63
45–49	207	279	1.35	1.69
50–54	114	204	1.79	1.84
55 +	132	251	1.90	2.09
All ages	2,221	2,424	1.09	1.33

a few minor exceptions, the proportions of never-married females and of ever-S.D.W. females are higher in the sample than in the adjusted urban white population. These differences may reflect the more active participation of single and previously married females, as compared with married females, in many of the organizations and other groups through which the majority of histories was collected. To some extent the higher proportion of ever-S.D.W. women in the sample may have resulted from a more complete recording of previous marriages by the staff of the Institute than was obtained in the national censuses. In each of the four educational groups distinguished in this report the

---

[4] The detailed tabulations of the 1940 census on marital status and fertility refer to native white women; those of the 1950 census to total white women. The errors introduced into the 1945 estimate by the use of these two sets of data were not considered to be substantial enough to require adjustment.

differences between sample and urban white population (adjusted for age) were in the same directions and of similar magnitude.

Live births. The number of live births reported by the 2,221 ever-married women in the sample was 2,424, averaging 1.09 per woman. This is a very low figure, but it should be remembered that only one fifth of these women had reached the end of the childbearing period, the median age being 34.9 years. Table 7 shows a distribution of ever-married women by age at interview, the numbers of live births reported by the women in each age group, the average number of births per woman, and comparative estimates for urban white females in 1945, adjusted to the distribution of the sample by level of education and marital status (married once, living with husband; or ever-S.D.W.). The average number of births per woman is consistently lower in the sample than in the adjusted urban white population. In most age groups the difference is comparatively small, about one tenth, but among the younger women it is fairly substantial. This situation should surprise no one, as mothers with small children tend to confine their activities to their own homes and are not easily reached except by a house-to-house canvass.[5] Again the lower fertility of the sample, as compared with the urban population (adjusted for age) is found on each of the four levels of education.[6]

In summary, then, the distribution of the sample by marital status and the numbers of live births reported by the respondents suggest patterns of behavior similar to those observed in the urban white population of the United States, taking into consideration the much higher educational attainment of the sample. Nuptiality (proportion married), stability of marriage, and marital fertility are, however, somewhat below the levels prevailing in approximately comparable segments of the general population.

---

[5] Most statistics in this book are based on the experience of all women who had passed the particular age groups to which these statistics refer. This procedure tends to minimize any distortion introduced by the failure to interview a sufficient number of young mothers.

[6] Additional comparisons between the white non-prison sample and estimates for urban white females in 1945 are presented in Chapter 4.

Table 8. Sample Description: Number of Females
For White Non-Prison Females
By Age, Marital Status, and Educational
Level at Interview

Age at interview	Total sample	Educational Level			
		0–8	9–12	13–16	17+
WHITE NON-PRISON FEMALES					

		Never Married			
11–15	34	14	20		
16–20	1,573	1	94	1,471	7
21–25	818	1	74	580	163
26–30	210		34	79	97
31–35	137	4	21	46	66
36–40	116	3	12	24	77
41–45	70	4	3	22	41
46–50	49	1		4	44
51+	65	5	12	8	40
Total	3,072	33	270	2,234	535
Per cent of total sample	58.0	0.6	5.1	42.2	10.1

		Married Once, Still Married			
11–15	1	1			
16–20	73	2	14	55	2
21–25	304		51	182	71
26–30	294	3	71	136	84
31–35	233	5	56	100	72
36–40	217	5	43	105	64
41–45	162	8	26	60	68
46–50	101	7	17	43	34
51+	82	10	25	25	22
Total	1,467	41	303	706	417
Per cent of total sample	27.7	0.8	5.7	13.3	7.9

		Ever Separated, Divorced, Widowed			
16–20	23	5	9	9	
21–25	51	2	20	23	6
26–30	89	2	29	44	14
31–35	124	1	49	43	31
36–40	125	7	38	49	31
41–45	119	9	24	46	40
46–50	91	7	24	26	34
51+	132	17	43	37	35
Total	754	50	236	277	191
Per cent of total sample	14.2	0.9	4.5	5.2	3.6

Table 9. Sample Description: Number of Females

For White Non-Prison Females

By Age at Interview, Marital Status at Interview, and Decade of Birth

Age at interview	WHITE NON-PRISON FEMALES				
		Decade of birth			
	Before 1890	1890– 1899	1900– 1909	1910– 1919	1920+
Never Married					
11–15					34
16–20				18	1,555
21–25				133	685
26–30			1	142	67
31–35			23	113	1
36–40			78	38	
41–45		12	57	1	
46–50		35	14		
51+	20	44	1		
Total	20	91	174	445	2,342
Per cent of total sample	0.4	1.7	3.3	8.4	44.2
Married Once, Still Married					
11–15					1
16–20					73
21–25				41	263
26–30			1	208	85
31–35			24	206	3
36–40		1	145	71	
41–45		17	144	1	
46–50		66	35		
51+	20	62			
Total	20	146	349	527	425
Per cent of total sample	0.4	2.8	6.6	10.0	8.0
Ever Separated, Divorced, Widowed					
11–15					
16–20					23
21–25				1	50
26–30				59	30
31–35			14	103	7
36–40			78	47	
41–45		11	108		
46–50		41	50		
51+	57	74	1		
Total	57	126	251	210	110
Per cent of total sample	1.1	2.4	4.7	4.0	2.1

Table 10. Sample Description: Number of Married Females
For White Non-Prison Females
By Age at Interview and Age at Marriage

	WHITE NON-PRISON FEMALES					
Age at interview	−15	16–20	Age at marriage 21–25	26–30	31–35	36+
−15	1					
16–20	4	92				
21–25	2	136	217			
26–30	3	98	223	59		
31–35	1	86	171	86	13	
36–40	3	67	165	75	27	5
41–45	1	49	130	72	16	13
46–50		35	90	39	19	9
51+		42	86	56	20	10
Total	15	605	1,082	387	95	37
Per cent of total married sample	0.7	27.2	48.7	17.4	4.3	1.7

Table 11. Sample Description: Number of Females

For White Non-Prison Females

By Age, Religious Devoutness, and Marital Status at Interview

WHITE NON-PRISON FEMALES

Age at interview	Protestant De-vout	Protestant Moder-ate	Protestant Inac-tive	Catholic De-vout	Catholic Moder-ate	Catholic Inac-tive	Jewish De-vout	Jewish Moder-ate	Jewish Inac-tive
Never Married									
11–15	9	6	4	2	1		1	2	8
16–20	330	301	132	89	20	16	58	282	345
21–25	205	180	133	66	19	17	11	64	120
26–30	41	48	57	27	6	7	1	4	24
31–35	25	29	38	11	4	4	1	3	20
36–40	26	32	35	7	1	4		3	9
41–45	17	11	24	5	1	3	1		8
46–50	13	15	17	1					2
51+	17	19	15	6		5	1		2
Total	683	641	455	214	52	56	74	358	538
Per cent of total sample	12.9	12.1	8.6	4.0	1.0	1.1	1.4	6.8	10.2
Married Once, Still Married									
11–15	1								
16–20	13	8	10	3		3	3	10	22
21–25	68	62	61	14	5	9	2	19	68
26–30	60	66	79	10	10	4	2	20	50
31–35	47	56	50	11	7	5	3	17	39
36–40	55	43	59	5	4	5	6	19	27
41–45	40	34	48	2	2	5	1	12	21
46–50	29	22	24	1	1	3	2	7	14
51+	20	16	15	3	1	2	3	5	17
Total	333	307	346	49	30	36	22	109	258
Per cent of total sample	6.3	5.8	6.5	0.9	0.6	0.7	0.4	2.1	4.9
Ever Separated, Divorced, Widowed									
11–15									
16–20	3	6	7	3	1	2	1		2
21–25	7	6	12	1	6	5		1	15
26–30	12	14	30	2	4	12		3	12
31–35	15	27	44	9	6	10		9	15
36–40	18	18	51	6	2	10	1	2	22
41–45	28	28	36	3	6	6		3	18
46–50	18	23	31	5	1	3		1	16
51+	35	27	37	10	4	5	2	2	19
Total	136	149	248	39	30	53	4	21	119
Per cent of total sample	2.6	2.8	4.7	0.7	0.6	1.0	0.1	0.4	2.2

Table 12. Sample Description: Number of Females

For White Non-Prison Females

By Age, Religious Devoutness, and Educational Level at Interview

WHITE NON-PRISON FEMALES

Age at interview	Protestant			Catholic			Jewish		
	De-vout	Moder-ate	Inac-tive	De-vout	Moder-ate	Inac-tive	De-vout	Moder-ate	Inac-tive
Educational Level 0–8									
11–25	5	7	2	6	1	3			3
26–45	12	4	4	12	6	7	1		6
46+	6	11	4	13	3	2	1	1	9
Total	23	22	10	31	10	12	2	1	18
Per cent of total sample	0.4	0.4	0.2	0.6	0.2	0.2	0.0	0.0	0.3
Educational Level 9–12									
11–25	85	39	49	27	16	10	2	19	34
26–45	69	93	105	33	24	23	4	22	54
46+	29	23	28	6	1	6	4	7	23
Total	183	155	182	66	41	39	10	48	111
Per cent of total sample	3.5	2.9	3.4	1.2	0.8	0.7	0.2	0.9	2.1
Educational Level 13–16									
11–25	501	483	257	125	32	29	70	343	483
26–45	179	158	208	25	10	21	6	43	112
46+	36	32	39	2	3	4	3	6	22
Total	716	673	504	152	45	54	79	392	617
Per cent of total sample	13.5	12.7	9.5	2.9	0.9	1.0	1.5	7.4	11.7
Educational Level 17+									
11–25	45	40	51	20	3	10	4	16	60
26–45	124	151	234	28	13	24	5	30	93
46+	61	56	68	5		6		1	16
Total	230	247	353	53	16	40	9	47	169
Per cent of total sample	4.3	4.7	6.7	1.0	0.3	0.8	0.2	0.9	3.2

Table 13. Sample Description: Number of Conceptions and Terminations For White Non-Prison Females By Marital Status of Females at Event, and Marital Status of Females Pregnant at Interview

Marital status at outcome and type of outcome	Marital status at conception			All statuses
	Single	Married	Previously married	
Single				
Live birth	20			20
Spontaneous abortion	19			19
Induced abortion	316			316
Pregnant at interview	2			2
Total conceptions	357			357
Married				
Live birth	45	2,341	8	2,394
Spontaneous abortion	4	626	0	630
Induced abortion	11	608	2	621
Pregnant at interview	2	72	1	75
Total conceptions	62	3,647	11	3,720
Previously Married				
Live birth	2	12	6	20
Spontaneous abortion	0	2	16	18
Induced abortion	0	6	124	130
Pregnant at interview	0	0	3	3
Total conceptions	2	20	149	171
All statuses				
Live birth	67	2,353	14	2,434
Spontaneous abortion	23	628	16	667
Induced abortion	327	614	126	1,067
Pregnant at interview	4	72	4	80
Total conceptions	421	3,667	160	4,248

Included as induced abortions are 68 therapeutic abortions.

Chapter 3

THE SINGLE WOMAN

There are few sexual problems that receive as much social attention and individual concern as pregnancy in the unmarried. Unlike certain preliterate cultures wherein a child under almost any circumstances is a welcome addition, our culture insists that a child be conceived in one and only one social situation, marriage, and born into a prefabricated structure of social relationships wherein the roles, duties, and obligations of relatives and neighbors are clearly defined. While society's conscious reaction to a pre-marital birth is usually expressed in terms of morality, there is an underlying and unexpressed cognizance that such a birth, as a practical matter, does not fit into the social structure and pattern. This pattern requires a marriage so that one can point out the child's father and his kin; so that society can demand that these relatives assist in the support of the child if this is necessary; so that in incorporating the child into itself, society will always have, to facilitate the process, known persons with known responsibilities. We might justly be accused of being less concerned with the child and primarily concerned with all the social machinery surrounding its conception, birth, and infancy. At any rate, our society makes no real provision for the unmarried parent and has developed various social sanctions to prevent and punish pregnancy in the unmarried.[1] These sanctions are omnipresent, religious as well as secular, and apply with special severity to persons of the middle and upper socio-economic levels. The inflexibility of these sanctions is such that an immature, headstrong girl who conceived during a spur-of-the-moment marriage that lasted but one week is in a more advantageous social position than an emotionally mature female with a conception resulting from a long engagement to a responsible man.

While society censures, sometimes brutally, the woman who bears a child outside of marriage, there is often an amused tolerance for the female who becomes pre-maritally pregnant but marries before the child is born. Many attitudes concerning sex have changed markedly within the past years, but the attitude toward unwed motherhood has not altered to any extent. In addition, our law insists that a pre-marital pregnancy, once begun, be carried to term. Legal sanctions against

---

[1] See Kingsley Davis 1939:232 for a thoughtful discussion of social taboos and illegitimacy.

30

bastardy and unmarried motherhood, while severe, are not so severe as those against induced abortion.

The unmarried are caught in a dilemma of our own making: on one hand there is the strong and basic sexual drive reinforced by the fact that society encourages the development of heterosexual interests and emotional involvements; on the other hand there is society's insistence that this must not lead to conception before marriage. At the same time our socio-economic structure is such that marriage must often be deferred for years. Our advertisements, drama, films, and literature insistently point out to girls the great goal: be beautiful, be alluring, be popular, have romance—yet do not allow these desirable accomplishments to lead to their logical conclusion until a marriage ceremony has taken place. To keep one's self and/or one's suitors at a high pitch of emotional and sexual excitement for five to ten years, from the beginning of dating to marriage, and meanwhile to abstain from coitus is, biologically speaking, a most unnatural as well as difficult task.

As is usually the case when social considerations conflict strongly with biological fundamentals and when society develops partially contradictory goals for its members, a large number of individuals depart from the social mores in practice although they may uphold them in theory. As we indicated in our volume, *Sexual Behavior in the Human Female,* roughly half of the women from the middle and upper socio-economic levels who married had had coitus prior to marriage. Although our data regarding females of the lower socio-economic level are inadequate, we know that the younger females of this group have an even greater incidence of pre-marital coitus.

The frequency of pre-marital coitus varies greatly; for the women in our sample who were having coitus it averaged about once in five or ten weeks among those under twenty and about once in three weeks for those over twenty. However, this coitus is ordinarily sporadic, occurring with some frequency for a period of time and then ceasing for weeks or months (1953:288–290). During such a period of coital activity the frequency is usually high enough to make pregnancy likely were it not for contraception. It should be noted at this point that according to present medical thinking there is a period of twelve to twenty-four hours' duration in each menstrual month when fertilization can occur.[2] The matter becomes one of statistical probability: at

---

[2] Rock and Loth 1949:68-69 in referring to fertilization state, "All this process, it is believed, must take place within twelve hours of ovulation . . . or at most twenty-four hours, for by that time the egg will have lost its susceptibility to fertilization." Fulton 1955:1221 makes an even stronger statement, "An ovum must be fertilized within a few hours after it leaves the follicle at ovulation. . . ."

a given frequency of coitus, and assuming random distribution, what are the chances that coitus will occur within a given twenty-four-hour period? If coitus averages once in two months, which is roughly the average frequency among females under twenty, there is only one chance in five during a year that it will occur during her fertile hours. A coital frequency of once in three weeks, the average for women of twenty-one and older, makes it an almost even chance that in one year coitus will occur once within the fertile period.

There is also the fact that pre-marital coitus is not randomly distributed, but is influenced by various factors, one of which is the periodicity of sexual arousal in some females. About 59 per cent of the females of our sample who had experienced sexual arousal recognized that they were more easily stimulated at certain stages of their menstrual cycles. Of these women only 11 per cent said they reached their peak of sexual drive at the midpoint between menstrual periods, when ovulation ordinarily occurs and the female becomes capable of conceiving. The great majority find themselves more easily aroused just before or just after menstruation, when they are least likely to conceive. Among females having a substantial amount of coitus the periodicity factor would be unimportant, but among women who are inclined to engage in coitus only at the time of their greatest arousal this factor would be of considerable importance.

While frequency of coitus is an obvious factor in whether or not a female becomes pregnant, there are numerous other factors, some of which are of prime importance.

1. There is evidence that adolescent females under seventeen are relatively sterile. Anthropologists have noted this so-called "adolescent sterility" in other cultures and it has received some attention in our own. It appears that the number of menstrual periods in which an egg is *not* released from the ovary (an anovulatory cycle) is much higher among young adolescent females than in older females.[3] Our present data cannot be utilized in examining this "sterility" since the factor of contraception cannot be excluded for a sufficient number of cases.

Of the 156 girls on whom we have detailed contraceptive information and who experienced pre-marital coitus within three years following their menarche, only 11 per cent failed to use contraceptives while 11 per cent used them occasionally and 78 per cent used them regularly. These girls had pre-marital conception rates in keeping with

[3] Carl Hartman first used the term "adolescent sterility" in 1931 in discussing reproduction in young monkeys. For a survey of evidence of its existence in young girls see Ashley Montagu 1946:57-141 and Dennis in Carmichael 1946:645. See Mazer and Israel 1951:66 for statement concerning ovulation in early adolescence.

those of all the girls of equivalent age whom we interviewed. Of 51 girls who married within three years following their menarche, 28 per cent used no contraceptives, 14 per cent used them occasionally, and 59 per cent used them regularly. Their marital conception rates are similar to those of our total married female sample of equivalent age.

2. The similar sterility of young males is even less well understood but nonetheless probable, and seems a matter of insufficient production of spermatozoa. Studies of experimental animals reinforce this assumption.[4] Extremely little work has been done on sperm counts of boys.[5] However, one of our collaborators has supplied data on four cases, all of whom had counts so low that they would be considered infertile. Because of contraception, our data are also inapplicable to a study of adolescent male "sterility."

3. Inasmuch as the great majority of females marry, and since the average age at first marriage in the United States is about twenty,[6] the reduction in fertility due to aging is but a minor factor in a study of conception among the unmarried. However, there are scores of other physiological factors that clinicians recognize, for example: the condition of the Fallopian tubes, the acidity of the vagina, the patency of the cervical os, and the permeability of the cervical mucus. In addition, a considerable number of factors may contribute to male infertility, such as defects in form or motility of the spermatozoa, low sperm counts, urethral acidity, and urethral or prostatic infections.[7]

4. The major factor aside from frequency of coitus is, of course, contraception. The extent to which contraception does or could reduce pre-marital pregnancies is at present impossible to ascertain precisely.

[4] See, for example, Webster and Young 1951:178.

[5] Older investigations of spermatogenesis in adolescent males are cited in G. Stanley Hall 1904 (1):419. Baldwin 1928 in checking morning urine samples of young boys found less than one quarter of his sample of 123 (ages 9-17) and less than half of those over 14 years showed sperm.

[6] Census data do not provide a figure for age at first marriage, but Glick 1955:4 fixes median age for all U.S. women at first marriage at 21.5 for 1940, and at 20.1 for 1950. Tietze and Lauriat 1955:164 in adjusting 1950 census data for educational level arrived at an average age ranging from 19.9 for 5 to 8 years' elementary schooling to 23.2 for 4 years or more of college. An average age of 20.2 years (first marriage, white females) from 19 reporting states in 1954 is provided by U.S. Vital Statistics, Special Reports 1956 (44):107.

[7] The complex nature of the factors involved in successful conception has been fully recognized only in the last 40 years. Early medical treatises on sterility such as Mondat 1844 were based on the principle that the "causes of sterility, as of fecundity, are situated in the organs destined for this purpose" (p. 11). Meaker's 1934 volume was a milestone in its summary of the progress in the clinical management of sterility and its emphasis on the multiple nature of its causation and the general division of responsibility between the sexes. For later findings in the field see such books as Simmons 1951, 1954, Harrison 1955, Farris 1956, and current issues of the journal *Fertility and Sterility*.

Often pre-marital coitus occurs under circumstances in which the regular use of an effective contraceptive is difficult and, more importantly, much pre-marital coitus is unpremeditated and impulsive. We have also recorded instances where one or both of the persons involved had determined not to have coitus and to strengthen this resolve omitted taking any contraceptive with them. Then when sexual arousal reached the point where caution was disregarded and the petting proceeded to coitus, no contraceptive was available.

One must also realize that many men are averse to the use of the condom, feeling that it interferes with sensation. Particularly at the lower socio-economic level this objection, coupled with the opinion that such mechanical devices are somehow unnatural, results in a minimal use of the condom. Furthermore, many women of this level are unaware of the vaginal diaphragm, nor is it easy for an unmarried female to go to a physician for a diaphragm fitting. Consequently, this group tends to rely more heavily upon less effective contraceptive measures such as douches, vaginal suppositories, and withdrawal.

In summary, it is obvious that in our culture there is a considerable amount of pre-marital coitus and, despite various voluntary or involuntary inhibiting factors, some of it results in pregnancy. It is with the incidence of such pregnancies and their outcome that the remainder of this chapter will be concerned.

In both tables and text we shall express our statistics in relation to three sorts of samples:

1. Total sample (total females). This consists of all our white non-prison females, regardless of whether they were single or married at the time of the interview or whether or not they had had pre-marital coitus. Figures relating to this sample show the magnitude of any given pre-marital phenomenon in a segment of the population such as devout Protestants or women of high school education, regardless of whether or not they subsequently married.

2. Single sample (total single females). This consists of all our white non-prison females who had never married prior to a specified age. Figures relating to this sample show the size of any given pre-marital phenomenon among the still unmarried segment of the population under consideration. In brief, these are females who, being single, are still eligible to have pre-marital experience in coitus and conception. In tables where the coital segment of this sample is given (Table 15, 20, 21) this segment is labeled "single females with coitus."

3. Coital sample (females with pre-marital coitus). This consists of all our white non-prison females who have had pre-marital coitus, regardless of whether or not they subsequently married. Such females,

since they have all been exposed to the possibility of pre-marital pregnancy, provide in many ways the best sample for an examination of the relation between pre-marital pregnancy and its outcome and various social factors such as religion, educational achievement, and age at marriage. An analysis of this sample shows simultaneously the effect of the amount of coitus and the effect of contraception. These two effects cannot, in this study, be analyzed separately.

PREGNANCY

RELATION TO AGE, TO MARITAL STATUS AT INTERVIEW, AND TO COITAL EXPERIENCE

As we have pointed out, our total sample of white non-prison females has certain limitations in comparison with the urban white population of the United States, hence it cannot be used *as a whole unit* to elucidate what has happened in the U.S. population; it approximates the socio-economic upper 20 per cent of the urban white population. Note, however, that when the sample is subdivided, as into educational or age at marriage categories, the findings can be applied to a much larger segment of the urban white population.

Accumulative experience. By the age of forty, which for most women is essentially the end of reproductive life, roughly 10 per cent of our total sample had had a pre-marital pregnancy, regardless of their ultimate marital status (Table 15).[8] This figure was reached gradually:

---

[8] There are several other studies reporting experience of pre-marital conception, but it should be kept in mind that the samples vary in important features such as source and method of obtaining data, and the age and marital status, as well as the educational attainment of the women reporting. The figures show a range of from 3.5 to 30 per cent of pre-marital conception experience to be compared to our Table 15 or Table 22.

Hamilton 1929:125, 133 cited 8 per cent of 100 married women as having experienced a pre-marital conception.

Dickinson and Beam 1934:33 found 4 per cent with pre-marital conceptions in their total sample of 500 single women.

Stix 1935:351 reported 35 pre-marital conceptions among 991 married women in a birth control clinic sample. If one assumes that 35 different women were involved, this gives a 3.5 per cent experience figure.

Raymond Pearl's monumental 1939 study provided fertility data on a sample of over 25,000 white obstetrical patients from 139 co-operating hospitals in the northeastern United States. Calculations made from Table 26, p. 181, fix the pre-marital conception experience of the married sample at 7.3 per cent. If we calculate the present data on the basis of fertile married females in order to make it comparable, we arrive at a 16.8 figure.

Brunner 1941:163 in a rather selective sample based on gynecology clinic records of 254 single females found 30 per cent had conceived pre-maritally.

Beebe 1942:61 recorded pre-marital conceptions as reported by 15 per cent of 1,165 married females enlisted for a contraceptive service in Logan County, West Virginia.

by age twenty, 3 per cent had become pregnant before marriage; by age twenty-five, 8 per cent; and by age thirty, 10 per cent.

While, as we have said, our total sample consists primarily of the upper fifth of the urban white population, it is nevertheless clear that pre-marital pregnancy is an enormous social phenomenon that has involved not merely a few unfortunates, but millions of women now living.

Immediately one asks what has happened to these women; are their lives blighted, can they reorient themselves in our society? The answer is: they get married either before or after the end of the pregnancy. We arrived at this interesting conclusion by examining our unmarried sample. In the total sample we have just discussed, at any given age some of the women were married and some were not. For example, of the 8 per cent who had experienced a pre-marital pregnancy *by* age twenty-six some had husbands *at* age twenty-six and some had not. By eliminating a female from our calculation of accumulative experience as soon as she married, we could compute the percentages of premarital pregnancy among the still unmarried females of our sample. Thus, for instance, the percentage given by age twenty-six is based upon women who had never married by that age.

The accumulative experience of pre-marital pregnancy among the women who remained unmarried is less than that of the total sample, at least until age thirty-three (Table 15). By age twenty, 2 per cent of the unmarried had become pregnant as opposed to 3 per cent of the total sample; by age twenty-five, 5 per cent versus 8 per cent; and by age thirty, 8 per cent versus 10 per cent. Obviously some of the women who conceived before marriage were getting married[9] and hence could not be counted any longer as unmarried females who had experienced pre-marital pregnancy. The great majority of these marriages were not, as one might presume, "shotgun marriages," but mar-

---

Whelpton in a discussion at the 1942 abortion conference cited 48 definite pre-marital pregnancies and 14 suspected ones among the 1,080 couples in the Indianapolis fertility study. If one uses the total figure and assumes different couples were involved, this would represent a 6.2 per cent pre-marital pregnancy experience. See Taylor 1944:37.

Lewis-Faning 1949:86 in the British Population Commission report on family limitation found a 17.5 per cent experience of pre-marital conception in a sample of over 3,000 married women.

---

[9] Legal recognition of such "forced" marriages is revealed by some state laws, which permit waiving the minimum legal age for marriage if the bride is pregnant at the time. This is true of the 1957 revision of the Indiana law, which permits the judge to use his discretion in such a contingency. According to Vernier 1931 (1):117 Arizona, Delaware, Michigan, and Ohio permitted marriage under age of consent when a court hearing disclosed that the girl was pregnant.

riages contracted after the pregnancy had ended. Of our 327 females who became pregnant while unmarried, only 63 married during their pregnancies—that is, 19 per cent (about one out of five). Looking at it another way 2.8 per cent of the total married sample were pregnant at time of marriage.[10]

After thirty, when nearly all the women who marry have married, the percentage of single females who have become pregnant exceeds slightly the percentage for the total sample. By age thirty-five the figure for the total sample is 10 per cent, while for those still unmarried at that age the figure is 11 per cent. The explanation seems to be this: before thirty, the females who had pre-marital coitus (some of whom conceived) were marrying more often than were those who had not had pre-marital coitus; this results in the percentage of females who had pre-marital pregnancies being greater in the total sample than in the single sample. However, as increasing age made marriage more difficult to achieve or less desirable, progressively fewer of the women with pre-marital coitus married: they remained single and thereby caused the percentage of single females who ex-

---

[10] Various other studies report on the incidence of pregnancy at time of marriage, but chiefly as evidenced by a live birth prior to a nine months' interval after the date of marriage. These figures provide a partial measure of pre-marital conceptions among married females. Such data include:

Sydenstricker 1932:26 reported 4 per cent of first births as occurring before six months of marriage in a group of 326 wives in Cattaraugus County, New York.

Landis et al. 1950:767 listed 3 per cent of 212 fertile wives of college students as reporting pregnancy at time of marriage.

Christensen 1953:57 by comparing marriage records and subsequent birth certificates of 1,531 couples in Tippecanoe County, Indiana, showed that 12 per cent of the wives were pregnant at marriage. He used the birth of a live child before seven months of marriage as an indication. An earlier similar study (1939) in Utah County, Utah, found that the wives in 11 per cent of 1,670 fertile married couples were pregnant at marriage.

European material reflecting the extent of pregnancy at marriage is plentiful. For example:

Gunzert 1953:78 in the official yearbook of Frankfurt a.M., reported 70 per cent of children born in the first year of married life as pre-maritally conceived.

Dück in Giese and Willy 1954:195 reported 32 per cent of over 2,500 Austrian brides in Innsbruck, Austria, as pregnant at time of marriage.

In Great Britain the Family Census of 1946 showed from 19 to 24 per cent of the women married during the period 1900-1940 gave birth to a child prior to eight and a half months of marriage. This included pre-marital births as well. See Glass and Grebenik 1954:141.

Henry 1951:431 recorded from 12 to 35 per cent of first births in four Czechoslovakian provinces as occurring before seven months of marriage.

Croog 1952:361, summarizing official data from Northern European countries up to 1948, reported from a fourth to a fifth of all the brides in Denmark, Finland, and Sweden pregnant at the time of marriage.

perienced pre-marital conception to increase and finally surpass that of the total sample. This is a matter of simple duration of exposure to the possibility of pre-marital conception. Women who marry late, after thirty, also tend to have begun pre-marital coitus at later ages, but by the time of marriage have accumulated more years of coital experience than those who marry at younger ages (Table 15).

From the foregoing data it is plain that pre-marital coitus, pre-marital pregnancy, and marriage are closely associated phenomena. To find out which, pre-marital coitus or pregnancy, is followed more often by marriage, we took our sample of college educated females and divided them into three groups: those without pre-marital coitus, those with pre-marital coitus who did not become pregnant, and those with pre-marital coitus who became pregnant. All three groups were subdivided according to age at the time of interview, and we calculated the percentage ever married by that age. The results are given in Table 14.

Table 14. Per Cent Ever Married

For College Educated Females

By Age at Interview and Pre-marital Experience

	COLLEGE EDUCATED FEMALES					
Age at interview	Never pre-marital coitus	Pre-marital coitus without conception	Pre-marital coitus with conception	Never pre-marital coitus	Pre-marital coitus without conception	Pre-marital coitus with conception
	Per cent ever married			Number of females		
21–25	19.3	42.2	43.6	659	327	39
26–30	56.3	65.2	65.9	206	207	41
31–35	62.3	73.2	74.4	151	164	43
36–40	68.6	73.4	70.5	137	169	44
41–50	79.9	70.3	76.1	244	172	46

It is evident that the occurrence of pre-marital coitus is strongly correlated with marriage and that whether or not coitus resulted in conception is unimportant in a purely statistical sense. From the point of view of the individual woman, the important inference to be drawn from these data is that a pre-marital pregnancy does not necessarily impede her subsequently marrying.

While there are advantages in analyzing groups of females without reference to whether or not they have had pre-marital coitus, we find that to include a large proportion of virgins in our analyses masks some of the differences that we have discovered to exist between various groups. Consequently we have also calculated the accumulative experience of pre-marital pregnancy for females who had pre-marital coitus. This calculation answers the question, "Of girls who do have coitus before marriage, how many become pregnant as a result?"

By age fifteen, some 6 per cent of the girls who had pre-marital coitus at or before that age had become pregnant; by age twenty, nearly 13 per cent; by age thirty, 21 per cent; and ultimately by the mid-thirties we find that of women who have had pre-marital coitus

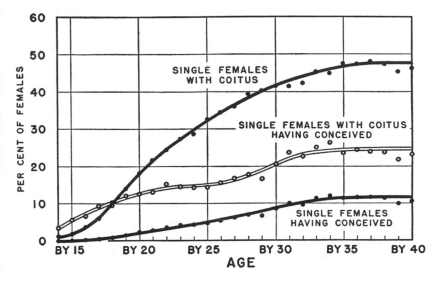

Figure 2. Accumulative Experience in Coitus and in Conception for Single Females and for Single Females with Coitus.

Data from Table 15.

and were still unmarried no less than one quarter had become pregnant at least once (Table 15, Figure 2). We hope that the hasty reader will not gain the impression that one quarter of the females with pre-marital coitus become pregnant; this is true only of the women who remained single into their fourth decade of life and who, in consequence, had been exposed to the possibility of pre-marital pregnancy many more years, on the average, than their younger sisters. Since most women marry and since most of them marry in their early twenties, it is more enlightening to state that of the females who have pre-marital coitus nearly one fifth become pregnant, the percentages for those who marry before age twenty-five ranging from 18 to 19 per cent (Table 16).[11]

---

[11] In a small sample of 28 married females who had had pre-marital coitus, Hamilton 1929:125, 133 found 8 cases (29 per cent) of pre-marital conception. In Dickinson and Beam 1934:33 a rather selective sample of 60

It should be noted, however, that in the course of a lifetime the females of our sample display about the same percentages of pre-marital pregnancies regardless of their marital status (Table 22). The never-married, the ever-married, the married-once, and the separated, divorced, or widowed all reveal similar percentages.

The majority of females who experienced a pre-marital pregnancy did so only once (81 per cent). In our sample 13 per cent became pregnant twice prior to marriage, 5 per cent three times, and 2 per cent four or more times.[12]

Age-specific rate. In computing the rate (frequency) at which the females of our sample conceived before marriage, we need to employ some unit of time. For our total sample, those married and unmarried, with and without pre-marital coitus, we have used as the unit of time the number of postadolescent years lived. For our single females we used as the unit of time pre-marital years; and for single females with pre-marital coitus we have used coital years. Rate is expressed in terms of the number of pre-marital conceptions per hundred of the relevant years.

Taking our total white non-prison sample (Table 20, first column) we see that between adolescence and age fifteen the rate is very small, but between ages sixteen and twenty there are 0.6 pre-marital conceptions per hundred years lived. The maximum rate, 1.1, is attained between ages twenty-one and twenty-five. Between twenty-six and thirty the rate drops to 0.8 and thereafter falls rapidly: 0.3 between thirty-one and thirty-five and 0.2 between thirty-six and forty. Since extremely few women experience two conceptions within a year, these rates per hundred years lived may also serve to show the percentage of women who pre-maritally conceive in any one year within the age-period. Thus the rate of 1.1 for age-period 21-25 means that, on the average, in any one year between ages twenty-one and twenty-five, 1.1 per cent of the women had a pre-marital conception. The rise of

---

single females with coital experience among a doctor's gynecologic patients showed a 33 per cent experience of pre-marital pregnancy. Brunner 1941:164 in a similar sample of 166 women reported 46 per cent pre-marital pregnancy experience.

[12] There are few reports on the frequency of pre-marital conceptions per single woman.

Hamilton 1929:125 indicated that one of his sample of 100 women had had "five illicit pregnancies," all of which were aborted before the third month. The other seven pre-marital pregnancies appear to have been reported by seven different females.

Auken 1953:253, in a report on 129 pre-marital conceptions among 106 Danish women, also found the large majority (83 per cent) with a single pregnancy, 12 per cent with two, and 5 per cent who had experienced three.

these rates reflects an increasing number of women having pre-marital intercourse, the maximum occurring between twenty-one and twenty-five when the most women were engaging in the pre-marital coitus that typically occurs just before marriage. The subsequent decline reflects the fact that they were marrying and hence were ineligible for a pre-marital conception.

The value of a figure concerning total females is that it indicates the incidence of a phenomenon in relation to the total population or any segment thereof. For example, the figure 0.8 given for age-period 26-30 means this: if one had a sample of primarily upper socio-economic level women (i.e., a sample comparable to ours) consisting of post-adolescent females, some of whom were married and some of whom were not, one would find that between ages twenty-six and thirty, 0.8 per cent of them experienced a pre-marital pregnancy.

Now turning to only those females who were unmarried during each of the age-periods involved (Table 20, second column), we find the rates of conception for the unmarried exceed the rates for the total sample, since the denominator for the total sample includes the women who married and were thereafter ineligible for a pre-marital conception. The increase in rate among the unmarried, reaching its maximum point between ages twenty-six and thirty, is probably the simple result of the increase in the percentage of unmarried females having coitus (1953:334); the following decrease is due to a complex of factors including aging, perhaps also a greater use of contraception, and the selected nature of the residual sample.

In dealing with these women with pre-marital coitus (Table 20, third column) we refine our analytical technique by discarding as our unit of measurement pre-marital years lived and substituting coital years: those years in each of which pre-marital coitus presumably occurred at least once. From adolescence to age fifteen there are four pre-marital conceptions per hundred years (i.e., in an average year between adolescence and age fifteen about 4 per cent of the girls with coitus were impregnated); between ages sixteen and twenty-five the rate stabilizes at about 7 per hundred; and then falls off to 6 between ages twenty-six and thirty, 3 between ages thirty-one and thirty-five, and 2 between ages thirty-six and forty. The relatively low figure for girls of fifteen or younger is explained by their low coital frequency: 0.1 per week as opposed to 0.2 to 0.4 for older women (1953:334). Since we know that the frequency of pre-marital coitus remains constant or slightly increases from age twenty-one to age forty, and that there is an increase in the proportion of pre-marital years that were coital years, the progressive decrease in conception rate beyond age twenty-five must stem from a more effective use of contraception as well as physiological decrease in fecundity.

Accumulative rate. The question of how often single females of a given age conceive has been answered in the discussion of age-specific rate; here we shall concern ourselves with the broader aspect of the matter: how frequently do women conceive pre-maritally within their reproductive lifetimes? What is the overall lifetime rate of pre-marital conception? Taking all females age thirty-six and older, i.e., women who are not likely to have any more pre-marital pregnancies, we find (Table 22) that in our sample there are 14 pre-marital conceptions for every hundred females. If we confine our attention only to those who had pre-marital coitus, the rate is 31 per hundred.

It is of interest to divide the latter group into those who married and those who had not married (at least by the time they contributed their case histories). The never-married exhibit a pre-marital conception rate of 29 per hundred while those who married have a higher rate of 32. This is understandable since pre-marital pregnancy sometimes forces marriage and also since sexually more responsive females are more apt not only to become pregnant but also to seek marriage successfully (Table 14).

Up to this point in this chapter we have been dealing with our entire single and coital samples of white non-prison females. At this point we shall turn to analyses with important sociological implications; we shall examine the relation between various social factors and reproductive behavior. In doing this, we shall deal primarily with our coital sample: all the females who have had pre-marital coitus.

RELATION TO AGE AT MARRIAGE

The age at which women marry has an effect upon the incidence of pre-marital pregnancy since it sets the limit to the number of years in which she may have pre-marital coitus. Conversely, of course, a pre-marital pregnancy sometimes provokes a hurried marriage.

Accumulative experience. Since, as we have shown in our volume on the female (1953:291 ff.), the bulk of pre-marital coitus tends to be concentrated in the years just prior to marriage, it is inevitable that the incidence and frequency of pre-marital pregnancy are also highest at that time, as shown later in Table 21.

Among our total sample of women who ultimately married, from 9 to 21 per cent conceived before marriage, the percentage rising with increased age at marriage. This increase is partly due to the increase, with age, in the proportion of females who have had pre-marital coitus and in the amount of such coitus (Table 16). While only about half the women who married by age twenty had had such coitus, some two thirds of those who did not marry until after age thirty had had this experience.

Of those with pre-marital coitus who married by age twenty, a total of 18 per cent were pregnant sometime before marriage; of those who married between twenty-one and twenty-five, 19 per cent; of those who married between twenty-six and thirty, 22 per cent; and of those who married after thirty, 31 per cent (Table 16).[13] In brief, the longer a woman delays marriage, while having coitus, the greater are her chances of incurring a pregnancy; this rather obvious fact is not surprising, but the magnitude of the percentages of those who do become pre-maritally pregnant is most unexpected.

A careful reader may note that the percentages given above are greater than those given in the accumulative experience for all females with pre-marital coitus (Table 15). The explanation is twofold. Obviously all women in this age-at-marriage study married, and pre-marital pregnancy sometimes leads to marriage either before or after the pregnancy ends. Secondly, and more importantly, our sample of all females with pre-marital coitus includes women who never married (up to the time they were interviewed), and among them is a higher proportion of sexually less responsive women who have a correspondingly lesser amount of pre-marital coitus and hence fewer pregnancies. Ultimately, however, the never-married tend to match the ever-married in percentage of females with pre-marital pregnancies (Table 22) as they accumulate more years of unmarried life.

Age-specific rate. Computing the rate (frequency) of pre-marital conception and expressing it in terms of the number of such conceptions per hundred coital years, one notes that the rates successively increase and reach their peaks in the age-period in which marriage occurred (Table 21). The rate is greatest for those who married between ages sixteen and twenty (14 per hundred coital years), and less for those who married later (about 12). This fits well with our knowledge that the majority of females who have pre-marital coitus have it with their fiancés, and that the frequency of coitus is usually higher with a fiancé than with another partner. One may say with consider-

---

[13] In contrast, however, the percentages of women who were pregnant at the time of their marriages is inversely related to the age at marriage. For the present sample, of the women married by age twenty, 4.8 per cent were pregnant, of those married at twenty-one to twenty-five years of age, 2.3 per cent were pregnant, and even fewer among those married at older ages. The same inverse relationship to age at marriage was reported by Christensen 1953:57.

able justification that approaching marriage is heralded by an increase in pre-marital coitus and pregnancy.[14]

Accumulative rate. Since accumulative experience revealed that the longer a woman delayed marriage the greater the probability of her becoming pregnant, it is not surprising to find that the rate of pregnancy is greater among those who marry later (Table 16). Thus we see that for every hundred girls with pre-marital coitus who married by age twenty there were 21 pre-marital conceptions, while among those who married after age thirty there were more than double that number of conceptions (44).

If one examines the total sample, which includes all females regardless of whether or not they had had pre-marital coitus, the same trend mentioned in the above paragraph is seen clearly.

The accumulative rates per hundred females are naturally somewhat higher than the equivalent percentages given under accumulative experience, since rates include those cases where a female had more than one pre-marital pregnancy. As one would expect, the older women are more apt than the younger ones to have had more than one pre-marital pregnancy.

RELATION TO EDUCATIONAL LEVEL

When we divide our females into several groups according to their formal education, we are not primarily searching for the effects of education upon individuals. The classification is made because actually educational level has proved to be our best single measure of an individual's socio-economic status in society. Our decision to use education as a measure of socio-economic status was confirmed by a series of exploratory calculations based on parental occupation: the results were essentially the same as those derived from educational level analyses. Nowadays with greater educational facilities and scholarships, educational level does not have as strict a correlation with socio-economic background as it had in years past, but it is still strong enough to allow us to think of the two as roughly equivalent. Thus we feel that our college educated sample represents rather accurately the upper socio-economic stratum, and our smaller high school educated sample roughly approximates the urban middle socio-economic stratum.

Accumulative experience. There is a negative correlation between educational level and pre-marital conception. Our small sample for

---

[14] A sudden increase in pre-marital conceptions during the four months preceding the date of marriage was shown in Christensen 1953:56. His cases were limited to pre-marital pregnancies that terminated in marriage.

those who had not gone beyond the eighth grade is insufficient for inclusion in Table 17 and for any but the most tentative statements. There is some indication that of those who had had pre-marital coitus as many, if not more, became pregnant before marriage as did females with high school education. However, there is also some reason to believe that the grade school educated conceived the bulk of these pregnancies during their teens, and thereby differ from the high school

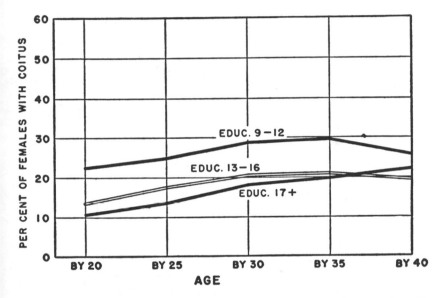

Figure 3. Accumulative Experience in Pre-Marital Conception for Females with Pre-Marital Coitus by Educational Level.

Data from Table 17.

educated. This is to be expected: by their middle or late teens these grade school females would have been out of school for some years leading more independent lives and possibly working.

Examination of Table 17 reveals that a higher percentage of the females with only a high school education had a pre-marital pregnancy than of those who went on to college and beyond. For example, by age twenty-five some 11 per cent of the high school educated had become pregnant before marriage, 8 per cent of the college educated, and 5 per cent of the females who eventually went into postgraduate work.[15]

---

[15] Pearl 1939:182 showed the highest per cent of pre-marital conception experience among his illiterate and elementary school educational groups. For these women, with a sample of over 15,000, he reported 10 per cent with pre-marital

This situation in part depends upon the proportions of girls in each educational category who had had pre-marital coitus, and the proportion is higher among the less educated. This is not the sole explanation, however, for by age thirty the proportions of those in both groups who had had pre-marital coitus were almost identical (nearly half), yet the less educated still showed higher percentages becoming pre-maritally pregnant.

When we turn to women with high school education (Grades 9-12), we see that about one quarter of the females with pre-marital coitus had had a pre-marital pregnancy by age twenty-five (Table 17, Figure 3). This percentage does not rise markedly in later ages. We suspect, but at present cannot demonstrate, that the grade school females would present equally high percentages.

The females who went to college but not on into postgraduate studies present a different picture. This we feel is not due to any influence exerted by colleges, but rather to the fact that most of them come from middle class and upper class environments. At any rate, we find that relatively few with pre-marital coitus had been pregnant in their teens (11-13 per cent). Bit by bit the percentages steadily increase until, by age thirty, 21 per cent have had this experience. Putting it another way, if one were to interview both married and unmarried college educated women aged thirty or more, all of whom had had pre-marital coitus at some time in their lives, one would learn that about one-fifth of them had conceived before marriage. While the college educated did not arrive at this 21 per cent level until well into their late twenties, the high school educated reached it in their teens and the grade school educated presumably reached it also in their teens.

The women who went beyond college into postgraduate work reveal a pattern essentially like that of the college educated, except that they tend to be a few percentage points lower by any given age up to thirty-five.

The differences in pre-marital conception experience between the educational groups shown in Table 17 and Figure 3 seem to stem from four sources. First, the less educated begin pre-marital coitus at an earlier age. Second, they have a higher frequency of pre-marital coitus prior to age twenty-one. Third and fourth, there appears to be a difference in the use of and/or the efficiency of contraceptives. For instance, the high school educated, college educated, and postgraduates

---

pregnancy experience. His total high school educated group of over 8,000 showed 8.2 per cent, while the total college sample (1,672 cases) showed a 3.6 pre-marital pregnancy experience. These figures compare well with ours.

display roughly the same number of coital years per female, yet differ markedly in conception experience and rates. In any case, the inverse relation between educational achievement and pre-marital conception is clear-cut.[16]

While these educational level differences stem from a number of factors, as we have seen,[17] the essential factor is the different attitudes held by the various socio-economic groups toward pre-marital pregnancy and sex in general (1948: Chapter 10).

Age-specific rate. When we compute rate of pre-marital conceptions per hundred coital years (years in each of which pre-marital coitus presumably occurred), again we find there are insufficient raw data for the grade school educated and hence we can compare only our other three educational groups (Table 21).

Up to age twenty-five, the higher the educational level, the lower the rates: between ages sixteen and twenty the high school educated have a rate of 10 as contrasted to 6 for the college educated and 5 for the women who later went into postgraduate work; between ages twenty-one and twenty-five the equivalent rates are 10 versus 6 and 5. Up to this point the high school educated were becoming pregnant roughly twice as often as the postgraduates. After age twenty-five the situation apparently changes and we now find the rate among the high school educated dropping to the level of, and even somewhat

---

[16] A similar inverse relationship, but based on occupational classification of the husband, was found in Christensen 1953:57. Lowest level of pre-marital pregnancy of wives at time of marriage (5 per cent) was in professional occupations, and highest (16 per cent) among laborers, with farm couples intermediate. An earlier study showed similar results.

Higher rates of pre-marital pregnancy among lower status groups (manual labor versus nonmanual) were also reflected in the British Family Census, in which live births prior to six and a half months of marriage were tabulated. Here the differences were greater than two to one. See Glass and Grebenik 1954:142-144.

For similar Swedish findings based on the criterion of family income see Sweden, Statistika Centralbryån, Folkräkningen den 31 December 1945, Vol. 7:2, p. 40, Table N.

De Wolff and Meerdink 1957:309 found similar results when comparing the percentages of first births that had been pre-maritally conceived in professional and laboring groups in Amsterdam, 1948-1955.

[17] While earlier marriage cannot be overlooked, it does not appear to be a primary factor in the differences in the pre-marital conception experience in the various educational levels, if one can assume that the findings of the British Family Census analysis on pre-marital conceptions terminating in live births would apply here. With their larger sample they were able to hold the age of marriage constant, but still found very strong differences as between occupational groups, with the live birth rate prior to six and a half months' duration of marriage from five to almost ten times as high in the manual workers group in comparison with the professional and salaried employees categories. See Glass and Grebenik 1954:143, 145.

below, the rates of the college and postgraduate groups; however, this may simply reflect a small sample size.

Converting rate per hundred coital years into percentage of females involved, as can be done in a situation such as this where in the vast majority of cases the women who conceived did so only once, we can say that between ages sixteen and twenty-five about 10 per cent of the high school educated with pre-marital coitus became pre-maritally pregnant as an annual average, 6 per cent of the college educated, and 5 per cent of the postgraduates. After age twenty-five the percentages apparently become about the same for all three educational groups, being at a 5 to 6 per cent level between ages twenty-six and thirty.

Accumulative rate. Considering first only those who had pre-marital coitus, we see that the educational level has a more pronounced effect at younger ages (Table 17). By age twenty, for example, there were 25 pre-marital conceptions for every hundred girls of high school education as opposed to 15 for those who attended or later attended college, and 12 for those who ultimately went into postgraduate work. By age thirty-five, essentially the end of pre-marital reproductive life, the respective rates are about 39, 28, and 29. The reduced rates after age thirty-five are the result of a generation change to be discussed subsequently.

The total sample, including those without as well as with pre-marital coitus, also illustrates the same relation between educational level and pre-marital conception, and the differences up to age twenty-five are even more pronounced in the total sample since a larger percentage of the less educated had had pre-marital coitus than had the better educated.

Our grade school educated are represented by too few cases to allow inclusion in the table, but such few cases strongly suggest that they have higher rates than any other educational group.

RELATION TO DECADE OF BIRTH

Let us see now how a female's chances of becoming pregnant before marriage are affected by still another factor: the decade in which she was born. The popular opinion, not without foundation in fact, is that various generations have been distinguished by somewhat different sexual conduct. Setting aside the perpetual human lament that the younger generation is always more unrestrained sexually, our earlier work has not only confirmed the obvious fact that over the years attitudes and behavior change, but has described the type and quantity of change (1953:298-302). We now face the question of what these changes have produced in terms of pre-marital pregnancy. We have approached this problem by dividing our females into groups according to the decade in which they were born.

Interpreting the statistics of this birth decade analysis proved most difficult. The span of time covered by the lives of the women of our sample includes two world wars, one great depression, and periods of prosperity, all of which are known to influence reproductive behavior. Furthermore, our decade groups do not synchronize with these historical events; for example, in our 1900-1909 birth decade a female born in 1900 passed through her more fertile years of twenty to thirty during prosperity, while a female born in 1909 lived through her more fertile years in the midst of a depression. Before discussing the statistical measurements, which are complex and, at points, seemingly contradictory, it is worthwhile to give a brief résumé of what seems to have occurred in connection with birth decade and reproductive behavior.

It would appear that among those with pre-marital coitus the percentage who became pregnant was about the same in birth decades 1890-1899 and 1900-1909, but increased somewhat among those born in 1910-1919; however, there was also another trend: of the women who did become pregnant, more of those born in the more recent decades had a second pre-marital pregnancy (Table 18). This situation explains why accumulative experience can remain constant or decrease with successive birth decades while accumulative rate can increase.

The females born in 1920-1929 constitute a separate phenomenon: in their teens they were singularly infertile, but after twenty they showed a sharp increase in the number who became pregnant and also in the frequency of pregnancy.[18] This reversal of behavior is quite explicable in the light of what we know of the fertility of married women: that there was a general decrease in the incidence and frequency of marital conceptions until the postwar "baby boom." This "boom" naturally was largely confined to females born since 1920, and hence the incidence

---

[18] At this point one might reason as follows: many females of our sample are college educated; the females of the 1920-1929 birth decade would be more likely than females of other birth decades to be of college age at the time our interviewing was done; therefore our 1920-1929 group contains more college educated females than the other decade groups and hence the figures represent educational level differences rather than decade differences. This reasoning, while apparently logical, is refuted by the fact that the educational level of the 1920-1929 females is virtually identical with that of the females belonging to other birth decades. By age twenty the median female born between 1920 and 1929 had 15.9 years of education, the median female born between 1910 and 1919 had 15.8, and the median female born between 1900 and 1909 also had 15.8 years of schooling. By age twenty-five the 1920-1929 group had somewhat less education than the other groups, the median female having had 15.7 years of education compared to 16.2, 16.4, and 16.5 for the other decade of birth groups.

of experience and rate figures for the 1920-1929 decade increased sharply. There was also what one could term a "marriage boom," and the proportion of younger people marrying increased considerably. We know that pre-marital conceptions are most frequent among females who subsequently marry, and that the bulk of such pregnancies occurs within roughly a two-year period prior to marriage. Consequently, we feel that the increase in experience and rate of pre-marital pregnancy among the females born between 1920 and 1929 can be considered the forerunner of the later "marriage boom" and "baby boom."[19]

Accumulative experience. Table 18 reveals that in our total sample there has been, by and large, a progressive increase with successive birth decades in the percentage of females who became pregnant before marriage. Most of the increase is due to the fact that the proportion of females having pre-marital coitus also increased from decade to decade. For example, by age twenty-five only 19 per cent of the women born between 1890 and 1899 had had pre-marital coitus, for the next decade the figure is 41 per cent, for the next decade 49 per cent, and for our most recent decade 55 per cent. This explains why the percentage of our total sample experiencing a pre-marital pregnancy by age twenty-five rose from 3 per cent to 11 per cent.

If we next confine our attention only to those women who had pre-marital coitus, we see that birth decades 1890-1899 and 1900-1909 are essentially alike, but that the percentage of women who became pregnant increases among those born in 1910-1919. The females born in 1920-1929 behaved as we previously described, manifesting a low percentage by age twenty and then presenting by age twenty-five a percentage equaling that of the previous decade of birth.[20] The differences are not great, never exceeding 4 per cent.

Age-specific rate. Table 21 shows a decrease in pre-marital pregnancies between ages sixteen and twenty of from 8 pregnancies per

---

[19] The positive relationship of pre-marital fertility and married fertility is recognized in Glass and Grebenik 1954:143 (Table 5) and in U.S. Vital Statistics, Special Reports 1950 (33):71, in which the rise of illegitimate births in relation to legitimate births in the last decade is discussed.

[20] Christensen 1953:57 also found decade variation in his study of pre-marital conceptions that terminated in marriage. His sample is only roughly comparable here, as it is based on marriages occurring during a three-year span of each of three decades rather than on decade of birth. His findings were:

        1919-1921   11.9 per cent
        1929-1931   14.8 per cent
        1939-1941   9.8 per cent

This would indicate a higher rate for the early depression period, which he suggested may have resulted from an increase in pre-marital contacts because of the retarding of marriages.

hundred coital years among the 1900-1909 females to 5 among the 1920-1929 females. Between twenty-one and twenty-five the trend is reversed (the 1920-1929 females now having a rate of 8, the 1910-1919 about 7, and the 1900-1909 only 6), presumably because of "marriage and baby boom" phenomena that influenced not only the 1920-1929 females, but also to some degree the younger 1910-1919 women. Between ages twenty-six and thirty the former trend toward a decrease with successive birth decades reasserts itself, but perhaps only because we do not have sufficient 1920-1929 females to tabulate in this 26-30

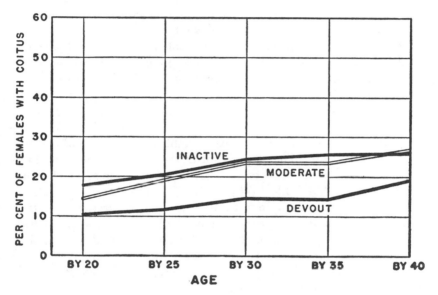

Figure 4. Accumulative Experience in Pre-Marital Conception for Protestant Females with Pre-Marital Coitus by Degree of Religious Devoutness.
Data from Table 19.

age-period. The caution necessary in drawing inferences from fairly small differences, such as some seen in age-specific rate, is emphasized when one notes that among the 1900-1909 females vagary of sample causes the rate to fall from 6 (ages 26-30) to 1 (ages 31-35) and then rises to almost 3 (ages 36-40, when fecundity is known to be less than at ages 31-35).

Accumulative rate. If again we confine our attention to only those females who had pre-marital coitus (since we know that a higher proportion of the women born in recent decades has had pre-marital coitus than of those born earlier), we see that by any age after twenty

there is a definite increase in the number of pre-marital pregnancies
(Table 18). By age thirty-five, for example, the 1890-1899 females had
had 28 such pregnancies per hundred females, the 1900-1909 women
had had 31 and the 1910-1919 women had had 40. This increase in pre-
marital pregnancy should give pause to those who feel a simple answer
to the problem can be provided by contraceptives currently available.

RELATION TO DEGREE OF DEVOUTNESS

In our volume on the female we found that degree of religious devoutness was a potent factor in female sexual behavior (1953:304 ff.).
Consequently it will be no surprise that reproductive behavior exhibits
a strong correlation with degree of devoutness.

Accumulative experience. Our Protestant sample reveals that fewer
of the more devout women experience pre-marital pregnancy. Obviously this hinges on the fact that proportionately fewer of them have
had pre-marital coitus. By age twenty, for instance, 16 per cent of the
devout Protestants had had coitus, 22 per cent of the moderately devout,
and 29 per cent of the religiously inactive. Yet when we consider only
those with coital experience we see that this is only a partial explanation. By age twenty some 18 per cent of the religiously inactive Protestants in our sample with pre-marital coitus had experienced a pre-
marital pregnancy (Table 19, Figure 4). From this age they build up
to a 24 per cent level by age thirty, and by the latter part of their
fourth decade of life 26 per cent have had at least one pre-marital
pregnancy. The percentage among the moderately devout is less,
reaching 15 per cent by age twenty; later in life the difference between
the inactive and moderately devout lessens. The devout Protestants
uniformly exhibit the lowest incidences of all: from a 10 per cent incidence by age twenty there is an increase to 14 per cent by age thirty,
and beyond that there is some evidence that a figure in the neighborhood of 19 per cent is reached by age forty. In brief, degree of
devoutness has a high negative correlation with the accumulative experience of pre-marital pregnancy.[21] One reason for this is the fact
that the religiously inactive have pre-marital coitus with greater frequency than the more devout (1953:343) and have experienced coitus
for more years.

---

[21] A difference in incidence of pre-marital pregnancy at time of marriage based on
the criteria of a religious versus a civil marriage ceremony, as shown in the
Christensen 1953 study, possibly bears on the present findings in regard to
religious devoutness. Among the couples with a registered first birth in the
five years following marriage, 21 per cent of the civil ceremony wives, as contrasted with 10 per cent of the religious ceremony wives, were pregnant at
the time of marriage.

Our Catholic and Jewish samples are too small for such subdivision but some experimental calculations show that the same correlation holds. We fortunately have enough religiously inactive Jewish women in our sample to permit calculation. It is noteworthy that up to age thirty they have a low incidence of experience,[22] between the moderately devout and the devout Protestants; but by age thirty-five their percentages become essentially like those of the moderately devout Protestants. Our small Catholic sample provides higher figures than those for Protestants and Jews, but the composition of the Catholic sample is such that direct comparison is not justified.[23]

Age-specific rate. Expressing the rate of pre-marital conceptions in terms of rate per hundred coital years we find that the rate between adolescence and age fifteen is extremely small in all our religious groups. After age fifteen, however, the negative correlation we have previously seen becomes apparent (Table 21). Between sixteen and twenty the inactive Protestants have a rate of 9 pre-marital pregnancies per hundred coital years, the moderately devout 6, and the devout 4. In the following age-period, 21–25, the equivalent rates are 7, 7, and 5. This is the age-period in which the rates for the moderately devout and devout are highest, whereas the inactive have their highest rate in the preceding age-period of 16–20. Between twenty-six and thirty the inactive maintain their former rate but the other two Protestant groups exhibit lower rates essentially like those they manifested between ages sixteen and twenty. All three groups have lower rates after age thirty.

The inactive Jewish females present rates essentially like those of the moderately devout Protestants: their initial rate (between ages sixteen and twenty) is 6 per hundred and in age-period 21-25 they reach 7.

Our Catholic females are too few to sustain an age-specific breakdown in terms of degree of devoutness.

Accumulative rate. Four groups are available for comparison: the three Protestant categories and the inactive Jewish. These rates con-

---

[22] Pearl 1939:181 did not calculate percentages of pre-marital conception experience for his religious categories of ever-married females, but Table 26, if summarized, shows a markedly lower figure for Jewish women, 1.5 per cent, as against 7.6 per cent for the Protestants. Since these data were based on the fertility histories of women who were obstetrical patients in metropolitan hospitals, they are not entirely representative, but the sample is large, over 14,000 for the two categories.

[23] The Pearl survey found no difference in the extent of pre-marital conception as between his Protestant and Catholic ever-married sample, both showing 7.6 per cent experience.

firm our earlier finding about the relation between pre-marital pregnancy and degree of religious devoutness (Table 19). By age twenty,
the inactive Protestants with pre-marital coitus had a rate of 21 conceptions per hundred females; the moderately devout 16; and the devout 10. By age thirty-five the rates were 38 for the inactive, 34 for the
moderately devout, and 16 for the devout. The religiously inactive
Jewish women again are similar to the moderately devout Protestants.
The total sample shows the same relations, the differences being exaggerated by the differing proportions of females who had pre-marital
coitus.

OUTCOME OF PREGNANCY

We have thus far examined pregnancy in the unmarried; now the
important question arises, what was the outcome of these pregnancies? It is with this that the remainder of the chapter will be concerned.

There are three possible outcomes or terminations of pregnancy:
live birth, spontaneous abortion (including stillbirth), and induced
abortion. We have defined our use of these terms in Chapter 2. From
the point of view of society and the pregnant woman herself there
is, besides the three types of outcome just mentioned, another important possibility: marriage prior to the termination of the pregnancy.
Consequently this is given the status of a separate category in some
of the tables.

We have at our disposal for analysis 270 females who account for
355 pregnancies that ended while the females were unmarried. Of
these pregnancies the great majority (316) terminated in pre-marital
induced abortion. From this simple enumeration of what data we have
available, it is obvious that we can say very little concerning either
live birth or spontaneous abortion among the unmarried. Actually this
deficiency, while regrettable, is not serious: other statistics are available for data on illegitimate births.[24] Furthermore, any statistics on

---

[24] *U.S. Vital Statistics, 1950* (1), 1954:93 (Table 6.28) shows from 1.6 to 2.4 per
cent of all white births as illegitimate during the years 1938-1950. The present
data (40 out of 2,434) calculates to 1.6 per cent.
   European levels of illegitimacy are cited as higher. Gille 1949:32 reported
that of the total births in 1936 to 1940, 12.6 per cent were illegitimate in
Sweden, 7.5 per cent in Finland, and 6.3 per cent in Norway. Croog 1951:
218 lists 8 to 9 per cent for Denmark. Gunzert 1953:79 in the official year
book for the city of Frankfurt a.M., Germany, reported 12 per cent of all
births as illegitimate. Percentages of illegitimate births to total births in various
countries for 1951 are cited in the French journal *Population* 1956:219:
England, 4.8 per cent; Austria, 16.5 per cent; France, 6.7 per cent; Italy,
3.4 per cent; Norway, 3.7 per cent; Holland, 1.4 per cent; Portugal, 11.5 per
cent; Sweden, 9.9 per cent; Switzerland, 3.5 per cent.

spontaneous abortion prior to marriage are necessarily deceptive owing to the prevalence of induced abortion: an unknown number of pregnancies that would otherwise have ended in spontaneous abortion were terminated by induced abortion. The major contribution our research can make is the analysis of pre-marital induced abortion, a subject that has been much discussed but about which very little has hitherto been known.

RELATION TO AGE AND TO MARITAL STATUS AT INTERVIEW

Accumulative experience. As we have indicated, the number of women who have a pre-marital live birth or spontaneous abortion is small. For our sample we calculate that in a lifetime 1 per cent or less of the women with pre-marital coitus have ever experienced either type of outcome.

Induced abortion, however, is a phenomenon of greater magnitude.[25]

---

[25] One source from which the not inconsiderable incidence of induced (and occasionally spontaneous) abortion in single females may be inferred is the summaries of hospital abortion cases in which the marital status of the patients is given. Since these studies deal with groups of females, all of whom are being given hospital care following an abortion, the figures cannot be compared to data from the present study. Thus we find:

Johnson 1931:781 reported over 14 per cent single women among 288 hospital abortion cases in Louisville, Ky.

Watkins 1933:162 listed 6 per cent unmarried abortion cases in a total of 341 abortion patients, half of whom were induced abortion cases, in an Oregon county hospital.

Witherspoon 1933:368 stated that of a sample of 200 cases in the New Orleans Charity Hospital, 14 per cent were unmarried, and all but four cases were "criminal abortions." One fifth of the single women were nonwhite.

Stewart 1935:873 found 9 per cent single women in an abortion series of 1,700 case records at Boston City Hospital, 1929-1932.

Peckham 1936:110 stated that single females accounted for 10 per cent of 2,287 abortion cases (about one third of sample was nonwhite) over a 38-year period at Johns Hopkins Hospital, Baltimore.

Simons 1939:841 found 12 per cent of 995 cases of hospital abortion were single women, over two thirds of whom were in for care following an admitted induced abortion, in a Minneapolis hospital.

Hamilton 1940:922 recorded that among 353 white abortion cases in a Bellevue sample, 8 per cent were single, and two thirds of these admitted induced abortion.

Tietze 1949:60, in reporting on a series of 363 illegal abortions, found 28 per cent of them were performed on single females.

Timanus stated that about half of his 3,000 illegal abortion cases were females up to the age of the twenties, and as few as 8 per cent were single among the cases past 40 years of age. See his statement at the Planned Parenthood 1955 Abortion Conference, Calderone 1958. (This book is in preparation, hence pagination cannot be supplied.)

The fact that single women are obviously more reluctant to seek hospital care following an abortion makes the figures cited in the hospital studies rather unreliable, as Tietze 1954:23 has pointed out.

In attempting to determine the percentage of females who ever experience a pre-marital induced abortion, we have examined the data on the women aged thirty-six and over who may be said to have completed their pre-marital reproductive lives. Our total sample of these women indicates that 8 per cent have experienced a pre-marital induced abortion. Of those women aged thirty-six or more who had pre-marital coitus prior to age thirty-six, some 18 per cent had had an induced abortion (Table 22).[26]

Sociologically, it is interesting to examine what relation exists between pre-marital induced abortion and subsequent marital status. Taking these same women, those thirty-six and older who had pre-marital coitus, we find that of those who never married (at least not prior to the interview) some 21 per cent had had an induced abortion; for those who married the figure is 17 per cent. This is not a great difference, and it would be unwise to draw moral inferences from it —especially since the same table (Table 22) would indicate that of women who married once and were still married at time of interview a higher proportion (18 per cent) had had pre-marital induced abortions than women whose marriages had broken up (16 per cent).

The relation of age to the percentage of pre-marital pregnancies that terminate in marriage is best illustrated in age-specific rates to be discussed later.

Accumulative rate. Still thinking in terms of lifetime experience and hence confining ourselves to women of thirty-six and over who had experienced pre-marital coitus, we found a rate of 26 pre-marital induced abortions per hundred women[27] (Table 22). Those who never marry have a slightly higher rate (27) than those who marry (25), but

---

Examples of similar European data are found in:

Davis 1950:129, in a 15-year survey of abortion cases in a London hospital, showed an 11.4 per cent incidence of single females among 2,665 abortion cases.

Bumm 1916:387 indicated that 15 per cent of one month's abortion cases in the University clinic, Berlin, were unmarried females.

Brezina and Reuterer 1935:324-325 found that one third of all reported abortion cases in Austria, 1929-1932, were single women.

Sutter 1950:86 reported 38 per cent of 1,414 induced abortion cases studied in a Paris hospital, 1946-1949, were single women.

---

[26] Hamilton 1929:125, 133 also reported an 8 per cent experience of pre-marital induced abortion for his sample of 100 married women.

Dickinson and Beam 1934:33 in their study of 500 single women, found 2.4 per cent had had an induced abortion. Our comparable figure is 2.6 per cent.

Brunner and Newton 1939:84, in a clinic sample of 345 single women, found 10 per cent had experienced an induced abortion.

[27] The Hamilton 1929 study (pp. 125, 133) showed a closely similar accumulative rate of 23.3 pre-marital induced abortions per 100 females with pre-marital coital experience, while the Davis 1929:21 findings calculate to a rate of 18 per 100. Three fourths of her total sample were college educated.

once again we see that the prevalence of pre-marital abortion is somewhat smaller among those who subsequently married and had their marriages break up (23). Why this should be true we do not know. Of some sociological interest is the fact that of the marriages forced, or at least hastened, by a pregnancy as many endured as dissolved.

The rates calculated for our total sample of women aged thirty-six and older are slightly less than half as great as those for women with coitus, since about 45 per cent of all women aged thirty-six and over had had pre-marital coitus.

Outcome ratio. In computing the relative proportions of live birth, spontaneous abortion, and induced abortion, one must deal with the number of terminated pregnancies rather than with the number of females involved. Taking all 355 pre-marital terminations in our sample (not merely those experienced by women aged thirty-six or more) we find that 6 per cent were live births,[28] 5 per cent were spontaneous abortions, and 89 per cent were induced abortions.[29] The social stigma attached to illegitimacy in this country is such that the vast majority of unmarried pregnant women will desperately seek and secure abortions.

At this point it is well to examine the outcome of pre-marital pregnancies that terminated in marriage. Our sample offers for inspection 64 pre-marital pregnancies that were carried into subsequent marriage. Two of these terminated after the short marriages broke up. Excluding two pregnancies that had not ended by the time of interview, of the remaining 60, 75 per cent ended in live birth, 7 per cent in spontaneous abortion, and 18 per cent in induced abortion. The

---

Dickinson and Beam 1934:33 reported a rate of 20 induced abortions per 100 single coital females, with a sample of 60 such women.

Bromley and Britten 1938:259 listed 5 per cent of 192 college women with pre-marital experience as having had induced abortions.

Brunner 1941:164 reported a 39.7 per cent induced abortion experience among 166 single clinic patients with pre-marital sexual experience.

[28] Auken 1953:253, in a sample of Danish women found almost a third of 129 pre-marital pregnancies with a termination in birth outside of marriage. See Croog 1951:218 for a discussion of the improved position of the unmarried mother in Denmark.

[29] Brunner 1941:165 showed an outcome ratio of 69 per cent induced abortions, and of 14 per cent spontaneous abortions, for 176 pre-marital conceptions reported by clinic patients, both single and now married. This appears to include pre-marital pregnancies carried into marriage. If one calculates an outcome ratio from Table 2, p. 164, of the 77 pregnancies of single women, one finds that 86 per cent resulted in induced abortion and 8 per cent in spontaneous abortion.

A fetal mortality ratio relating to illegitimate births is provided in U.S. Vital Statistics, Special Reports 1956 (42):354. These data are based chiefly on late fetal deaths, however, and thus are not comparable to the present induced or spontaneous abortion data.

difference between the 6 per cent live births of those who did not
marry and the 75 per cent live births of those who did is in itself
sufficient commentary on the strength of the social sanctions against
illegitimacy.[30]

Age-specific outcome ratio. These age-specific ratios (Table 27)
clearly demonstrate that older females resort more and more to
induced abortion and have correspondingly fewer live births.[31] For
example, between adolescence and age twenty some 6 per cent of the
pregnancies end in live birth, 3 per cent in spontaneous abortion, 69
per cent in induced abortion, and 21 per cent in subsequent marriage;
but after age twenty-five, live births account for but 3 per cent, spontaneous abortion for 5 per cent, induced abortion for 86 per cent, and
subsequent marriage for the remaining 6 per cent. This reflects the
difficulty experienced by young females, especially those under
twenty-one, in obtaining an induced abortion; older women find it
somewhat easier. It is also clear that older women are less inclined,
or perhaps less able, to enter into a forced marriage.

From a demographic point of view it is interesting to examine what
proportion of pre-marital pregnancies ended in live birth and what
proportion were "wastage" *regardless of whether or not the woman
married before the end of her pregnancy.* The lower portion of Table
27 reveals that live birth decreases markedly with age, falling from 23
per cent of the pregnancies incurred between adolescence and age
twenty to 8 per cent of the pregnancies incurred after twenty-five.

RELATION TO AGE AT MARRIAGE

Accumulative experience. The age at which a woman marries exhibits a strong and consistent correlation with the incidence of induced

---

[30] It is of interest here to observe the role that pre-marital pregnancies play in the
total fertility of certain European countries. In Denmark, Sweden, and Finland we find that during the years 1945-1948 from a fourth to a fifth of the
marriages are followed by a birth within six months. These births represented
over 10 per cent of the total legitimate births in Denmark and Finland, and
14 per cent of them in Sweden in 1947. See Croog 1952:361, 363.
    In the fertility analysis of the British Family Census, Glass and Grebenik
1954:142 reached the following conclusion: "Hence looked at both in its
relation to total fertility and in terms of its incidence among married women,
pre-nuptial conception cannot be regarded as 'abnormal,' or as the expression
of 'immorality' on the part of a small section of the population. On the contrary, it is substantial in its incidence and is associated with marriages which,
by definition, lasted until Census date. Moreover, it has a long historical tradition. There is statistical support for the view that pre-nuptial conceptions are
a quite important feature of the family in Britain . . ."
[31] Williams and Thorner 1956:223 showed that among white births in Florida,
1953, only 15 per cent of the illegitimate, in contrast to 27 per cent of the
legitimate, were to mothers 30 or older.

abortion prior to marriage (Table 23). This could have been anticipated since we have already seen that the longer females with pre-
marital coitus delay marriage, the more likely they are to become
pregnant, and we also know that the vast majority of pre-marital
pregnancies terminates in induced abortion.

Of our total sample of ever-married females, including those with
and without pre-marital coital experience who married by age twenty,
roughly 4 per cent had an induced abortion before marriage; approximately 20 per cent of those who married after age thirty had this

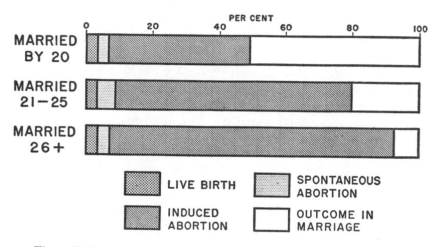

Figure 5. Outcome of Pre-Marital Conception by Age at First Marriage.
Data from Table 28.

experience. This dramatic jump is due in part to an increase, with
increased age at marriage, in the proportion of women who had pre-
marital coitus.

Among only those with pre-marital coitus, the lowest incidence of
pre-marital abortion, 7 per cent, is in the group of females who marry
between adolescence and age twenty. The percentage increases as the
age at marriage increases until among those who marry at and after
age thirty-one the incidence of induced abortion reaches nearly 30
per cent. These percentages, as expected, partly parallel those of accumulative experience of pre-marital pregnancy: for instance we saw
(Table 16) that 31 per cent had conceived before marriage: therefore
it is no surprise to find that 30 per cent had pre-marital induced abortions (Table 23). A larger discrepancy exists between the pregnancy
experience and the induced abortion experience of females marrying

at younger ages, but this is because more of the younger females marry while pregnant and hence become ineligible to experience a pre-marital induced abortion: while 18 per cent of those who married by age twenty had conceived before marriage, only 7 per cent had had induced abortions.

Accumulative rate. The rates (Table 23), as expressed in terms of the number of pre-marital abortions per hundred women with pre-marital coitus, show the same trend that was manifested in accumulative experience. Those who married between adolescence and age twenty had a rate of about 9 abortions per hundred females. With each succesive age-at-marriage group the rate is greater, ultimately being about 40 per hundred women among those who married after age thirty.

Outcome ratio. Table 28 and Figure 5 show that age-at-marriage groups differ primarily in the proportion of pregnancies that are ended by induced abortion and in the proportion of pregnancies that are carried into subsequent marriage. For the three age-at-marriage groups the percentage of pregnancies ending in pre-marital live birth is the same (3 to 4 per cent) and, with one inexplicable but rather small exception, the percentage of spontaneous abortion is the same. However, those who married by age twenty had the smallest proportion of pregnancies terminating in induced abortion (43 per cent) and the largest proportion carried into marriage (51 per cent).[32] Those who married between ages twenty-one and twenty-five ended 71 per cent of their pregnancies in induced abortion, while 20 per cent were resolved in marriage. Among those who married after age twenty-five, some 86 per cent of the pregnancies were deliberately aborted and only 7 per cent were carried into a subsequent marriage.

In brief, it seems clear that with increasing age at marriage there is an increase in pre-marital induced abortion and a corresponding decrease in the proportion of pre-marital conceptions carried into marriage.

RELATION TO EDUCATIONAL LEVEL

Accumulative experience. Our total sample indicates that in a lifetime about 8 per cent of the women who went beyond grammar school experienced a pre-marital induced abortion. Those of grammar school

---

[32] Glass and Grebenik 1954:141 (footnote 2) show in both their data and those of the Registrar General's for Great Britain a much higher incidence of live births prior to eight and a half months' duration of marriage for the females with younger ages at marriage. Thus for the females marrying under twenty, the rates were about three times as great as they were in any age period past twenty-five.

education exhibit a lower figure, 6 per cent, which is in keeping with our impression that this group is more inclined to permit pregnancy to continue than are females of the middle and upper socio-economic levels where illegitimate births are less socially acceptable. This impression will be discussed in more detail in Chapter 6.

Taking women of thirty-six and over who have had pre-marital coitus prior to age thirty-six, we find comparison can be made only for the high school, college, and postgraduate groups. Since we have

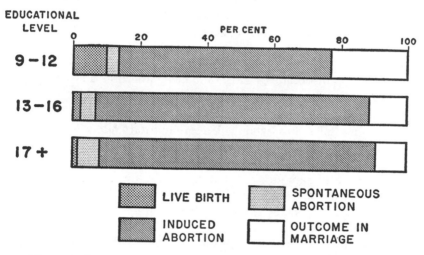

Figure 6. Outcome of Pre-Marital Conception by Educational Level.
Data from Table 28.

demonstrated that the incidence of pre-marital pregnancy is inversely related to educational level, Table 24 comes as no surprise. Twenty-two per cent of the females who went into but not beyond high school had at least one induced abortion, 18 per cent of the college educated females, and 17 per cent of the postgraduate females.

Accumulative rate. Using the same sample as defined above, one finds that the high school educated have a rate of 31 induced abortions per hundred females with pre-marital coitus, while the college and postgraduate females have a lower rate, 24 and 26 respectively. The fact that the postgraduate rate is slightly higher than the college rate is probably meaningless in view of our sample size (Table 24).

Outcome ratio. In comparing the high school educated, college educated, and postgraduate females, the high school educated are seen to have the largest proportions of pre-marital live births (10 per cent) and pregnancies resolved in marriage (23 per cent); conversely, they have the smallest proportion of induced abortion (63 per cent). Our general knowledge of the mores and behavior of the lower socio-economic stratum leads us to feel that the grade school educated would exhibit an even greater proportion of pregnancies ending in pre-marital live birth. The college educated and postgraduate groups are alike in that about 2 per cent of their pregnancies ended in birth and 82 to 83 per cent in induced abortion; however, a somewhat larger proportion of the pregnancies of the college educated was carried into subsequent marriage—12 per cent as against 9 per cent for the postgraduate group (Table 28, Figure 6).

RELATION TO DECADE OF BIRTH

The relation of decade of birth to induced abortion is essentially the same as the relation of decade of birth to pre-marital pregnancy.

Accumulative experience. By age twenty the percentage of females with pre-marital coitus who had a pre-marital induced abortion is essentially the same (12 per cent) for those born in the years 1900–1909 and 1910–1919 (the decade 1890–1899 cannot be utilized at this point because of sample size), but definitely lower (7 per cent) for women born in the decade 1920–1929 (Table 25). By age twenty-five a trend becomes visible: the percentage of females who had a pre-marital induced abortion increases with each successive decade of birth from 1890 to 1919. The 1920–1929 group still is below the two preceding birth decade groups but the difference is now small—just as in incidence of pre-marital pregnancy the 1920–1929 group tended to "catch up" with its predecessors. The fact that its percentage rises from 7 per cent by age twenty to 11 per cent by age twenty-five suggests that it may eventually equal or surpass the percentages for the earlier groups; but unfortunately we do not have sufficient data to calculate beyond age twenty-five for the 1920–1929 females.

Beyond age twenty-five the same trend persists: each successive decade includes a greater percentage of members who have had induced abortions. By age thirty, 14 per cent of the 1890–1899 females had had this experience; 16 per cent of the 1900–1909 females; and 19 per cent of the 1910–1919 females. By age thirty-five, decades 1890–1899 and 1900–1909 also show, inexplicably, an identical per cent of 17, but the 1910-1919 females manifest the surprisingly high figure of 24 per cent.

The trend toward an increase in induced abortion followed by a decrease shown by females of birth decade 1920–1929, is more consistent and striking when one examines our total sample, but this consistency is partly because with each successive decade more women have had pre-marital coitus.

Accumulative rate. These data (Table 25) on the number of induced abortions per hundred females present even more clearly the same situation one sees in accumulative experience; an increase in rate with each successive birth decade except for those born between 1920 and 1929. And once again this group shows signs of eventually achieving a rate comparable to or in excess of the rates established by the women of the 1910–1919 decade. In connection with this last statement one should recall that there are many hidden factors involved in our decade-of-birth analyses, a complication that is particularly true of the 1920–1929 birth decade. A comparison of accumulative experience with rate indicates also that with each successive birth decade up to 1919 there was a slight but growing tendency for women to have more than one induced abortion. This trend does not, evidently, persist among the 1920–1929 females.

Outcome ratio. Our decade-of-birth analysis in Table 28 reveals over the years these salient features: an increase in the proportion of pre-marital pregnancies ending in live birth before marriage, an increase in the proportion of pregnancies carried into marriage, and a corresponding decrease in the proportion of induced abortions. It is true that up to and including birth decade 1910–1919 induced abortion increased in absolute frequency but the relative proportion declined because the frequency of pre-marital conception increased even more. Also, a greater number of these more recent conceptions were carried into marriage or ended in live birth prior to marriage.[33] Proportionately, induced abortion fell from 82 per cent among the 1900–1909 group to 68 per cent among the 1920–1929 group.[34]

The apparent increase in the proportion of spontaneous abortions among the women born in 1920–1929 is probably fortuitous since only seven spontaneous abortions are involved. Although the number of cases is small, it appears that the increase in the proportion of live

---

[33] The increase in number of pre-marital live births is indicated in U.S. Vital Statistics, Special Reports 1950 (33):74, which showed an increase in the rate of births to single white women from 7 per thousand (ages 15-44) in 1940 to 12 in 1947.

[34] Dickinson and Beam 1934:33, in material that was largely gathered in the early 1900's, found eight births and 12 abortions in their sample of 20 pre-marital pregnancies.

Lewis-Faning 1949:169 in the British survey on family limitation found a decade difference in percentage of induced abortions among pre-nuptial conceptions terminating in marriage. Since a high percentage of these resulted in live births, the induced abortion ratio was low, only 0.6 for those marrying before 1930, and 1.3 for those marrying after 1930.

births took place among the females of decade 1910–1919 and was maintained by the females of decade 1920–1929. One may speculate that this unexpected development stemmed from three things: within the past thirty years induced abortion has been given more attention in newspapers and magazines, which have pointed out its hazards and ill effects; there has also been, in general, an increase in the amount of legislation against abortion and a greater enforcement of the abortion laws; and thirdly, within the same period there has been an increase in homes for unmarried mothers, in adoption services, and in the revision of birth certificates so that illegitimacy is concealed.

RELATION TO DEGREE OF DEVOUTNESS

To take our 421 pre-marital pregnancies and impose upon them a multiple breakdown into three major religions, each containing three categories of degree of devoutness—a total of nine divisions—and then further subdivide by type of outcome, is to reduce many of the ultimate samples to the vanishing point. All that can reasonably be done is to deal with the three Protestant categories and one Jewish category, these being numerically large enough for treatment.

Accumulative experience. When we confine ourselves as usual to women thirty-six and older so as to examine completed pre-marital reproductive lifetimes, it is clear that degree of religious devoutness rather strongly influences the incidence of pre-marital induced abortion, just as we saw that it also influenced the frequency of pre-marital coitus. Twenty-one per cent of the inactive Protestant women with pre-marital coitus had induced abortions, 19 per cent of the moderately devout, and 10 per cent of the devout (Table 26). The closeness of the inactive and moderately devout, which is also observable in other types of sexual behavior, strengthens our belief that many of our moderately devout participate in religious activities for social reasons, but are intellectually and emotionally equivalent to our non-devout category. The inactive Jewish have an induced abortion figure of 17 per cent, which is in keeping with their customary tendency to be more nearly like moderately devout than inactive Protestants; we shall see this same phonemenon in accumulative rate.

Essentially the same picture is seen in our total female sample, except that the figures for the moderately devout tend to be more truly intermediate than they were in the sample of women with pre-marital coitus. This discrepancy between the relative positions of the moderately devout in the total versus the coital sample may be explained as follows: in the total sample the intermediate position of the moderately devout reflects the fact that by age thirty-five, 33 per cent of the devout had had pre-marital coitus, 44 per cent of the moderately devout, and 57 per cent of the religiously inactive (Table 19).

Accumulative rate. Using the sample described above, Table 26 reveals that the inactive Protestants have about 32 induced abortions per hundred females with pre-marital coitus, the moderately devout 29, and the devout 12. The inactive Jewish females have a rate of 28.

Outcome ratio. While sample size does not permit a thorough investigation, the data we do possess suggest that the greater the degree of devoutness the smaller is the proportion of pregnancies ended by induced abortion (Table 28). Seventy-nine per cent of the pregnancies of all our religiously inactive Protestants were aborted in contrast to 69 per cent for the moderately devout and 65 per cent (based on only 37 pregnancies) for the devout. There is also some indication that the devout women are more apt to marry when they discover they are pregnant than are the religiously inactive.

SUMMARY

Our white non-prison females when taken as a unit correspond to the socio-economically upper 20 per cent of the U.S. population. Ultimately one tenth of this group, which includes those without as well as those with pre-marital coitus, had a pre-marital pregnancy regardless of their subsequent marital status. By age twenty-one, 4 per cent of all females had conceived while unmarried and 13 per cent of those who had had pre-marital coitus. Of those who conceived, four fifths had only one conception. Pre-marital coitus, pre-marital pregnancy, and marriage, it is apparent, are closely associated phenomena, the first two becoming more prevalent as marriage approaches. There is evidence that more women with pre-marital coitus, including those who became pregnant, marry than women without pre-marital coitus. Of those in our sample who had a pre-marital pregnancy, 19 per cent married while pregnant.

Of the pre-marital pregnancies that ended before marriage, 6 per cent were live births, 5 per cent spontaneous abortions, and 89 per cent induced abortions. Of our 2,221 ever-married females, almost 3 per cent were pregnant when they married.

The age at which a woman marries is clearly a powerful factor in influencing pre-marital reproductive behavior. Roughly half to two thirds of all females in the sample who had married had had pre-marital coitus, the percentage increasing with increased age at marriage. Fewer of those who marry at younger ages have pre-marital conceptions than those who marry later; this is true even in the sample consisting solely of females who had pre-marital coitus.

Induced abortion is commoner among women who marry later. Of those who conceive before they marry, more of those who marry young carry their pre-marital conceptions into marriage; females who marry at older ages do so much less often.

Educational level, our measure of socio-economic status, permits us to extend our findings to a considerable segment of the urban white U.S. population. There is a negative correlation between educational achievement and pre-marital pregnancy: the better educated are seen to have fewer pre-marital pregnancies, even when the sample is confined to those with pre-marital coitus. This appears to be due to a differential use of contraceptives and to the fact that the less educated had more years of coitus during their pre-marital life. The differences disclosed by a study of educational levels are derived in the final analysis from the different attitudes (mores) held by the various socio-economic groups toward pre-marital coitus and pregnancy.

Because more of them became pregnant before marriage, there is a greater incidence of induced abortion among the less educated; but in terms of ratio, a higher proportion of their pregnancies end in live birth or are carried over into marriage than is true of the better educated.

A decade-of-birth study is extremely complex, but one may say it shows that over the years there has been an increase in pre-marital pregnancy. The post-World War II "marriage boom" is reflected by a sudden increase in pre-marital pregnancy, especially among the women born between 1920 and 1929—once again demonstrating that pre-marital coitus, conception, and subsequent marriage are closely associated.

While there has been an increase in the number of induced abortions and the percentage of females having them, there has also been a trend for a larger proportion of pre-marital pregnancies to end in live birth and to be carried into marriage. This trend is in part due to the relative youthfulness of the women born in the more recent birth decades; young females encounter more difficulty in securing induced abortions and are also more apt than older women to marry when pregnant before marriage.

Finally, our study showed that the degree of religious devoutness exerts an unequivocal effect on reproductive behavior. The more devout women have fewer pre-marital pregnancies, and this is true even when one studies only those women who had coitus. Likewise, induced abortion is less prevalent among the more devout.

Table 15. Accumulative Experience: Pre-marital Conception

For Total Females, Total Single Females, and
Single Females with Coitus

By Age

BY AGE	TOTAL FEMALES, TOTAL SINGLE FEMALES, AND SINGLE FEMALES WITH COITUS					
	Total females	Total single females	Single females with coitus	Total females	Total single females	Single females with coitus
	Per cent of females with conception experience			*Number of females*		
14	0.1	0.0	3.4	5,271	5,268	58 (1.1%)
15	0.1	0.1	5.9	5,258	5,244	102 (1.9)
16	0.3	0.3	6.5	5,230	5,191	201 (3.9)
17	0.7	0.6	9.6	5,065	4,971	303 (6.1)
18	1.4	1.0	9.6	4,625	4,426	459 (10.4)
19	2.3	1.7	12.1	4,068	3,713	519 (14.0)
20	3.3	2.3	12.6	3,589	3,066	554 (18.1)
21	4.3	2.8	13.0	3,200	2,463	537 (21.8)
22	5.3	3.7	15.2	2,921	2,031	501 (24.7)
23	6.2	4.1	14.9	2,730	1,679	456 (27.2)
24	6.8	4.2	14.5	2,561	1,392	399 (28.7)
25	7.5	4.7	14.5	2,416	1,166	380 (32.6)
26	8.0	5.4	15.7	2,270	980	337 (34.4)
27	8.3	6.2	16.9	2,148	839	307 (36.6)
28	8.9	7.0	17.7	2,039	742	294 (39.6)
29	9.3	6.7	16.8	1,916	652	262 (40.2)
30	10.1	8.6	20.6	1,823	569	238 (41.8)
31	10.4	10.0	23.9	1,737	511	213 (41.7)
32	10.4	9.8	22.9	1,629	451	192 (42.6)
33	10.6	11.5	25.1	1,535	419	191 (45.6)
34	10.2	12.0	26.6	1,436	384	173 (45.1)
35	10.2	11.3	23.6	1,329	337	161 (47.8)
36	10.4	11.7	24.5	1,242	299	143 (47.8)
37	9.9	11.6	24.0	1,128	268	129 (48.1)
38	9.8	11.3	23.9	1,048	239	113 (47.3)
39	9.2	10.0	21.9	958	210	96 (45.7)
40	9.3	10.7	23.1	871	196	91 (46.4)

Table 16. Accumulative Experience and Rate: Pre-marital Conception For Total Females and Females with Pre-marital Coitus By Age at Marriage

TOTAL FEMALES				FEMALES WITH PRE-MARITAL COITUS			
−20	Age at marriage 21–25	26–30	31+	−20	Age at marriage 21–25	26–30	31+
Per cent of females with conception experience							
8.7	9.6	11.9	20.5	18.2	18.9	21.6	30.7
Conceptions per 100 females							
9.8	11.5	19.1	29.5	20.5	22.6	34.7	44.3
Per cent with coitus				*Years of coitus per 100 females*			
47.9	50.7	55.0	66.7	163	258	477	836
Number of females							
620	1,082	387	132	297	549	213	88

Table 17. Accumulative Experience and Rate: Pre-marital Conception For Total Females and Females with Pre-marital Coitus By Educational Level

BY AGE	TOTAL FEMALES			FEMALES WITH PRE-MARITAL COITUS		
	Educational level			Educational level		
	9–12	13–16	17+	9–12	13–16	17+
	Per cent of females with conception experience					
20	6.7	3.2	1.9	22.2	13.4	10.6
25	10.8	7.7	4.9	24.9	17.4	13.3
30	13.2	9.7	8.3	28.7	20.5	18.0
35	11.2	9.8	9.4	29.7	21.0	19.8
40	8.0	8.1	9.2	25.9	19.6	22.0
	Conceptions per 100 females					
20	7.6	3.6	2.0	25.1	15.1	11.6
25	13.9	9.9	6.3	31.9	22.4	16.9
30	17.6	12.7	11.4	38.1	26.7	24.8
35	14.6	13.1	14.0	38.6	28.1	29.4
40	8.0	9.6	14.0	25.9	23.2	33.3
	Per cent with coitus			*Years of coitus per 100 females*		
20	30.2	24.0	17.5	249	225	251
25	43.5	44.3	37.1	350	312	348
30	46.1	47.5	46.2	435	416	442
35	37.8	46.8	47.5	557	510	571
40	31.0	41.3	41.9	585	659	615
	Number of females					
20	672	1,682	1,134	203	403	198
25	527	897	894	229	397	332
30	393	638	699	181	303	323
35	267	449	530	101	210	252
40	174	271	358	54	112	150

Table 18. Accumulative Experience and Rate: Pre-marital Conception For Total Females and Females with Pre-marital Coitus By Decade of Birth

BY AGE	TOTAL FEMALES				FEMALES WITH PRE-MARITAL COITUS			
	Decade of birth				Decade of birth			
	1890–1899	1900–1909	1910–1919	1920–1929	1890–1899	1900–1909	1910–1919	1920–1929
	Per cent of females with conception experience							
20	1.7	3.7	4.6	3.0		18.0	17.4	11.5
25	3.3	7.0	9.4	10.9	17.1	17.1	19.1	19.6
30	5.5	10.5	14.0		22.0	21.0	24.0	
35	7.2	11.3	17.7		24.3	21.6	28.3	
40	7.5	12.4			24.3	24.9		
	Conceptions per 100 females							
20	1.9	4.1	5.2	3.5		19.9	19.6	13.1
25	3.6	9.3	12.0	13.0	18.6	22.9	24.4	23.4
30	6.1	14.4	18.6		24.2	28.8	32.0	
35	8.3	15.9	25.3		28.0	30.5	40.4	
40	9.4	16.1			30.6	32.2		
	Per cent with coitus				*Years of coitus per 100 females*			
20	9.9	20.8	26.7	26.4		245	239	225
25	19.3	40.7	49.2	55.4	329	335	326	346
30	25.1	50.0	58.3		418	441	415	
35	29.5	52.0	62.7		507	549	521	
40	30.7	50.0			650	578		
	Number of females							
20	363	774	1164	1185		161	311	313
25	363	774	989	193	70	315	487	107
30	363	772	580		91	386	338	
35	363	711	158		107	370	99	
40	362	410			111	205		

Table 19. Accumulative Experience and Rate: Pre-marital Conception
For Total Females and Females with Pre-marital Coitus
By Religious Devoutness

BY AGE	TOTAL FEMALES				FEMALES WITH PRE-MARITAL COITUS			
	Religious devoutness				Religious devoutness			
	Protestant			Jewish	Protestant			Jewish
	Devout	Moderate	Inactive	Inactive	Devout	Moderate	Inactive	Inactive
Per cent of females with conception experience								
20	1.6	3.2	5.1	3.7	10.2	14.5	17.8	12.4
25	3.5	7.4	10.6	8.1	11.5	19.2	20.4	17.4
30	4.7	10.8	13.9	10.0	14.3	23.5	24.4	19.7
35	4.7	10.4	14.8	10.3	14.4	23.8	25.9	22.8
40	5.1	10.3	13.8	4.3	19.3	27.0	26.0	
Conceptions per 100 females								
20	1.6	3.5	6.1	4.3	10.2	15.7	21.2	14.3
25	4.1	9.3	13.9	10.1	13.4	24.1	26.8	21.9
30	5.5	14.5	18.9	14.1	16.5	31.7	33.1	27.6
35	5.4	14.9	21.4	15.4	16.3	34.1	37.5	34.2
40	5.5	13.8	19.4	4.3	21.1	36.5	36.6	
Per cent with coitus					Years of coitus per 100 females			
20	16.0	22.2	28.9	29.9	221	242	262	205
25	30.4	38.4	51.9	46.3	294	341	354	312
30	33.0	45.8	57.1	51.0	391	453	452	394
35	32.9	43.8	57.1	45.1	485	608	559	501
40	26.3	37.9	53.0	35.0	649	623	620	
Number of females								
20	796	776	896	538	127	172	259	161
25	516	528	690	335	157	203	358	155
30	403	400	524	249	133	183	299	127
35	316	288	392	175	104	126	224	79
40	217	195	247	117	57	74	131	

Table 20. Age-Specific Rate: Pre-marital Conception

For Total Females, Total Single Females, and Single Females with Coitus

By Total Years Lived, Total Pre-marital Years, and Years with Pre-marital Coitus

AGE PERIOD	TOTAL FEMALES, TOTAL SINGLE FEMALES, AND SINGLE FEMALES WITH COITUS						
	Total years	Pre-marital years	Pre-marital years with coitus	Total years	Pre-marital years	Pre-marital years with coitus	Per cent of pre-marital years with coitus
	Conceptions per 100 years			*Number of years*			
11–15	0.0	0.0	3.9	26,386	26,366	204	0.8
16–20	0.6	0.7	6.8	22,577	21,367	2,036	9.5
21–25	1.1	1.8	6.7	13,828	8,731	2,273	26.0
26–30	0.8	2.2	5.7	10,196	3,782	1,438	38.0
31–35	0.3	1.2	2.8	7,666	2,102	930	44.2
36–40	0.2	1.1	2.3	5,247	1,212	572	47.2
41–45	0	0	0	3,248	723	312	43.2

Eight conceptions before age 16 were reported by the sample of females aged 16 and older.

Table 21. Age-Specific Rate: Pre-marital Conception
  For Single Females with Coitus
  By Age at Marriage
  By Educational Level
  By Decade of Birth
  By Religious Devoutness

AGE PERIOD	SINGLE FEMALES WITH COITUS							
	Age at marriage				Age at marriage			
	16–20	21–25	26–30	31–35	16–20	21–25	26–30	31–35
	Conceptions per 100 coital years				*Number of coital years*			
16–20	13.8	6.1			392	759		
21–25		12.2	4.6			632	541	
26–30			12.1	*5.2*			297	*212*

AGE PERIOD	Educational level			Educational level		
	9–12	13–16	17+	9–12	13–16	17+
	Conceptions per 100 coital years			*Number of coital years*		
16–20	9.6	5.9	5.0	481	1,044	458
21–25	9.8	6.4	5.1	437	941	849
26–30	*5.3*	6.2	5.7	*226*	471	705
31–35		3.0	3.0		263	542
36–40			2.3			341

AGE PERIOD	Decade of birth			Decade of birth		
	1900–1909	1910–1919	1920–1929	1900–1909	1910–1919	1920–1929
	Conceptions per 100 coital years			*Number of coital years*		
16–20	8.2	7.6	4.9	355	682	1,034
21–25	5.9	6.8	8.1	663	970	471
26–30	6.3	4.9		650	576	
31–35	1.3			525		
36–40	2.5			324		

AGE PERIOD	Religious devoutness				Religious devoutness			
	Protestant			Jewish	Protestant			Jewish
	Devout	Moder-ate	Inac-tive	Inac-tive	Devout	Moder-ate	Inac-tive	Inac-tive
	Conceptions per 100 coital years				*Number of coital years*			
16–20	3.5	5.7	8.7	5.9	317	421	653	375
21–25	5.2	7.1	6.9	7.4	324	494	856	325
26–30	*3.0*	5.9	7.1		201	340	551	
31–35		*1.9*	4.0			*216*	377	
36–40			*2.9*				*240*	

Table 22. Accumulative Experience and Rate: Pre-marital Conception and Outcome

For Total Females and Females with Pre-marital Coitus, Aged 36 and Older at Interview

By Marital Status at Interview

MARITAL STATUS AT INTERVIEW	TOTAL FEMALES AND FEMALES WITH PRE-MARITAL COITUS, AGED 36 AND OLDER AT INTERVIEW							
	Con-cep-tion	Induced abor-tion	Con-cep-tion	Live birth	Spont. abor-tion	Induced abor-tion	Outcome in marriage	Number of females
	Total females							
	Per cent of females with experience		*Rate per 100 females*					
Total sample	10.3	8.0	14.1	0.5	0.4	11.5	1.7	1,329
Never married	9.7	9.3	13.0	0.7	0	12.3	...	300
Ever married	10.5	7.6	14.4	0.5	0.5	11.3	2.1	1,029
Married once, still married	11.4	8.2	15.5	0.4	0.9	12.1	2.1	562
Ever S.D.W.	9.4	6.9	13.1	0.6	0	10.3	2.1	467
	Females with pre-marital coitus							
Total sample	23.0	17.8	31.4	1.2	0.8	25.7	3.7	595
Never married	21.5	20.7	28.9	1.5	0	27.4	...	135
Ever married	23.5	17.0	32.2	1.1	1.1	25.2	4.8	460
Married once, still married	25.2	18.1	34.3	0.8	2.0	26.8	4.7	254
Ever S.D.W.	21.4	15.5	29.6	1.5	0	23.3	4.9	206

Excluded were pregnancies occurring at age 36 or later.

In each marital classification, nearly identical percentages of women reported pre-marital coitus (44–45 per cent).

Table 23. Accumulative Experience and Rate: Pre-marital Induced Abortion
For Total Females and Females with Pre-marital Coitus
By Age at Marriage

	TOTAL FEMALES			FEMALES WITH PRE-MARITAL COITUS			
	Age at marriage				Age at marriage		
−20	21–25	26–30	31+	−20	21–25	26–30	31+
Per cent of females with induced abortion experience							
3.5	6.4	9.3	19.7	7.4	12.6	16.9	29.5
Induced abortions per 100 females							
4.2	8.1	16.0	26.5	8.8	16.0	29.1	39.8
Number of females							
620	1,082	387	132	297	549	213	88

Table 24. Accumulative Experience and Rate: Pre-marital Induced Abortion For Total Females and Females with Pre-marital Coitus, Aged 36 and Older at Interview By Educational Level

	TOTAL FEMALES			FEMALES WITH PRE-MARITAL COITUS			
	Educational level				Educational level		
0–8	9–12	13–16	17+	0–8	9–12	13–16	17+
Per cent of females with induced abortion experience							
6.0	8.2	8.2	7.9		21.8	17.6	16.7
Induced abortions per 100 females							
7.2	11.6	11.4	12.3		30.7	24.3	25.8
Number of females							
83	267	449	530	*32*	101	210	252

Table 25. Accumulative Experience and Rate: Pre-marital Induced Abortion For Total Females and Females with Pre-marital Coitus By Decade of Birth

BY AGE	TOTAL FEMALES				FEMALES WITH PRE-MARITAL COITUS			
	Decade of birth				Decade of birth			
	1890–1899	1900–1909	1910–1919	1920–1929	1890–1899	1900–1909	1910–1919	1920–1929
Per cent of females with induced abortion experience								
20	0.8	2.6	3.1	1.9		12.4	11.6	7.3
25	1.4	5.0	6.8	6.2	7.1	12.4	13.8	11.2
30	3.6	7.9	11.0		14.3	15.8	18.9	
35	5.0	8.7	15.2		16.8	16.8	24.2	
40	5.5	9.5			18.0	19.0		
Induced abortions per 100 females								
20	1.1	3.0	3.7	2.2		14.3	13.8	8.3
25	1.7	7.2	9.2	7.3	8.6	17.8	18.7	13.1
30	4.1	11.8	15.3		16.5	23.6	26.3	
35	6.1	13.2	22.2		20.6	25.4	35.4	
40	6.6	12.9			21.6	25.9		
Number of females								
20	363	774	1,164	1,185		161	311	313
25	363	774	989	193	70	315	487	107
30	363	772	580		91	386	338	
35	363	711	158		107	370	99	
40	362	410			111	205		

Table 26. Accumulative Experience and Rate: Pre-marital Induced Abortion
For Total Females and Females with Pre-marital Coitus,
Aged 36 and Older at Interview
By Religious Devoutness

TOTAL FEMALES				FEMALES WITH PRE-MARITAL COITUS			
Religious devoutness				Religious devoutness			
Protestant			Jewish	Protestant			Jewish
Devout	Moderate	Inactive	Inactive	Devout	Moderate	Inactive	Inactive
Per cent of females with induced abortion experience							
3.2	8.3	12.2	7.4	9.6	19.0	21.4	16.5
Induced abortions per 100 females							
3.8	12.8	18.1	12.6	11.5	29.4	31.7	27.8
Number of females							
316	288	392	175	104	126	224	79

Table 27. Age-Specific Outcome Ratio
For Pre-marital Conceptions
By Age

AGE PERIOD	PRE-MARITAL CONCEPTIONS				
	Type of pre-marital outcome			Outcome in marriage	Total conceptions
	Live birth	Spontaneous abortion	Induced abortion		
	Per cent			*Per cent*	*Number*
−20	6.2	3.4	69.2	21.2	146
21–25	4.6	5.3	74.3	15.8	152
26+	3.4	5.0	85.7	5.9	119
Total	4.8	4.5	75.8	14.9	417*
	Outcome irrespective of marital status				
−20	22.6	4.1	73.3		146
21–25	16.6	6.6	76.8		151
26+	7.5	5.8	86.7		120
Total	16.1	5.5	78.4		417†

*Excluded were four conceptions: two that were reported by single females pregnant at interview, and two that were conceived before marriage but terminated in a post-marital status.
†Excluded were four conceptions not terminated at time of interview.

Table 28. Outcome Ratio

    For Pre-marital Conceptions

    By Marital Status at Interview

    By Age at Marriage

    By Educational Level

    By Decade of Birth

    By Religious Devoutness

CATEGORIES	PRE-MARITAL CONCEPTIONS				
	Type of pre-marital outcome			Outcome in marriage	Total conceptions
	Live birth	Spont. abortion	Induced abortion		
	Per cent			Per cent	Number
Marital status at interview					
Never married	8.3	5.0	86.7	. . .	121
Married once, still married	2.9	5.7	70.8	20.6	175
Ever S.D.W.	4.1	2.4	70.7	22.8	123
Age at marriage					
−20	3.3	3.3	42.6	50.8	61
21–25	3.2	5.6	71.0	20.2	124
26+	3.5	3.5	85.9	7.1	113
Educational level					
9–12	10.1	3.7	63.3	22.9	109
13–16	2.4	4.3	81.7	11.6	164
17+	1.6	6.2	82.9	9.3	129
Decade of birth					
1900–1909	1.6	4.8	81.7	11.9	126
1910–1919	6.2	3.1	76.5	14.2	162
1920–1929	6.5	7.5	67.7	18.3	93
Religious devoutness					
Protestant devout	*8.1*	*8.1*	*64.9*	*18.9*	*37*
Protestant moderate	5.6	3.3	68.9	22.2	90
Protestant inactive	5.1	5.1	79.1	10.7	178
Jewish inactive	0	3.5	84.2	12.3	57

Chapter 4

THE MARRIED WOMAN

Marriage is a social device for regulating heterosexual activity, preventing socially disruptive competition, and establishing the mutually advantageous responsibilities of the spouses and their offspring. It is and has been for millenniums the foundation of human social organization. A biological family can exist without marriage, but a family as a part of human society requires the social sanction that we call marriage. Marriage in some form has been practiced by all human groups of which we have knowledge, and ordinarily the vast majority of adults in any such group are or have been married. In our own society nearly 90 per cent of the individuals ultimately marry.

An essential aspect of marriage is reproduction. In many preliterate cultures and ancient civilizations there were few tragedies greater than an infertile marriage. Humanity has been almost obsessed with fertility: the fertility of the fields, the fertility of animals, and above all the fertility of marriage. The economic motivation is obvious, and even in our present society wherein children are not the economic asset they once were, they still represent insurance against the loneliness and destitution that may accompany old age. This universal interest in human fertility as well as having permeated the general mores, has become a part of many religions. Societies that otherwise insist upon a monogamous and lasting marriage will, if the marriage proves infertile, permit second wives, concubines, divorce, or adoption. In the United States refusal to procreate can be grounds for annulment.[1]

Consequently, whatever can be learned about marital pregnancy and its outcome is of extreme importance and interest not only to the individual but also to our society and to humanity itself.

PREGNANCY

RELATION TO AGE AND TO MARITAL STATUS AT INTERVIEW

Our contribution to the existing body of data on marital pregnancy will be modest, but unique in that we shall deal with all marital con-

---

[1] Ploscowe 1955:60-61 states, "The concealment of a desire not to have children is a fraud that goes to the essence of the marriage contract." He adds that such fraud constitutes grounds for annulment.

ceptions; nearly all previous studies have had to approach conception indirectly through examination of live birth data.[2]

Accumulative experience. While ultimately 80 per cent of our sample of ever-married women became pregnant while married (Table 32), this figure was not achieved until the end of reproductive life. By age twenty nearly one third of the married females had become pregnant; by age twenty-five, slightly more than half; by age thirty, roughly two thirds; by age thirty-five, about three quarters; and finally in the fifth decade of life the 80 per cent level is reached.

Since our sample contains a comparatively high proportion of women who have been separated, divorced, or widowed, accumulative experience was computed separately for those who had married once and were, at time of interview, still married. The percentages for this married-once group are slightly below the percentages for the ever-married sample until age twenty-five and slightly above thereafter, ultimately reaching 83 per cent.[3]

While over a lifetime roughly 20 per cent of our sample of women never conceived during marriage, this does not mean that they were entirely infertile; some of them had pre-marital pregnancies, others had a pregnancy after their marriages had terminated. Among women of forty-six and older, 16 per cent of the ever-married and 14 per cent

---

[2] Important exceptions to this are the Indianapolis study of fertility by Whelpton and Kiser, and the National Health Survey of 1935-1936 analyzed by Kiser in 1942 for group differences in urban fertility. Other studies of total pregnancies have been based largely on the previous pregnancies of groups of women with nontypical fertility levels. These include studies of birth control clinic patients, patients of gynecologists or obstetricians, or hospital confinement cases.

Vital statistics data on live births and on fetal deaths could theoretically be combined to make a total pregnancy figure, but the fetal death reports are only partial and chiefly for those late in pregnancy. A few studies of sexual behavior have provided data on total pregnancies of a more general sample. The present data will be compared to findings in pertinent previous studies, but the differences in samples and interviewing techniques must be kept in mind.

[3] Other reports on the proportion of women who fail to become pregnant in marriage vary from 3 to 22 per cent, depending upon the sample. The estimate of 10 to 15 per cent used by Hellman in Cecil 1951:347 is typical. Some data include a distinction between voluntary and involuntary sterility. For example, Brunner and Newton 1939:84 found 3.4 per cent of involuntary sterility among 4,500 married women; Kiser 1939:63 reported 7 per cent from a New York City sample; Brunner 1941:162 cited 9 per cent from his married women patients; and Whelpton and Kiser 1950 (2):335 concluded that 9.8 per cent of the 1,080 couples surveyed in the Indianapolis study were unable to become pregnant. Total sterility generally comparable to the present data would include 16.5 per cent in the Katharine Davis 1929 study, 23 per cent cited by Brunner 1941, and 16.3 per cent in the Whelpton and Kiser survey. The latter was limited to Protestant women with unbroken marriages.

of the married-once had never become pregnant either in or out of marriage. This percentage is higher than that of the women who married young (between ages sixteen and twenty), of whom only 9 per cent failed to conceive at least once in their lifetimes. Even this cannot be taken as a definitive figure for sterility, since we cannot determine certain hidden factors such as the fecundity of their male partners and the skill and consistency with which contraception was employed.

Age-specific rate. Table 38 presents the number of conceptions per hundred years of marriage occurring within given age-periods. Between ages sixteen and twenty there were 22 conceptions per hundred marital years, but the greatest fertility is in age-periods 21-25 (24) and 26-30 (24). After age thirty there is a rapid decrease in the conception rate: following an initial drop to 16 at ages 31-35, the rate is halved (8) in the subsequent age-period 36-40, and more than halved (2) in the following age-period.[4] The above rates can, of course, be expressed as percentages of females involved. Thus, for example, one can say that in an average year between ages sixteen and twenty, 22 per cent of these young wives became pregnant.

The decrease in conception rate following age thirty is due in part to contraception, practiced by those who felt their families sufficiently large, and in part to a slightly lower frequency of coitus (1953:394). The extent and rapidity of the decrease also suggests that lessened fecundity resulting from aging is also involved. The aging of the reproductive system leads ultimately to menopause which, while often dramatic in its symptoms, is simply the recognizable result of a previously less evident decrease in fecundity.

In our volume on the female (1953:736) we noted that, in our sample, menopausal symptoms began at a median age of forty-six, although in some women they began as early as thirty-three. Thus one can expect that there will be a small number of women beginning menopause in their thirties, and that the number will increase vastly as women live into their fifth decade of life. One must also realize that prior to the advent of the recognizable symptoms of menopause there

---

[4] Pregnancy rates by duration of marriage rather than by age were shown in Stix 1935:354 and Beebe 1942:108. The figures are not comparable with the present data since they are drawn from more fertile groups, but they show similar trends in lessening rates with time. The Stix data covering from the first five years of marriage to 15 years or more of duration show rates from 68 to 18 pregnancies per hundred years of exposure.

Tietze et al. 1950b:345 found age and duration of marriage both strong factors in lowering fecundity when they measured it by length of time required to conceive. They demonstrated that duration of marriage was more important than age in lengthening the period required.

is a period of near-sterility that may vary in duration from many months to some years.[5]

Part of the decrease in the fecundity of the women of our sample is attributable to the various pelvic operations that are performed much more often from the thirties on. Typical of these are the removal of cystic ovaries, removal of all or part of the uterus, and surgery upon the oviducts (Fallopian tubes). It is in the later years that an appreciable number of women have their oviducts cut or tied to preclude further pregnancies. A minor factor, but one worth note, is the general policy among physicians to postpone pelvic operations or X-ray treatment for younger females until they have reached their thirties.

The fact that the conception rate is slightly less between ages sixteen and twenty than between ages twenty-one and thirty probably reflects the use of contraception: few teen-age wives of the upper socio-economic level (who constitute the bulk of our sample) are desirous of a pregnancy at that age. This is particularly true of wives who are in college or whose husbands are in college. The essential identity of the rates for age-periods 21-25 and 26-30 has no meaning in terms of fecundity; a likely explanation is that a considerable number of women who marry at ages 23-25 delay beginning a family for a few years and hence their conceptions fall in the 26-30 age-period.

Computing rates for women who married once and were still married at the time they were interviewed, we find that prior to age twenty-five their conception rates were lower than those of the women whose marriages had ended. This is rather unexpected and the underlying reasons are not wholly clear. However, we do know that the separated, divorced, or widowed are, as a group, somewhat older than the women in our married-once group, and since we also know that within a given age-period women born in earlier decades conceived more often than women born in subsequent decades, this may be at least a partial explanation. The median age at interview was 39.9 for the

---

[5] Whitehead 1848:216 in an early British study on abortion and sterility, reported that 42 was the median age of the final pregnancy of 38 married women although the average age of final menses was 47.5.

Most data on the relationship of sterility to later ages in women is based on births rather than on pregnancies, and since there appears to be a high loss among pregnancies in older women (see notes 22 and 23, this chapter) these figures give a somewhat distorted picture of ability to conceive at later ages. For example, U.S. *Vital Statistics 1955* (1), 1957:220 shows only about one tenth of one per cent of all births in 1955 as occurring to women 45 and older. Davis 1952:847, cited only two deliveries to women of 47 and 48 among 100,000 at the Chicago Lying-in Hospital. On the other hand, while Tietze 1957:91 showed sharply increasing sterility with age among 209 of the highly fertile Hutterite women, 1.4 per cent of the confinements occurred to women 45 or older.

separated, divorced, or widowed (S.D.W.) and 32.5 for the married-once. In addition, the S.D.W. women of our sample have a median age at marriage of 21.8, whereas the married-once have a median of 23.4, and we shall subsequently see that youthfulness and conception are closely related.

Accumulative rate. The number of marital conceptions per hundred women achieved by a given age is shown in Table 32. These rates are not in themselves too meaningful since in this table we have not held constant such powerful factors as age at marriage and educational level, but the general trend is worth noting. Our sample of married females of twenty or under averaged less than one conception for every two women (rate of 42 per 100). By age twenty-five the average is nearly one conception for every one woman (92); and by the end of reproductive life it would seem that there are about five marital conceptions for every two women (266).[6] As we noted earlier, the women whose marriages eventually terminated were more fertile before age twenty-five than women who had one marriage and remained married, the former having by age twenty-five a rate of 103 conceptions per hundred females in contrast to the latter's 84. After age twenty-five the reverse is true.

Extra-marital conception. As everyone since dim antiquity has known, or at least suspected, some wives conceive by men other than their husbands. In this study we have not ordinarily differentiated such extra-marital conceptions from the marital conceptions, since the former are numerically insignificant and since the conceptions and outcomes were legally within wedlock. Of our 2,221 ever-married women, 26 reported a total of 32 pregnancies known or believed to have been the result of extra-marital coitus. Of course there must be an

---

[6] Several other studies show accumulative marital conception rates. Davis 1929:10 reported a rate of 229 per 100 for the 985 women answering this item. Two thirds were college educated, and they had been married an average of almost 11 years.

Dickinson and Beam 1931:264 showed a 167 rate for the women under forty, and a 224 rate for those over forty at report.

Hudson and Rucker 1945:542 found an average of 3.11 pregnancies (a 311 rate) among 250 married patients of completed fertility.

The question of average total fecundity if the possibility of pregnancy is uncontrolled by contraception has received considerable attention. For a woman who marries at twenty, it was fixed at 12 pregnancies by Whitehead 1848. Stix and Notestein 1940:32, Table 10, placed the figure at 14 pregnancies from their New York City data. Whelpton and Kiser 1950 (2):319 estimated 4.5 pregnancies per Indianapolis woman, under thirty at marriage, married 12 to 15 years. Tietze 1952 set it at almost 12 conceptions for a woman marrying prior to age eighteen, based on Canadian census data from rural areas of Catholic Quebec.

additional number of extra-marital conceptions not recognized as such even by the women involved; these conceptions make a study of the frequency of extra-marital conception correspondingly unreliable.

The 26 women who conceived extra-maritally are in terms of education and religious affiliation similar to our total sample of ever-married women.

Of the 32 pregnancies, 4 were conceived by wives aged twenty-one to twenty-five, 6 by wives twenty-six to thirty, 13 by wives thirty-one to thirty-five, 5 by wives thirty-six to forty, and 4 by wives aged forty-one and over. The terminations of these pregnancies will be described later.

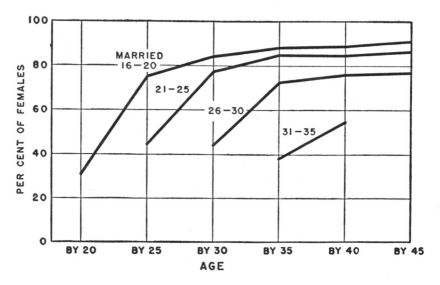

Figure 7. Accumulative Experience in Marital Conception by Age at First Marriage. Data from Table 33.

RELATION TO AGE AT MARRIAGE

Just as age at marriage is a potent factor in pre-marital reproductive behavior because it limits the time available for pre-marital activity, so it also determines how much of the fecund span of life is contained within marriage. Consequently, it is once again of primary importance.

Accumulative experience. This calculation (Table 33, Figure 7) reveals two phenomena: the decrease of fertility (and presumably fecundity) with age and, as a lesser phenomenon, the voluntary postponement of marital conception.

By the end of reproductive life 91 per cent of the females who married between ages sixteen and twenty had become pregnant in marriage; of those who married between ages twenty-one and twenty-five the equivalent percentage is 86; of those who married between ages twenty-six and thirty, only 77 per cent conceived; and of those who married between ages thirty-one and thirty-five, the percentage apparently does not reach 60. These relative differences exist not only at the end of reproductive life, but at any age.[7] The importance of age at marriage is emphasized when one notes that by age twenty-five the percentage of our youngest-marrying group who had become pregnant is almost as great as the percentage achieved over a lifetime by those who married between twenty-six and thirty, and probably greater, we would assume, than the percentage that would be achieved by those marrying after age thirty.

The question of the postponement of marital conception appears to be involved, in that for each age-at-marriage group the greatest percentage increase in pregnancies occurs in the five years immediately following the age-period in which the women married. For example, by age twenty only 31 per cent of those who married between ages sixteen and twenty had conceived, but by age twenty-five the figure is 75 per cent. In similar fashion those who married between twenty-one and twenty-five leap from 44 per cent by age twenty-five to 77 per cent by age thirty. Of course, not all this increase is attributable to postponement of conception; some of it results from the fact that some women married near the end of their age-period and had less time in which to become pregnant in that age-period. This sort of methodological artifact does not occur in the subsequent calculations for older ages: for example, when in connection with those who married between ages sixteen and twenty, we refer to the percentage who had conceived by age twenty-five, we are referring only to the women who had completed their twenty-fifth year of life.

Age-specific rate. Table 39, bearing out the conclusions drawn from the data on accumulative experience, shows that in three of the four age-at-marriage groups the conception rate reaches its maximum in the five years following the age-period in which the marriage occurred. The exception is seen among the women who married between ages thirty-one and thirty-five, who reach their maximum rate during the age-period in which they married. Apparently the progressive deterioration of the female reproductive system precludes their maximum rate from falling in to the next five-year period. Also, these late-marrying

---

[7] Beebe and Geisler 1942:3 reported that of a group of 382 rural Kentucky wives whose average age at marriage was 18.2 years, only 4 per cent had never been pregnant.

women are, as a group, in a hurry to conceive, which again would tend to make the maximum rate fall in the age-period of their marriage. Women marrying at younger ages realize that they have ample time in which to reproduce and hence are more prone to delay pregnancy, particularly if they or their husbands are in college.

The factor of contraception makes it difficult to draw inferences concerning fecundity. While it strongly influences both accumulative rate and age-specific rate, it has less effect on accumulative experience, since the majority of married women voluntarily try to become pregnant at least once. We made some fruitless efforts to evaluate the role played by contraception through comparing married females with unmarried females having pre-marital coitus, holding age constant. In doing so, however, we made what to us is a rather interesting discovery. Confining our attention to females aged sixteen to twenty, we find the age-specific conception rate is 22 conceptions per 100 coital years for the married (Table 39) and 14 for the unmarried who will marry by age twenty (Table 21). In other words the conception rate of the married is not even twice that of the soon-to-be married. Several factors are involved in this high pre-nuptial conception rate. Engaged couples have pre-marital coitus more often than those who are not engaged, and doubtless an engaged couple would be more inclined to "take a chance" when contraceptives were not at the moment available. Furthermore, some of the marriages of these females under twenty-one were forced: of the 297 who had pre-marital coitus, 54 conceived, and of these, 30 married while pregnant. Some of these 30 marriages might not have taken place were pregnancy not involved.

Accumulative rate. This rate mirrors what we saw in accumulative experience: the women who married at younger ages have, by any given age, a higher conception rate than those who married at older ages. Table 33 indicates that in our sample those who marry between ages sixteen and twenty-five have experienced, as a lifetime average, about three marital pregnancies each; those who marry between ages twenty-six and thirty, two; and those who marry between ages thirty-one and thirty-five have had but one marital pregnancy.

The relative infrequency of pregnancy within the age-period in which marriage occurred, followed by a dramatic increase during the following five years, is seen in accumulative rate even more vividly than it was in accumulative experience. For example, of those who married between sixteen and twenty, the rate by age twenty is forty-one; by age twenty-five it is 160: the rate has quadrupled, and is greater than the rate attained over a reproductive lifetime by those who married after age thirty. A dramatic increase is also seen among the women who married between twenty-one and twenty-five, and twenty-six and thirty—the rates almost triple. Among those who married between ages thirty-one and thirty-five, the rate somewhat more than doubles. As we pointed out in our discussing of accumulative experience, part of the initial increase is the result of our method of calculation.

RELATION TO EDUCATIONAL LEVEL

Before examining the relation between pregnancy and the degree of formal education we must point out that our educational groupings

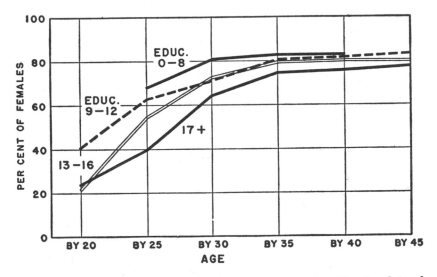

Figure 8. Accumulative Experience in Marital Conception by Educational Level. Data from Table 34.

differ slightly from those of the U.S. Census (see Census Comparison, Chapter 2).

Accumulative experience. Table 34 and Figure 8 indicate that there is a negative correlation between the amount of education and the percentage of married women in our sample who have become pregnant by a given age. That is to say, the less education a woman has the more likely she is at any age to become pregnant. The differences are sometimes not great, especially by older ages, but the trend is clear. For example, by age forty some 83 per cent of the women with grade school education have been pregnant, 82 per cent of the women with high school education, 80 per cent of those with college education, and 76 per cent of those who had postgraduate work.

Age-specific rate. Here, where rate is expressed in number of conceptions per hundred marital years, it is evident that early in life the less educated are more fertile (Table 40). Within age-period 21-25, the grade school educated had 35 conceptions per hundred years; the high school educated, 26; the college educated, 24; and the postgraduate women, 17. Between thirty-one and thirty-five, both the college and the postgraduate women exceed in rate the other two educational groups. This reversal in trend was anticipated since we know that the better educated tend, in our sample, to marry somewhat later. The fact that the postgraduate women have the highest rates in age-periods 31-35 and 36-40 suggests their tendency to marry late and then to hasten to reproduce; also postgraduate women who marry at younger ages are more inclined than females of other educational groups to delay marital conception until they or their husbands have completed their educations and attained some degree of economic security.

Accumulative rate. The computation of the number of marital pregnancies per hundred married females (Table 34) reveals clearly the negative correlation we have discussed. The accumulative nature of this computation accounts in part for the fact that the correlation does not disappear in the older ages but continues to the end of reproductive life.[8] Thus, for example, we see that by age twenty-five there were 163 conceptions per hundred females of grade school education, 115 for the high school group, 87 for the college, and 58 for the postgraduates; by age forty-five these differences are still apparent, the figures being respectively 363, 284, 265, and 219. Examining experience and age-specific rate (described previously), it is clear that during the most fecund years of life considerably more of the less educated were becoming pregnant; this initial "head start" of the less educated prevents the college educated and postgraduate women from subsequently "overtaking" them in terms of accumulative rate.

RELATION TO DECADE OF BIRTH

The relation of decade of birth to conception, a subject of considerable complexity when we examined it in connection with premarital conception, is seen more clearly in terms of marital conception.

Accumulative experience. In general, Table 35 indicates that with each successive birth decade a smaller percentage of married females become pregnant by any given age, but it also reveals that the females

---

[8] Stix and Notestein 1940:184-185 showed higher rates of conception among wives of manual workers than among wives of white collar workers, both in the total sample and when classified according to contraceptive practices. When conception was tabulated by duration of marriage, the differences between occupational groups were also evident.

born between 1920 and 1929 depart from this trend. By age twenty-five, beginning with decade -1889, the percentages run 67 per cent (-1889), 63 per cent (1890-1899), 57 per cent (1900-1909), 46 per cent (1910-1919), and then the 1920-1929 group reverses the trend with 61 per cent. This figure may represent the postwar "baby boom," on which we commented earlier and which has impressed social scientists as well as the public at large. There are not in our sample enough 1920-1929 women to let us make comparisons beyond the age of twenty-five; but women over twenty-five in the 1910-1919 or 1900-1909 decade groups always have a lower incidence of pregnancy than women in the prior decade groups.

Since age at marriage was demonstrated to be an important factor, we made an additional calculation holding age at marriage constant (Table 37). While this procedure necessarily reduced sample size and hence the stability of the figures, it in general confirmed our previous findings. The presumed effects of the "baby boom" show up vividly in the 1920-1929 group and also among the 1910-1919 females aged between thirty-one and thirty-five—i.e., when they were living between 1941 and 1954, the period during which the "boom" began.

Age-specific rate. This measurement (Table 41) confirms once more our generalization that there was a progressive decline in marital conceptions until the "baby boom" phase following World War II. This is evident in our 1920-1929 group between ages twenty-one and twenty-five. However, the conditions that contributed to this sudden flare-up of fertility also influenced older women: at ages twenty-six to thirty and thirty-one to thirty-five the rates of the women born 1910-1919 exceed those of the prior birth decade group. This is in keeping with what we have said, since from twenty-six to thirty the 1910-1919 women would be living between 1936 and 1949, and their ages from thirty-one to thirty-five would coincide with the years from 1941-1954. Part of each period falls within the "baby boom" phase. Some of the women born in 1910-1919 had emerged childless from the depression and were ready to have children when the economic situation improved.

Accumulative rate. The same pattern that emerged from accumulative experience is again visible here. With each successively more recent birth decade the number of marital conceptions per hundred females, by any given age, is steadily smaller, with one exception. This exception again consists of the females born between 1920 and 1929. Up to age twenty they conform to this trend, but by age twenty-five they have reversed it (Table 35). For example, by age twenty-five the women born before 1890 had experienced 169 conceptions per hundred females; the women born between 1890 and 1899 had had 110; those born between 1900 and 1909, 91; those born between 1910 and 1919,

75; but the 1920-1929 females provided a rate of 116 per hundred. Following age twenty-five, sample size still precludes the use of the 1920-1929 group, but (as in accumulative experience) the rate of the most recent decade available for comparison is always less than the rates of prior decade groups.

Translating rates into their simplest terms, it would seem that the women born before 1890 had, in their lives, an average of slightly over three pregnancies apiece;[9] the women born in 1890-1899 had almost

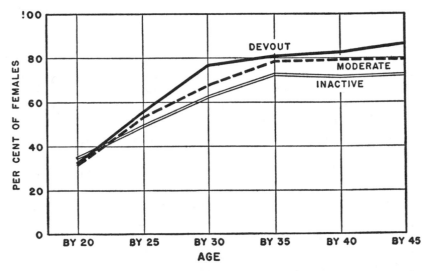

Figure 9. Accumulative Experience in Marital Conception for Protestant Females by Degree of Religious Devoutness.

Data from Table 36.

three; and the women born in 1900-1909 had two. Predicting from our sample, the women born in 1910-1919 should ultimately have an average of two (or slightly fewer) pregnancies. For the 1920-1929 decade our data permit no prediction.

RELATION TO DEGREE OF DEVOUTNESS

The effect that the degree of religious devoutness has on sexual behavior (and its reproductive consequences) is strongest where religiously taboo behavior is involved. Not surprisingly it is a factor of less consequence when one examines sexual behavior sanctioned or encouraged by the church.

---

[9] This figure is matched in a comprehensive study of pregnancy levels in New York City as gathered from early records from the Sloane Hospital for Women. Harris and Gunstad 1936:150 reported that the records on 6,390 women showed a pregnancy rate of 351 for the period 1890-1921.

Accumulative experience. Taking first the Protestant sample, we find the interesting fact that as far as pregnancy experience is concerned there are only minor differences between the devout, moderately devout, and religiously inactive groups during the younger ages. However, bit by bit, the differences between the groups increase until by age forty-five as many as 86 per cent of the devout group had become pregnant, 79 per cent of the moderately devout, and 73 per cent of the inactive (Table 36, Figure 9). Why these differences exist we do not wholly know; the Protestants, as a group, make no great issue of contraception, and there seem to be no real differences in the frequency of marital coitus (1953:398). Furthermore, the median age at marriage is the same for these groups and there seem to be no significant differences in educational level. However, the differences may in part result from the differences in the proportions of the separated, divorced, or widowed (S.D.W.) contained in the three categories of devoutness. The S.D.W. women display in later life conception rates lower than those of the women who married once and remained married. Thus the fact that the devout have higher marital conception rates in later life is probably owing to their having the lowest proportion of S.D.W. women—37 per cent (at age thirty-one and over) compared with 42 per cent for the moderately devout and 50 per cent for the religiously inactive.

The Jewish sample provides some unexpected results. By age twenty, only 19 per cent of the inactive religious group had conceived as contrasted to 32-35 per cent of the equivalent Protestant group. This is probably because our young Jewish sample contains a relatively large proportion of women who were in college at the time they were interviewed, and because our Jewish sample as a whole tends to be even more urban than our Protestant and Catholic samples. Yet by age 25 and thereafter the percentage of inactive Jewish women who became pregnant essentially equals that of the devout Protestants. Again, the explanation seems to derive in part from the proportions of S.D.W. women in the samples. As we said earlier, the Jewish group has fewer S.D.W. women than the Protestants. Thus we would anticipate low accumulated experience in younger life followed by a progressive increase in later life. This expectation is fulfilled, but we are still left with the fact that religiously inactive Jewish women by age twenty have far fewer pregnancies than the devout Protestants, despite the fact that the proportions of S.D.W. females are the same in both groups. Our only explanation is that given above; in our sample, the Jewish women were more urban and had a greater number of their members in college at the time of interview. Our less extensive sample of moderately devout Jewish women provides results similar to those derived from moderately devout Protestants. The seeming disclosure that a greater percentage of inactive Jewish women than of the moderately devout had experienced a marital pregnancy is probably a vagary of sample. There are too few cases in our Catholic sample for an analysis of degree of devoutness.

Age-specific rate. In examining the number of marital conceptions occurring within a given five-year age-period, it would seem that degree of religious devoutness ceases to be an influential factor after age thirty-five. Before thirty-five, the more devout women display higher rates than the less devout. The differences, while consistent, are not large (Table 42).

Accumulative rate. This calculation showing the number of marital conceptions per hundred females by a given age clearly illustrates the relation of degree of religious devoutness to marital pregnancy (Table 36). From age twenty-one on, among the Protestants, the more devout have consistently higher rates. By the end of reproductive life the devout exhibit an accumulative rate of 274; the moderately devout, 269; and the religiously inactive, 222.[10] This same trend holds true among our Jewish sample. Insufficient cases preclude an intra-Catholic comparison.

The puzzling fact that by age twenty the devout Protestants were less fertile than the religiously inactive cannot be explained unless one assumes that the devout who married before twenty tended to marry nearer twenty than did the inactive, and hence more of their conceptions occurred after that age. However, this may be a vagary of small sample.

Extra-marital conception. The 26 women of our sample who reported that they conceived, while married, by males other than their husbands are unlike our total sample of married women in one other respect: they are, as a group, irreligious. Twenty of them reported that they never attended church or synagogue, five did so very rarely, and only one attended regularly. By our definition, therefore, 25 of the 26 fall in the category of religiously inactive, and one in the devout category. There were no extra-marital conceptions reported by the moderately devout.

---

[10] The finding of the Indianapolis fertility study on the common factor, which operates between traditionalism (as expressed here in degree of devoutness) and size of family desired, is possibly reflected in the present data. The relation was most pronounced when the wives' attitudes were used as a measure and in the more extreme categories of traditionalism. See Freedman and Whelpton in Whelpton and Kiser 1952 (3):696.

OUTCOME OF PREGNANCY

There are, of course, three possible terminations of pregnancy: (1) live birth, the birth of a living embryo that is, in addition, sufficiently developed to live outside the uterus; (2) spontaneous abortion, the involuntary loss of any embryo regardless of age (stillbirths are included); (3) induced abortion, wherein the embryo of any age is intentionally killed within the uterus or expelled before it is old enough to live outside the uterus. Legal therapeutic abortions and illegal induced abortions are considered together. One could also label these three types of outcome as: live birth, involuntary pregnancy wastage,[11] and voluntary pregnancy wastage.

This section on outcome will be based upon only those women whose conceptions ended within marriage: our sample contains 3,645 such instances. The 22 marital pregnancies that terminated after the marriage no longer existed will be treated subsequently in the section on post-marital life. Pregnancies conceived outside marriage but terminated in marriage are included; these are numerically few: 60 were pre-marital conceptions (two such conceptions had not ended and hence are excluded here), and 11 were post-marital conceptions that ended in a following marriage.

RELATION TO AGE AND TO MARITAL STATUS AT INTERVIEW

Accumulative experience. Our sample of females who had ever married indicates that in their reproductive lifetimes about three quarters of them experienced a live birth,[12] one quarter had a recognizable spontaneous abortion,[13] and one fifth to one quarter had had an

---

[11] Raymond Pearl first suggested the use of the term "reproductive wastage" in 1932. He defined it as "the total loss to fertility in reproductive processes begun but never brought to successful termination." See Pearl 1939:87.

[12] The 1950 U.S. Census showed from 18 to 21 per cent of childlessness among urban, white married women, ages 40 to 59 at enumeration. See U.S. Census, 1950, Special Reports, *Fertility*, 1955:19-21. Glick 1957:83 estimated that this figure may drop to 10 per cent in 10 more years.

  Closer to the present figure is that in the Katharine Davis study 1929:10, 20. Her largely college educated group showed 78 per cent as having experienced a live birth.

  Groups only slightly if at all affected by contraceptive practices such as the French Canadians and Hutterites show lower levels of sterility, ranging from 3.5 to 6 per cent. See Eaton and Mayer 1953:236; Lorimer *et al.* 1954:28-30 (reviews various studies including the analysis of childless marriages by Kuczynski 1938); Tietze 1957:90.

[13] Accumulative experience of spontaneous abortion is reported by Brunner and Newton 1939:84, who found 31 per cent of a sample of over 3,000 fertile women had experienced a spontaneous abortion. Brunner 1941:162 calculated a 20 per cent total of such experience among 727 married patients.

induced abortion[14] (Table 43). The percentage of women who had
had live births increased rapidly up to age thirty and more slowly thereafter. In contrast, the percentage of women with induced abortions increased slowly until the early thirties and thereafter remained essentially the same. The percentage of women who experienced spontaneous abortion rose rapidly until age thirty and continued to increase
more slowly thereafter. All this simply means that after the more fertile
years of life when all types of outcome increase, a few (4 per cent) of
the women in their late thirties and older had their first babies, a very
few had their first induced abortions, and a small number (6 per cent)
had their first spontaneous abortions.

Age-specific rate. Table 48 gives the number of live births and spontaneous and induced abortions per hundred years of marriage at different age-periods. From sixteen to twenty there are 14 live births per
hundred marital years; the number increases up through age-period
26 to 30 and thereafter declines rapidly.[15] The spontaneous abortion
rate fluctuates from about 3 to 4 per hundred married years until after
age-period 31-35, and then it also decreases rapidly. Induced abortion,
on the other hand, is at its maximum (nearly 7) in the years between
sixteen and twenty and consistently decreases thereafter, falling to less
than one per hundred years of marriage after age thirty-five.

As we have previously stated, the age-specific rate may also be used
to approximate the percentages of women involved in any one year

---

[14] The percentage of women who have ever experienced an induced abortion varies
more widely from sample to sample than either of the other two terminations
of pregnancy. Surveys report such varying figures as the following:

Davis 1929:20, 77 found 11.2 per cent of 826 fertile married women and
9.3 per cent of all married women who had experienced induced abortion.
Two thirds of this sample were college educated women.

Stix 1935:352 reported 35 per cent of 991 of New York City birth control
clinic patients had resorted to an induced abortion at least once. The repre-
sentativeness of this sample is strongly discounted in Stix and Wiehl 1938:623,
where it is designated as not typical of clinic patients in other cities or of
married women in general.

Brunner and Newton 1939:84 found a 15 per cent accumulative experience
of induced abortion among 3,216 women who had been pregnant (99 per
cent of this sample were married).

Brunner 1941:162 reported that 31 per cent of 727 married patients had
had at least one induced abortion.

Whelpton and Kiser 1950 (2):211 cited 1.8 per cent of an adjusted sample
of 1,977 couples as reporting illegal abortion experience in Indianapolis.

[15] This coincides with the generally accepted female fertility curve. See, for example, Siegler 1944:21; Lorimer et al. 1954:25 ff.; Henripin 1954:67-70.

U.S. Vital Statistics provides data on adjusted age-specific birth rates for
all married women for 1950-1955. Births per hundred women drop quickly
from younger ages. See U.S. Vital Statistics, 1955 (1), 1957: Introduction,
p. lxxi.

within an age-period. Thus one may say that 7 per cent of the married women aged sixteen to twenty had an induced abortion during any given year of this period.

Considerable differences exist between the married-once and those who were subsequently separated, divorced, or widowed (S.D.W.). Induced abortion was much more prevalent among the S.D.W. wives; in many cases the women must have foreseen or suspected the ultimate end of their marriages and hence were reluctant to bear children.[16] From our interviews, it is our impression that induced abortion is usually a by-product of, not a cause of, the breaking up of marriage. The reader will recall that we are discussing here outcome within marriage, not outcome subsequent to the dissolution of marriage. If we were to exclude the widowed from the S.D.W. sample, the prevalence of induced abortion would be shown to be appreciably greater.

Accumulative rate. The increase in the rates of the various outcomes is even more interesting than the rates themselves (Table 43). By age twenty there were 27 live births per hundred married females; this rate more than doubles by age twenty-five, nearly doubles again by age thirty, and thereafter increases at a slower pace, ultimately reaching 166 by the end of reproductive life.[17] The rates for spontaneous abortion behave in similar fashion: more than doubling, then nearly doubling, and then increasing more slowly. By age twenty there were five spontaneous abortions per hundred women, and at the end of reproductive life there were 52. Induced abortion, on the other hand, always increases more gradually, eventually rising from 13 by age twenty to 50.[18] Until the mid-thirties the rate of induced abortion exceeds that of spontaneous abortion; thereafter the two rates are essentially the same.

In comparing the once-married women with the ever-S.D.W. women,

---

[16] The finding in the Katharine Davis study (1929:77) of a difference in induced abortion experience as between "happy wives" (9.1 per cent) and "unhappy wives" (24 per cent) is partial substantiation of the differences shown here in the marital abortion rates of the married-once and S.D.W. wives.

[17] Davis 1929:10 showed a closely similar 177 rate per 100 for her largely college educated group of 991 wives. See Table 30 for a comparison between live birth rates of our sample and those of census.

[18] Stone and Hart 1932:20 cite a rate of 53 induced abortions per hundred women in an early sample of 2,000 women from the records of the Newark, N.J., Maternal Health Center.

Stix 1935:352 found a rate of 69.2 induced abortions per hundred women in her total sample of 991 birth control clinic patients.

Hamilton 1940:925, in reporting on a sample of women who were in Bellevue Hospital as abortion patients, found a rate of 30 previous induced abortions per hundred women. Their average age was nearly 28 years.

it is clear that the latter have a markedly lower live birth rate and a
higher induced abortion rate. Because of their higher conception rate
during the younger years of life, the ever-S.D.W. also display a higher
spontaneous abortion rate despite their high induced abortion rate.
However, during their thirties the once-married exceed the S.D.W.
in spontaneous abortion—which may be the by-product of their higher
live birth rate. Women who attempt to carry their pregnancies to term
rather than to abort them will naturally have higher spontaneous abortion rates. Also the married-once have, as a group, been married longer
than the S.D.W. and hence more of them were still married during
later life when spontaneous abortion is more likely to occur.

Age-specific outcome ratio. Table 52 shows the proportions of live
births, spontaneous and induced abortions within given five-year age-
periods.[19] After an initial 60 per cent in age-period 16-20, live births
build up until they account for 69 per cent of all outcomes between
ages thirty-one and thirty-five. In the next five years the proportion falls
to 64 per cent. Our few cases beyond age forty suggest that the proportion of live births is much less than it was between thirty-six and forty.[20]

Spontaneous abortion terminates 12 per cent of the pregnancies
within age-period 16-20 and thereafter increases, eventually accounting
for slightly more than one fifth of the pregnancies between ages thirty-
six and forty.[21]

---

[19] Other studies covering the proportions of total pregnancies resulting in live birth
with few exceptions use an over-all figure rather than an analysis by age
periods. These studies show a range of from 60.7 per cent reported in Brunner
1941:165 to the 88 and 89 percentages of the Indianapolis study and Pearl's
survey. In general they are somewhat higher than the present results. For
example:

	Per cent
Davis 1929:10, 20	78.0
Stone and Hart 1932:17	77.0
Kopp 1933:Appendix, Table 8	71.5
Stix 1935:351	69.4
Taussig 1936:25	70.0
Harris and Gunstad 1936:150	75.8
Abramson 1936:447	82.5
Dewees acc. Stix 1938:575	82.8
Stix and Wiehl 1938:622	81.0
Collins acc. Stix and Notestein 1940:77	84.5
Hudson and Rucker 1945:542	77.0

[20] Stix 1935:354 in a tabulation by years of married life showed a sharply decreasing percentage of pregnancies terminating in live births up to 15 years of
marriage, and a slight increase thereafter. This was based on a birth control
clinic sample.

[21] Because spontaneous abortions are of medical interest, there is extensive material
on their prevalence. Over 40 studies have been examined, and can be summarized thus:
Over-all figures range from 7 to 20 per cent, the lower figures occurring in

Induced abortion, if plotted graphically, represents something between a U and a J curve. Between sixteen and twenty it accounts for 28 per cent of the pregnancies, declining thereafter to 12 per cent between ages thirty-one and thirty-five, and rising slightly between ages thirty-six and forty. On the slim basis of 46 terminated pregnancies experienced by married women aged forty-one to fifty, the proportion of induced abortion seemingly increases markedly.[22]

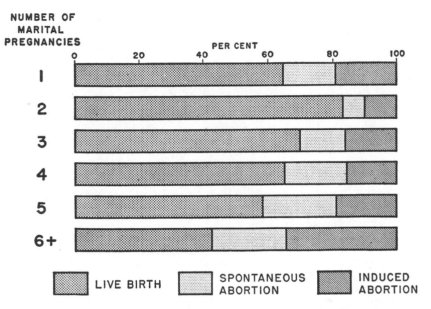

Figure 10. Outcome of Marital Pregnancy by Number of Times Pregnant. Based on Females Aged 36 and Older at Interview and Married by Age 30.

Data from Table 51.

samples in which induced ratios are high. Some of the highest ratios show in artificial insemination series, where early spontaneous abortions would be likely to be observed, as in Barton in Harrison, 1955:103.

The studies showing spontaneous losses by age of wife or by duration of marriage indicate higher percentages of loss early and late in the reproductive period. See Brunner and Newton 1939:86,88; Brunner 1941:169; Tietze et al. 1950a:1349; Erhardt and Jacobziner 1956:832.

[22] The source material on induced abortion ratios to pregnancies has been well summarized in Tietze 1954:20. The range of the studies is from none in two sources to the 23.8 per cent in Stix and Wiehl 1938. Studies on this subject are full of disclaimers of trustworthiness, and admit underreporting of induced abortions with few exceptions. See, for example, Whelpton in Taylor 1944, Stix and Notestein 1940.

Mehlan 1955:4 cited 14 to 19 per cent outcome ratio for illegally induced

The high proportion of induced abortion between ages sixteen and twenty presumably reflects the undesirability of having children while economically insecure or before the spouses feel they are ready for the responsibilities of parenthood. The terminal increase in abortion after age thirty-five represents chiefly unwanted pregnancies incurred by those who feel their families sufficiently large.

The two assumptions contained in the paragraph above have been tested to a certain extent by calculating the outcome ratios for women according to the number of marital conceptions they had experienced (Table 51, Figure 10). We find that among our ever-married women aged thirty-six and older those who had conceived once intentionally aborted 19 per cent of these first pregnancies; those who had been pregnant twice aborted 10 per cent of their pregnancies; those pregnant three and four times aborted 16 per cent; those who had conceived five times aborted 19 per cent; and those pregnant six or more times ended over one third (34 per cent) of their pregnancies by induced abortion.[23] These findings agree with our age-specific outcome ratio data and substantiate our belief that induced abortion is commonest among the youthful who have been married a short time and who wish to delay having children and among those who feel their families are already large enough. Our data does not permit us to tabulate type of outcome by order number of pregnancy.

The women who married once and were still married at time of

<hr>

abortions, 1946-1954, for East Germany. These estimates were based on an extensive survey by doctors of over 7,000 women.

The increase in ratios at later ages or with duration of marriage is confirmed in Brunner and Newton 1939:87 and Brunner 1941:170 (age); Brunner and Newton 1939:88 and Stix 1935:354 (duration of marriage). According to the latter two reports, 40 to 65 per cent of the pregnancies coming after 20 years of married life are intentionally aborted.

One of the first accounts of abortion records on a sample of U.S. women was printed in the *Zeitschrift für Sexualwissenschaft* in 1927. See Pirkner 1927:17-18. This note from abroad appearing in a German periodical was lacking in details, but indicated that data had been recorded on abortions among 1,655 women registered with the New York Birth Control Clinic under Dr. Hannah Stone's direction. Items referred to were number of prior pregnancies and induced and spontaneous abortions, religious affiliation, economic status, and nationality.

<hr>

[23] Data on the effect of a higher number of pregnancies on the outcome ratios of spontaneous and induced abortions in relation to live births can be derived from several other studies. For fifth and subsequent pregnancies Kopp 1933: Appendix Table 30 showed 25 per cent induced abortion, Stix and Notestein 1940:82-83 reported almost 50 per cent, and Whelpton and Kiser 1950 (2): 312 listed 18.4 per cent. The live birth ratios diminished correspondingly, ranging from 45 per cent (Stix and Notestein) to 67 per cent (Whelpton and Kiser) for fifth and subsequent pregnancies. Spontaneous abortions showed less marked effects.

interview display a higher proportion of live birth and a lower proportion of induced abortion than women who had been separated, divorced, or widowed. It is interesting to note that while Table 52 is based upon all the marriages of the S.D.W. women, the above statement is still true if one examines only their first marriages. However, we found that the S.D.W. women whose first marriages lasted into their thirties and forties had, at that point, outcome ratios essentially the same as those of the married-once group at the same age. This is to be expected. S.D.W. women who remarry show in their subsequent marriages a slightly greater tendency to have induced abortion than they did in their first marriages.

Extra-marital outcome. All the 32 conceptions resulting from extramarital coitus ended within the marriage during which they occurred. How they ended is rather interesting: 22 in induced abortions (one being therapeutic), 5 in spontaneous abortions, and 5 in the birth of children who were reared in the home. Of the 5 live births, 4 were to wives between thirty-one and forty, the other to a woman of twenty-three. In 2 of the 5 cases the husband was aware that he had not fathered the child.

RELATION TO AGE AT MARRIAGE

We have seen that age at marriage is an important factor in the frequency of conception, both pre-marital and marital. Now we shall examine its effect on the outcome of marital conceptions.

Accumulative experience. Eventually, about three quarters of the women who married between ages sixteen and twenty had a live birth and roughly four fifths of those who married between twenty-one and twenty-five. However, the difference here may be only a seeming one, since the number of cases in the 16-20 group is small beyond age forty and the accumulative experience drops, which suggests some sample vagary in this instance. It would be safer to say that roughly 80 per cent of the women of both age-at-marriage groups ultimately had a live birth. After twenty-five, the effect of physiological aging becomes evident: of the females who married between ages twenty-six and thirty, about 70 per cent had a live birth, while the figure for those who married between ages thirty-one and thirty-five is 46 per cent by age forty and probably would never exceed 50 per cent even if sufficient cases were available to extend the calculation to older ages.[24]

---

[24] Similar trends in increasing childlessness with later age at marriage have been shown in various other surveys.

U.S. Census 1950, Special Reports, *Fertility*, 1955:56-57, gives clear evidence on this point.

Spontaneous abortion relates to age at marriage in a most interesting way. Heretofore it has seemed to have a simple positive correlation with age—the older the women were, the more of them aborted spontaneously. While this remains true as a generalization, it is now evident that spontaneous abortion can be strongly influenced by several factors besides age, multiparity undoubtedly being one of them. This is made clear when one notes that the percentage of women who had a spontaneous abortion is lowest among the women who married between ages thirty-one and thirty-five. Only approximately half as many of these women aborted spontaneously as did the women of the other age-at-marriage groups. This is largely because, having been married for a shorter time, fewer of this group had conceived than of the women who married at younger ages. This duration of marriage factor also influences other types of outcome.

Induced abortion is progressively less common in each successive age-at-marriage group. Of the women who married between sixteen and twenty, over one third had an induced abortion; of those who married between twenty-one and twenty-five, one quarter; and of those who married later only about 15 per cent. Again, the differences are primarily a function of the number of years the women had been married. However, as we shall see in the age-specific outcome rate where duration of marriage is held reasonably constant, this factor does not wholly explain the differences that exist between the various age-at-marriage groups.

Age-specific rate. Within the age-period in which marriage occurred, there are no real differences in the rates of live birth of the various age-at-marriage groups. Spontaneous abortion varies from 3 to 5 per hundred years of marriage: i.e., 3 to 5 per cent of the women in any one year had spontaneous abortions. However, the rates for induced abortion reveal a strong trend, falling from 7 among those who married between ages sixteen and twenty to 4 among those who married between twenty-one and twenty-five, to 3 among those married between twenty-six and thirty, to 1 among those who married between ages thirty-one and thirty-five (Table 48).

With increasing age at marriage we again see a decline in induced

---

The pertinent data from the extensive British Family Census were given by Glass and Grebenik 1954:96.

Henry 1953 analyzed census material from European sources concerning childlessness. See Chapters 4 and 5.

See also Kiser and Whelpton 1944:81-82. Childlessness in the household survey in Indianapolis ranged from 9.3 for wives married at 17-19 years of age to 57 per cent for those married between 32 and 34.

abortion during the following age-period and a seemingly unimportant variation in spontaneous abortion. On the other hand, there is a consistent decrease in live births, which drop from 19 in our youngest age-at-marriage group to 8 in our oldest.

The same pattern obtains in the second and third age-periods following the age-period in which marriage occurred. In brief, with increasing age at marriage there is in general a reduction in both live birth rate and induced abortion rate.

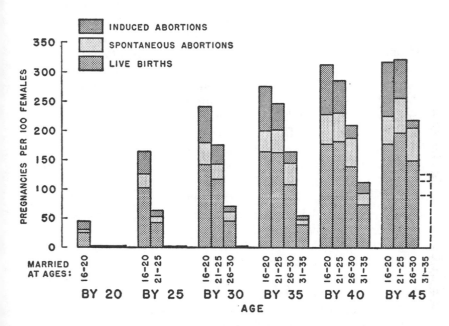

Figure 11. Accumulative Rate of Birth and Abortion in Marriage by Age at Marriage.

Data from Table 44.

Accumulative rate. While, by virtue of having married earlier, the females who married between sixteen and twenty exhibit higher live birth rates by any age up to thirty-five, those who married between twenty-one and twenty-five ultimately have a greater number of live births (Table 44, Figure 11). This is most surprising. Previous demographic experience would lead us to expect those who married youngest to have had the largest number of live births by the end of reproductive life. In our analysis, however, we see that they had an ultimate rate of 178 live births per hundred women, while those who married be-

tween twenty-one and twenty-five had 197 live births.[25] This is not the
result of any eleventh-hour activity by those who married between
twenty-one and twenty-five. If one holds duration of marriage roughly
constant by examining the age-period following that in which marriage
occurred, the age-period following that, and so on (reading the table
diagonally) without regard for chronological age, one sees that the
rates for those who married between twenty-one and twenty-five always
exceed the rates of the younger marrying group. For example, in the
age-period following the one in which marriage took place the rates
are 102 for those who married between ages sixteen and twenty and 119
for those who married between twenty-one and twenty-five.

If one compares the accumulative marital conception rates of the
females who married between sixteen and twenty with the rates of
those who married between twenty-one and twenty-five in the same
way we did above (ignoring chronological age and comparing them by
approximate duration of marriage), one again sees that the rates for the
women who married between twenty-one and twenty-five always
slightly exceed the rates for those who married between sixteen and
twenty. Hence our problem concerning live birth rate is evidently
linked with the same problem in conception rate. One probable explanation for both problems is that on an average those who married
between sixteen and twenty had by any given time (not by a given
age) fewer years of marital life than those who married later. For
example, we can assume that of those who married between sixteen and
twenty most married nearer age twenty than age sixteen; let us assume
the average age of marriage to have been 19. This means that by the
end of the five-year age-period following the age-period in which the
marriage occurred, these women had an average of seven years of
marriage. Now of those who married between twenty-one and twenty-
five we can assume that the majority married between twenty-one and
twenty-three; let us say the average age of marriage was twenty-two.
This means that by the end of the five-year age-period following the
age-period in which the marriage occurred, this group had an average
of nine years of marriage. Obviously a group of women with nine years
of marital life should have experienced more marital conceptions and
live births than a group with an average of seven years of marital life.

Another factor also merits attention. In other studies the females

---

[25] Extensive analysis has been made of the effect of tardy marriages on the birth
rates of the women involved. For illustrative material see: U.S. Census, 1950,
Special Reports, *Fertility*, 1955:56-57; Henry 1953 (using data from a wide
variety of countries studied in detail the effects of age at marriage on fertility,
Chapters 4 and 5); Glass and Grebenik 1954:97, Table 28; Henripin 1954:
70ff.

who married by age twenty were largely of the lower socio-economic level, where live births are more frequent than in the middle and upper socio-economic levels. Our sample of females who married between sixteen and twenty contains proportionately fewer of the lower socio-economic level and hence provides lower birth rates.

The effects of aging are seen among those who married after age twenty-five:[26] the women who married between ages twenty-six and thirty produced 150 live births per hundred females, and those who married between thirty-one and thirty-five had produced 73 by age forty and their eventual rate would presumably not exceed 90 (Table 44).

Spontaneous abortion rates follow, in general, the same pattern as live birth rates.

The accumulative rate of induced abortion is greater among females who marry at younger ages; this holds true whether one compares the age-at-marriage groups by a given age or whether one compares them on the basis of number of marital years lived. The extremely high induced abortion rate of those who married young is largely because these women had more than one abortion. For example, we see that by age forty-five about 38 per cent of those who married between sixteen and twenty had had induced abortions, and that they accounted for 92 abortions per hundred females: i.e., these women who had experienced induced abortion averaged 2.4 abortions per woman. In contrast, one sees that the women who married between twenty-six and thirty, or later, and had induced abortions, had an average of only 1.3. While the lessening of fecundity with increasing age partly explains this relation between age at marriage and induced abortion rate, it by no means explains it wholly: a real difference in behavior is involved, as will become apparent when outcome ratios are examined.

Age-specific outcome ratios. The proportions of pregnancies ending in each of the three types of outcome within given five-year age-periods show an increase in the proportion of live births with increasing age at marriage. This trend is, however, muted beyond age twenty-five by the inevitable increase in spontaneous abortion (Table 53). Thus we see that as an over-all average, 61 per cent of the pregnancies of women who married between ages sixteen and twenty resulted in live

---

[26] Truex 1936, in a study of size of 691 families covering three generations, stated that in all series the women who were over 30 years of age at marriage showed the smallest average families.

Whelpton and Kiser 1943:232 revealed sharply lowered total live births among late-marrying wives. Rates ranged from 366 per hundred wives married under seventeen to 69 for those married between twenty-nine and thirty-one years of age. These women were forty to forty-four years old at report.

birth; 68 per cent for those who married between twenty-one and twenty-five; 67 per cent for those who married between ages twenty-six and thirty; and 63 per cent for those who married between ages thirty-one and thirty-five. Holding the number of years married more or less constant, as explained in the discussion of accumulative rate, it is still evident that the women who married after age twenty had a greater proportion of their pregnancies end in live birth than those who married between ages sixteen and twenty.

Spontaneous abortion also tends to increase proportionately with increased age at marriage. On the average, 16 per cent of the pregnancies of women who married between ages sixteen and twenty were thus aborted (this is increased by the inexplicably high figure at age-period 26-30), 16 per cent for those who married between twenty-one and twenty-five, 23 per cent for those who married between ages twenty-six and thirty, and 27 per cent for those who married between ages thirty-one and thirty-five.

The proportion of conceptions terminated by induced abortion decreases with increasing age at marriage. This is true not only at any given age, but also when one compares the groups on the basis of duration of marriage. For example, no less than 29 per cent of the pregnancies of those who married between ages sixteen and twenty were aborted during the same age-period, whereas the comparable figures for the other age-at-marriage groups are 18 per cent and 13 per cent respectively. For the women who married between ages thirty-one and thirty-five (whose outcomes are numerically too few for an analysis by five-year periods) there is evidence that the proportion of induced abortion in this first marital period is in the vicinity of 9 per cent.

Taking over-all averages for all ages, 23 per cent of the conceptions of our youngest age-at-marriage group ended in induced abortion as against 16 per cent and 10 per cent for those who married at older ages.

It would appear that those who marry young and who at younger ages have many years of potential reproductive life ahead feel that they can "afford" abortion; those who marry late place a higher value upon their conceptions. The increase in abortion noted in the third age-period after the one in which marriage occurred (i.e., after at least ten years of marriage), reflects unwanted pregnancies among those who felt their families already complete.

RELATION TO EDUCATIONAL LEVEL

Accumulative experience. Table 45 and Figure 12 indicate that with greater education there is a progressive tendency for fewer women to have live births. This tendency is marked up to age twenty-five and is still visible to a lesser degree thereafter. Obviously some of this is the direct result of the fact that the better educated females were in school at an age when the less educated no longer were, but there is also evidence of some delay in childbearing at ages when all the women had presumably completed their educations.

By age twenty-five, some 65 per cent of the married women of grade school education had had a live birth in contrast to 54 per cent of the high school educated, 44 per cent of the college educated, and 28 per cent of the women who went into postgraduate work. While the differences become less with increasing age, we find that by the end of the reproductive life 81 per cent of the grade school women have had a live birth as opposed to 71 per cent of the postgraduate women. The women of high school and college education occupy an intermediate position between these two extremes. This picture in general parallels that seen in accumulative experience of conception.

If we limit our sample to women of completed fertility, the relation of live birth experience to educational level is the same and, moreover, agrees well with census-derived data (see Table 29).

Table 29. **Census Comparison: Accumulative Experience,
Live Birth**

**For Ever-Married White Non-Prison Females of
Completed Fertility (Age 46 and Over), Compared
with Estimate for Urban White Females in 1945,
Adjusted to Age Distribution of Sample**

By Educational Level

EDUCATIONAL LEVEL	EVER-MARRIED WHITE NON-PRISON FEMALES		ESTIMATE FOR URBAN WHITE FEMALES
	Number	*Per cent*	*Per cent*
0–8	*41*	*80.5*	82.7
9–12	109	75.2	77.2
13–16	130	73.1	75.5*
17+	124	71.0	71.6*
Total	404	73.8	75.5†

*13–15 and 16+ years.
†Adjusted also to the distribution of the white non-prison sample by educational level.

The percentage of women who experienced spontaneous abortion seems less strongly linked to educational achievement. There is a general tendency for fewer of the better educated to have a spontaneous abortion,[27] but this is in part a result of the fact that fewer of them had

[27] The significance of nutritional factors during pregnancy in relation to spontaneous abortion and stillbirth is stressed by Sutherland 1949:64 ff., who summarizes seven studies relating to this problem. It undoubtedly is of some

become pregnant by a given age. Confining attention to the end of reproductive life (i.e., the experience of married women by age forty-five), one sees that roughly one third of the women of high school education or less had had at least one spontaneous abortion and approximately one quarter of those who went into college or beyond had had similar experience. For some inexplicable reason, our sample of high school educated appears to be more prone to abort spontaneously than other educational groups.

The percentage of women with induced abortion is, as it was with other types of outcome, generally in keeping with the percentage who became pregnant; this matter of proportion will be taken up subsequently. In general, the trend is for a higher percentage of the less educated to have experienced induced abortion. This is clear up to age twenty-five, but thereafter the trend is sometimes obscured, the high school educated and the college educated occasionally reversing their relative positions. However, by any age past twenty, the grade school women always have the highest percentage and the postgraduate women the lowest percentage.

Age-specific rate. Up to a point, this rate bears out the findings of our accumulative experience data. Table 49 shows that up to age twenty-five the less educated have a larger number of live births per hundred years of marriage. This may also be translated into the percentage of women involved: a higher percentage of the less educated have a live birth in any given year up to age twenty-five. After age twenty-five, the rates of live birth no longer reflect any consistent differences between the grade school educated, the high school educated, and the college educated; the postgraduate women display the highest live birth rates in age-periods 31-35 and 36-40.[28] To a considerable degree these educational level differences stem from differences in age at marriage, the grade school educated marrying earliest and the postgraduate women marrying latest.

Spontaneous abortion appears less strongly correlated with educational level. Prior to age twenty-five it follows the pattern of live birth, being most prevalent among the less educated. After age twenty-

importance in the incidences of abortion at different income or educational levels, and more so during periods of economic hardship.

[28] Grabill 1955:91 cited census data consistent with the educational trends in our sample. College women under age thirty reported fewer children under age five both in 1940 and 1950; and while college women reporting at age thirty and older in 1940 still showed this inverse relationship, the better educated women reporting at age thirty in 1950 showed higher numbers of children under five per 1,000 women than did the women of grammar and high school education.

five the fluctuations in the rate of spontaneous abortion are not especially meaningful.

Induced abortion rates (or percentage of women involved during a given year) are negatively correlated with educational achievement: the greater the amount of education, the lower the induced abortion rate. The high school educated and the college educated are not dissimilar in rate, but the postgraduates, in nearly every case, are the lowest.

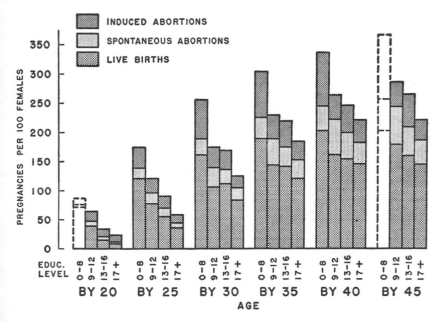

Figure 12. Accumulative Rate of Birth and Abortion in Marriage by Educational Level.

Data from Table 45.

One other trend is seen throughout all levels of education: in all groups for which we have adequate data the abortion rates decrease with age.

Accumulative rate. The number of live births per hundred females shows a strong and consistent correlation with educational level: the higher the educational level, the fewer the live births.[29] The differ-

---

[29] A large body of material, including several census reports, is available on differential fertility by educational levels, or by the roughly comparable criteria of economic, occupational, or social class. In general, the inverse relationship to number of live births noted here is shown in these studies. Typical of them are the following:

ences are marked at younger ages and diminish later, but even by age forty-five they are substantial (Table 45). Taking the extremes of our educational scale for illustrative purposes, we see that by age twenty-five there were about 119 births per hundred grade school women and only 36 births per hundred postgraduate women. By age forty-five the equivalent figures are 202 versus 147.[30]

Table 30. Census Comparison: Accumulative Live Birth Rate

For Ever-Married White Non-Prison Females of Completed Fertility (Age 46 and Over), Compared with Estimate for Urban White Females in 1945, Adjusted to Age Distribution and Marital Status (Married Once, Living with Husband, or Ever S.D.W.) of Sample

By Educational Level

EDUCATIONAL LEVEL	EVER-MARRIED WHITE NON-PRISON FEMALES		ESTIMATE FOR URBAN WHITE FEMALES
	Number of females	*Live births per 100 females*	*Live births per 100 females*
0–8	*41*	*202.4*	276.3
9–12	109	179.8	198.1
13–16	130	160.0	173.1*
17+	124	146.8	157.0*
Total	404	165.6	184.3†

*13–15 and 16+ years.

†Adjusted also to the distribution of the white non-prison sample by educational level.

Dunlop 1914 demonstrated that high fertility is associated with occupations of least skill and lowest economic status in Scotland.

Hart 1922 covered rural and urban groups from the Iowa census of 1915.

Notestein and Kiser 1935:34-36 used occupational status of the husband to compare fertility levels among unskilled workers, skilled workers, and business and professional classes.

Tietze 1943 found similar results when tested by income, education, and level of occupation.

Burgess in Taylor 1944:119-123 (economic level and education), Coogan 1946:43 (education levels among Catholic families in Florida), Dinkel 1952 (occupational levels), and Tietze and Grabill 1957:7 (education and occupation) all point in the common direction. The last study cited showed that such differentials have been substantially reduced during 1940-1950.

---

[30] Whelpton and Kiser 1943:253 reported sharp differences in live birth rates to women of varying educational levels in the Indianapolis Household Survey of over 41,000 wives. Rates of children born per hundred wives were: grade school, 210; high school, 133; college, 101. In contrast to these over-all figures, a further analysis in Whelpton and Kiser 1950 (2): 381-393 showed a direct relationship between fertility and socio-economic status in the couples who

When only women who have completed their reproductive lives are considered, the birth rate of the less educated is still distinctly greater than that of the more educated. This is shown in Table 30 where a comparison with census-derived data is also made.

While our rates for the high school educated, college educated, and postgraduate females compare rather favorably with the census rates, being only 10 per cent lower, there is a large discrepancy between our rate and the census rate for the grade school educated. This reflects the fact that our grade school sample does not represent the grade school educated of the general population as adequately as our better educated sample represents the better educated in the United States. A discussion of the nature of our grade school educated sample will be found in Chapter 7.

Ignoring for the moment the grade school educated, we find that the greater the amount of education, the lower the rate of spontaneous abortion, as one would expect in view of the live birth rates. The high school educated, by the end of reproductive life, had 66 such abortions per hundred women, the college educated 50, and the postgraduates 40. The grade school educated have lower rates than the high school educated, but this is because the grade school women have high induced abortion rates; they artificially abort a considerable number of pregnancies that would have, if given time, spontaneously aborted.

Induced abortion relates strongly with educational level. Even when one takes into account the differences in conception rate, it is evident that the grade school females in our sample are much more given to induced abortion than the other groups. Thus by age forty the grade school group had 93 induced abortions per hundred females—an average of almost one abortion per female—while the other groups had but 38 to 47 induced abortions. The differences between the induced abortion rates of the high school and college women are relatively small. The postgraduate women display definitely lower rates of induced abortion.

Age-specific outcome ratio. By and large, the differences in the percentages of pregnancy that end in live birth are not great between the various educational groups (Table 54). However, in a few instances some marked differences exist. In age-period 16-20, the college women had only 47 per cent of their conceptions result in live birth whereas the high school educated had 63 per cent. In age-period 36-40 the

---

were able to number and space their children as planned. The rates for the group reported were low, but the direct relationship was clearest when the husband's income was used as a measure, although rental value, net worth, occupation, education, and social status showed the same trend.

college educated show a striking reduction in the proportion of their pregnancies that terminate in birth (55 per cent), this being the result of a greatly increased incidence of spontaneous abortion coupled with an increase in induced abortion. But aside from these instances, which may be fortuitous, the proportion of pregnancies resulting in birth tends, in all groups, to range between 60 and 70 per cent.[31]

It would appear that the grade school educated have fewest spontaneous abortions because of their relatively high percentage of pregnancies artificially aborted. The high school educated and the college females show the anticipated increase of spontaneous abortion with age; by age-period 36-40 roughly one quarter of the conceptions of these two groups end in spontaneous abortion.[32] The increase is less evident among the postgraduate women, the rise being only from 16 to 19 per cent.

In the age-periods 21-25 and 26-30 (Table 54), a high proportion of the grade school educated have induced abortions—24 per cent and 29 per cent respectively; the data from Table 45 for these women at older ages would lead us to believe that a high abortion ratio continues throughout their reproductive lives.

The high school, college, and postgraduate groups are alike in having in their initial age-period a high percentage of induced abortion followed in subsequent age-periods by lower percentages. This undoubtedly reflects the fact that pregnancies are unwelcome while one is completing one's education or before one has become economically established. The difference is especially dramatic among the college educated who in age-period 16-20 aborted 36 per cent of their conceptions; the figure falls to 20 per cent in the next age-period, and lower yet (16 per cent) in the following one. Between ages twenty-one and thirty-five the percentages for the high school and college educated women are not dissimilar, but prior to twenty-one and after thirty-five the college group has considerably the higher figures.[33] The

---

[31] This figure is close to the 72.7 per cent of live births in the Brunner and Newton 1939 study in which the sample was confined to grade school and high school educated women with low income levels. See p. 90.

[32] Pearl 1939:228 found only minor differences in educational levels in regard to spontaneous abortion, except for a small illiterate group, which showed 11.7 per cent, the highest ratio.

Stix and Notestein 1940:79-80 found no differences as between educational attainment groups.

[33] Other studies are not consistent in their findings regarding variations in induced abortion ratios between educational level groups.

Stix and Wiehl 1938:624 showed the lowest percentage of induced abortions for lowest income groups. Pearl 1939:228 found only slight differences but the lower educational groups were somewhat higher than the college educated. Stix and Notestein 1940:79-80 found no differences in two occu-

postgraduate women had, in general, fewer of their pregnancies artificially aborted.

RELATION TO DECADE OF BIRTH

This particular factor, which previously proved complicated to analyze, once again presents some problems. One cannot assume that any great physiological differences existed between the women of different birth decades; but it is obvious that depression, periods of prosperity, wars and a legion of other factors strongly affected their reproductive characteristics. For example, one might expect a woman born in 1889 to regard induced abortion differently from a woman born in 1920. However, though our expectations of finding clear and simple decade differences were disappointed by the powerful and changing influences exerted by historical conditions, we have been able to define and describe with reasonable clarity the long-term trends.

Accumulative experience. Table 46 shows that with successive decades a smaller percentage of women had a live birth by any given age until this trend was suddenly reversed by the "baby boom" after World War II. The reversal is, of course, most evident among the females of our most recent decade of birth: 1920-1929. Whereas the percentage of women who had a live birth by age twenty-five fell from 54 per cent (pertaining to the women born before 1890) to 38 per cent (the figure set by women born 1910-1919), the 1920-1929 women, by twenty-five, had a live birth rate of 54 per cent. The same factors that produced the "baby boom" among the younger married women also influenced women in their late twenties and early thirties; note that among the females of birth decade 1910-1919 the decline in the percentage who have live births has been checked by age thirty-five.

Until recently, the percentage of married women born in successive decades who had a spontaneous abortion was diminishing, since more of them were having induced abortions and fewer of them were becoming pregnant (Table 35). However, when the 1920-1929 group began the "baby boom," the percentage of women who had a spontaneous abortion rose markedly, since the percentage who became pregnant also rose. The same holds true for the 1910-1919 women at a correspondingly older age.

---

pational classes, white collar and manual workers. Kiser 1942:236 found the highest ratios of *total* pregnancy loss among the lowest income groups in the data he analyzed from the 1935-36 National Health Survey, but no distinction was made between spontaneous and induced abortion. In his analysis by educational levels he reported the opposite results.

Induced abortion shows a somewhat different trend. One sees a marked increase with each successive birth decade, from 1890 to 1909. However, among the women born between 1910 and 1919 the percentages are lower, and this is true also of those born between 1920 and 1929.[34] Among the 1910-1919 women some of the reduction in abortion reflects merely the fact that, up to age twenty-five, they had fewer conceptions than the women of earlier birth decades; and after twenty-five, apparently, they simply did not resort so often to induced abortion. By the time they were twenty-five, the 1920-1929 females were in the "baby boom" era and were keeping their pregnancies. In brief, it would seem that induced abortion increased and then in our last generation of women (born 1910-1930) decreased.

Age-specific rate. The rates of live birth mirror what we saw in accumulative experience; during the birth decades through 1900-1909 there was a decrease in rate, but the trend was reversed by the women of birth decade 1920-1929 and by the women in their late twenties and thirties of birth decade 1910-1919 (Table 49).

Spontaneous abortion rates follow, in a somewhat less clear fashion, the same pattern.

The rates of induced abortion in relation to birth decade are more difficult to describe. There was an increase among the women born up to 1899; among women up to age twenty-five the increase continued through decade 1900-1909, but thereafter the younger women show somewhat lower rates. After age twenty, the 1910-1919 and the 1920-1929 women display the lowest rates of all. One gains the general impression of an increase followed by a decrease, the decrease being delayed at younger ages.

Accumulative rate. Our calculations under this heading show the same trend: the number of live births per hundred married women decreased with successive birth decades until the recent "baby boom"

---

[34] An alarm over a supposed steady increase in induced abortion experience is reflected in many of the discussions of the subject. Olson, for example, in 1943:672 wrote of an "increase by an appalling percentage" during the last several decades. Simons 1939:84 cited an increase of 180 per cent in Minneapolis during the first three years of the depression. Although Millar 1934:303 did not see any major change in Cincinnati during 1918-1932, he cited slightly higher levels of induced abortion in the depression periods 1921-1922 and 1930.

Dr. Morris Fishbein claimed an increase of 20 to 40 per cent in over-all induced abortions in the two years following Pearl Harbor. See *Time*, March 6, 1944, p. 60.

In England the Ministry of Health and Home Office Abortion Committee Report of 1939 concluded that there had been "an increase in the prevalence of criminal abortion" in recent years. See p. 13.

when the trend was reversed, especially by the women born between 1920 and 1929 (Table 46). The women of birth decade 1910-1919 who were in their thirties at the time of the "boom" also responded to the same socio-economic stimuli and reversed the trend, but to a lesser degree. By age twenty-five, a point at which we can compare all five of our birth decades, one sees the rate fall from the 92 mark set by those who were born before 1890 to 51 among the women born between 1910 and 1919, and then rebound to 86 among the women born from 1920 to 1929.[35]

A subsidiary but interesting observation may be made from Table 46. The 1920-1929 women more than trebled their live birth rate between ages twenty and twenty-five, whereas the women of the preceding birth decade (1910-1919) failed to treble their rate and the women of 1900-1909 did not even double theirs.

Spontaneous abortion follows a pattern similar to live birth: a general decrease in rate with successive birth decades until the 1920-1929 women and the older 1910-1919 women reverse the trend.

The information concerning induced abortion provided by accumulative rate does not correspond too well with what we saw in accumulative experience, but agrees with the trends seen in our age-specific rate. It is evident that among the women of birth decades 1910-1919 and 1920-1929 there was a definite decrease in rate of induced abortion.

Age-specific outcome ratio. These figures show no clear relationship between birth decade and the proportion of marital pregnancies ending in live birth or spontaneous abortion (Table 55). However, the women born before 1890 spontaneously aborted an unusually high proportion of their pregnancies.

On the other hand, induced abortion manifests some meaningful and interesting variations. The depression of the 1930's resulted in a larger proportion of pregnancies that were artificially aborted. Note that the maximum proportion within each birth decade occurs in the age-period coinciding with the depth of the depression: 1890-1899, age-period 31-35; 1900-1909, 21-25; and 1910-1919, 16-20.

The consistent influence of the subsequent "baby boom" is evident among the 1920-1929 females in age-period 21-25 and among the 1910-1919 women beyond age twenty-six: the proportion of induced abortion decreased and that of live birth increased.

---

[35] The reversal of a long-term decline in U.S. birth rates and average family size has received wide attention. The various factors contributing to this phenomenon have been discussed in: U.S. Bureau of the Census, *Current Population Reports*, Series P-20, April 1947, No. 18 and April 1954, No. 65. Whelpton 1954b and 1956; Grabill 1955; Mayer and Klapprodt 1955; Statistical Bulletin, Metropolitan Life, October, 1956; Tietze and Grabill 1957:7.

Calendar time outcome ratio. By taking the decade in which a woman was born and her age when her pregnancy ended, we were able to devise a table showing pregnancy outcome ratios within particular periods of calendar time, and also the conception rates for these same periods (Table 31). The calendar year designated is the mid-point

Table 31. Outcome Ratio

For Pregnancies Terminated in Marriage

By Calendar Time

Type of outcome	PREGNANCIES TERMINATED IN MARRIAGE					
	1925	1930	1935	1940	1945	1950
	Per cent					
Live birth	61.9	62.4	64.8	68.1	69.6	70.2
Spontaneous abortion	14.5	13.3	16.9	18.4	18.1	19.4
Induced abortion	23.6	24.3	18.3	13.5	12.3	10.4
Number of outcomes	827	1,074	1,282	1,372	1,070	423
	Conceptions per 100 years of first marriage					
Marital conception rate	18.9	16.3	13.9	14.4	17.3	18.1

of a ten-year period; owing to the way in which the raw data were punched for mechanical tabulation, the periods overlap and this fact mutes the differences to some extent. From this table one can see that the proportion of live births has steadily increased while induced abortion has decreased.[36] The depression is marked here by a reduced conception rate.

RELATION TO DEGREE OF DEVOUTNESS

The degree of religious devoutness or the tenets of any religion could be expected to influence the outcome of pregnancy primarily in terms of permitting or opposing induced abortion. All the religions with which we are here concerned condemn such abortion, but the effect of this attitude upon a woman's behavior depends, of course, upon how devout she is.

Accumulative experience. Among Protestants the negative correla-

[36] Two other studies show a calendar time increase in induced abortion ratio but neither of them carries over far enough to parallel the trend in the present data. Stix 1935:358 presented an analysis of induced abortion ratios by periods from 1905 to 1932, and concluded that during the preceding 25 years there had been a "marked increase in the proportion of pregnancies terminated by illegal abortion." This sample was drawn from birth control clinic patients in New York City. Lewis-Faning 1949:169 found an increase also in British data based on wives married prior to 1930 and those married after.

tion between degree of devoutness and incidence of induced abortion is uniform and clear: a higher percentage of religiously inactive women have had an induced abortion, by any age, than have the devout. The moderately devout occupy an intermediate position (Table 47). By the end of life, between one quarter and one third of the religiously inactive Protestant women had experienced an induced abortion as compared to one seventh of the devout. Live birth, as a result, has a positive correlation with devoutness.

The same situation evidently obtains among the Jews, although they differ from the Protestants in having (after age twenty) higher percentages of women who have experienced induced abortion and live birth. The Jewish figures for these two outcomes are usually about 10 percentage points above the corresponding Protestant figures. Thus, for example, by age forty-five some 74 per cent of the religiously inactive Jewish women had had a live birth and 39 per cent an induced abortion; equivalent Protestant figures are 64 per cent and 29 per cent.

Although the data are insufficient for inclusion in the tables or for accurate comparison, it is clear that a vast difference exists between devout and inactive Catholics, especially with reference to induced abortion. In live birth experience, the devout and inactive Catholics are not dissimilar to the devout and inactive Protestants or Jews; in terms of spontaneous abortion the devout Catholics exhibit very low figures while the inactive possess very high ones, precisely the reverse of what one would logically expect. The percentage of devout Catholics with induced abortion experience is extremely low and of the religiously inactive rather high.

Age-specific rate. The more devout females had more live births per hundred years of marriage than the less devout or, putting it another way, a higher percentage of devout wives in an average year had a live birth. In the more fertile years of life, from ages twenty-one to thirty, devout Protestants had a rate of about 19 live births per hundred marital years as opposed to 13 or 14 for the religiously inactive (Table 50). While our Jewish and Catholic samples are too small for an age-specific calculation with three categories of devoutness, our scant data suggest that the same situation obtains.[37]

---

[37] The relation between the outcome of pregnancies and the degree of religious devoutness has been only tentatively explored. Burgess in Taylor 1944:118-119 pointed out the lack of analysis of fertility on the basis of nominal and active church affiliation. Using his own material on the parents of 1,000 engaged couples he showed that devoutness of religion was positively associated with the average number of children in a family. This finding is related to that of the Indianapolis study in regard to the tie between traditionalism and fertility. (See footnote 10, this chapter).

In general the rate of spontaneous abortion also shows a positive correlation with degree of devoutness.

Induced abortion is more common among the less devout. It is interesting that the moderately devout Protestants are nearly identical with the religiously inactive in their induced abortion rates between ages twenty-six and forty—only before twenty-six are the rates for the inactive markedly higher. To take one example, between ages twenty-

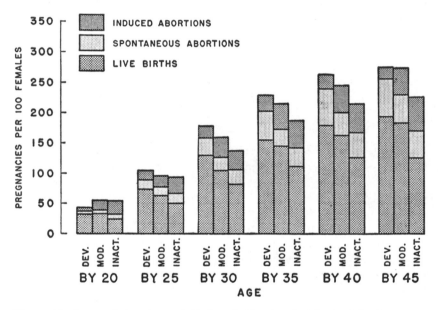

Figure 13. Accumulative Rate of Birth and Abortion in Marriage for Protestant Females by Degree of Religious Devoutness.

Data from Table 47.

one and twenty-five the devout have a rate of 3 such abortions per hundred married years (i.e., 3 per cent of the women in any one year), the moderately devout 4, and the inactive, 6. Between forty-one and forty-five the trend is reversed; this is probably fortuitous.

Accumulative rate. This measurement confirms again the basic pattern: the devout, irrespective of religious affiliation, have the highest rates of live birth and the lowest rates of induced abortion (Table 47,

---

Coogan 1946:19-22 found slightly higher fertility as measured by births among the more devout wives in a survey of Catholic women in a Florida diocese. Devoutness was tested by attendance at mass, by whether or not they made their Easter duty, and the frequency with which they received communion.

Figure 13). By the end of reproductive life the devout Protestant wives had 194 live births for every hundred females, the moderately devout, 183, and the religiously inactive, 126.

Among the Protestants the rates of spontaneous abortion are, as expected, also higher for the devout. This also appears to be true among the Jews. The Catholic sample is too small to give trustworthy figures.

Induced abortion rates are greater among the less devout, and in many instances the differences are extreme when the devout are compared with the inactive. Without exception, the induced abortion rates

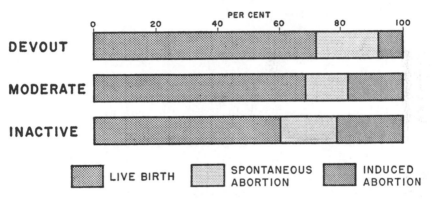

Figure 14. Outcome of Marital Pregnancy for Protestant Females by Degree of Religious Devoutness.

Data from Table 56.

are, by any age, greatest for the religiously inactive and least for the devout. The moderately devout occupy an intermediate position, but their rates are closer to those of the inactive than to those of the devout. This relation between induced abortion and devoutness is largely the result of the religious injunctions against abortion, which in the minds of some is synonymous with murder. However, it is also probable that the devoutly religious desire more offspring than do the religiously inactive.

Age-specific outcome ratio. The best test of the effect of religious devoutness is seen in Table 56 and Figure 14, where the proportions of the types of outcome are given. Live birth unquestionably accounts for a larger proportion of the pregnancies of the devout than of the religiously inactive. An over-all average shows that 72 per cent of the conceptions of devout Protestants end in live birth as compared to 60 per cent of the conceptions of the inactive.

Spontaneous abortion shows little relation to degree of devoutness.

The effect of religious devoutness is most striking in terms of induced abortion. While 8 per cent of the marital pregnancies of devout Protestants were artificially aborted, the moderately devout aborted 17 per cent and the inactive 21 per cent. The inactive Jewish sample was 24 per cent. Among the Catholics, our small sample would indicate that the devout abort many fewer of their pregnancies than do the inactive. There are few instances where the power of religion is more dramatically illustrated than here, where it motivates a woman to retain an unwanted pregnancy despite economic, social, and possibly even medical contraindications, and not only to endure months of discomfort but also to accept the ensuing years of child care.[38]

MARRIAGE AND REPRODUCTIVE BEHAVIOR

While this chapter and the chapters immediately preceding and following make it plain that the vast majority of pregnancies and terminations occur within marriage, it is desirable to present this fact explicitly and in some detail. In order to present the information in a lifetime perspective, and to avoid the problems resulting from the fact that our sample contains proportionately too many young unmarried females, we have derived the data below only from women aged thirty-six and older at the time they were interviewed (Table 57). In brief, we are dealing with the reproductive behavior of women who have completed or nearly completed their fertile years of life.

Of all the pregnancies reported by our total sample of white nonprison females aged thirty-six and older, 89 per cent were conceived in marriage; 90 per cent were terminated in marriage. Even greater are the percentages of live births and spontaneous abortions: 99 per cent of the former and 96 per cent of the latter occurred within wedlock. However, of our total of 708 induced abortions only 65 per cent were had by married women.[39] If one limits the sample of women aged thirty-six and over to ever-married women, or even to women married once and still married, the percentages given above are altered only slightly.

---

[38] In support of the present findings is the analysis by Freedman and Whelpton in Whelpton and Kiser 1950 (2):424-426, which shows the relationship of the degree of religious interest and of the planning of children. Tables 1 and 2 indicate in Protestant wives a high positive relation between religious faith and lack of pregnancy planning. Those wives reporting an intensive religious interest experienced a relatively large number of births in excess of the last wanted child.

[39] It is of interest to compare these findings to the range of percentages of single and married women represented in reports of hospitalized abortions. See footnote 25, Chapter 3.

Since the better educated are so strongly overrepresented in this total sample, it is necessary to subdivide by educational level. As far as conceptions are concerned, slightly over 90 per cent of the conceptions of the grade school, high school, and college educated women aged thirty-six and older were within marriage. The somewhat lower percentage (85) for the postgraduate women is largely the result of their having had more years of unmarried life. Marriage includes about 99 per cent of the live births among the women of all educational categories, and from 92 to 98 per cent of all spontaneous abortions. Induced abortion presents a different picture: the percentage of induced abortions within marriage decreases with increasing education. Among the grade school educated of our sample 85 per cent of all induced abortions were experienced by married women; the equivalent figures for the high- school educated are 71, for the college educated 68, and for the postgraduate women 52 per cent. Although the public is accustomed to think of induced abortion as a desperate resort primarily of the unmarried, actually it is clear that the vast majority of illegal abortions are performed upon married women.

SUMMARY

Our white non-prison married women, taken as a unit, approximate the socio-economic upper 20 per cent of the urban population, but include an overrepresentation of women who have been separated, divorced, or widowed. Ultimately 80 per cent of the ever-married women became pregnant while married, and averaged about three pregnancies each. In any one year an average of between one quarter and one fifth of the wives between ages sixteen and thirty conceived; after age thirty fertility rapidly decreased.

In the course of a lifetime three quarters of the women had a live birth, one quarter experienced spontaneous abortion, and between one quarter and one fifth had an induced abortion. Live birth accounts for three fifths to two thirds of all marital conceptions at any age up to forty; spontaneous abortion ends only about one pregnancy in ten in early life but increases until in late reproductive life about one fifth of all conceptions spontaneously abort. Induced abortion is most prevalent at younger ages when, presumably, the couples do not feel ready to have children: over one quarter of the conceptions of the young wives were deliberately aborted. Later induced abortion becomes less common but shows a tendency to increase in late life when many couples feel their families are sufficiently large. Induced abortion in marriage is commoner among women who later are separated, divorced, or widowed: marital trouble and instability are thought to be causative factors in induced abortion.

Age at marriage is an important factor in reproductive behavior since it determines the number of fecund years within marriage. The later a woman marries the less apt she is to become pregnant; also she will, on the average, have fewer pregnancies than a woman who marries at a younger age. Delaying marital conception is common, but the delay is not long: the maximum conception rate occurs in the five-year period following the five-year age-period in which the marriage took place.

About 80 per cent of those who marry before age twenty-six experience a live birth; the percentage drops rapidly among those marrying later. The proportion of pregnancies that end in spontaneous abortion is greater among those who marry at older ages; the proportion terminated by induced abortion is greater among those who marry at younger ages.

Analyses indicate that the better educated tend to postpone and limit the number of their conceptions when they are young; hence the less educated surpass them during this period of life in the percentage of wives with conception experience and in the number of conceptions. Later in life, however, the better educated exceed the less educated in conception rate: the former cease their procrastination while the latter have largely completed their families and are now limiting their conceptions. Despite this reversal, in the course of a lifetime fewer of the better educated become pregnant, and they have fewer pregnancies each.

Primarily because fewer of them become pregnant, the percentage of wives who have experienced birth, spontaneous abortion, and induced abortion is smaller among the better educated. The less educated not only have more live births but have them earlier in life. In terms of absolute number, the grade school educated have the most induced abortions and the postgraduate women the least. However, the college educated have a high proportion of the pregnancies they incur during college age aborted; thereafter the induced abortion ratio is roughly the same for the high school educated and the college educated, with the postgraduate women reporting somewhat lower figures. Our fragmentary data on the grade school educated suggest that they probably have a larger proportion of induced abortions, at any age, than do the women of the other educational groups.

Decade of birth presents a more complicated picture. In general one can say that there was a trend toward a decrease in the number of marital conceptions and in the number of women who conceived until the recent post-World War II "baby boom," when this trend was halted and reversed. The depression of the 1930's lowered the conception rate and it did not return to its predepression level until after World War II.

Live births, like conceptions, tended to decrease among the women of successive birth decades until the "baby boom." Induced abortion showed an increase that was checked by the women born in and after 1910. But during the depression years in the 1930's the proportion of pregnancies that were artificially aborted rose among all wives of reproductive age.

Studying the proportions of marital pregnancies that ended in birth, spontaneous abortion, and induced abortion from roughly 1925 to 1950, we see an over-all slow increase in the proportion of live births and spontaneous abortions, and a corresponding decrease in induced abortions.

Degree of religious devoutness displays a strong and consistent relation to marital reproduction: more of the devout females conceive and they conceive more often than the religiously inactive. Similarly, greater religious devoutness correlates positively with live birth and negatively with induced abortions: relatively few devoutly religious women will have an induced abortion.

Table 32. Accumulative Experience and Rate: Marital Conception
For Ever-Married Females
By Marital Status at Interview

BY AGE	EVER-MARRIED FEMALES								
	Marital status at interview			Marital status at interview			Marital status at interview		
	Ever married	Married once, still married	Ever S.D.W.	Ever married	Married once, still married	Ever S.D.W.	Ever married	Married once, still married	Ever S.D.W.
	Per cent of females with conception experience			Conceptions per 100 females			Number of females		
20	31.7	25.4	36.8	42.4	30.2	52.2	523	232	291
25	53.9	52.0	56.5	91.9	83.8	102.8	1250	714	536
30	70.0	72.0	67.6	161.5	164.7	157.5	1254	699	555
35	78.4	82.0	74.2	214.2	223.8	203.1	992	534	458
40	79.3	82.4	76.1	247.4	262.8	232.2	675	336	339
45	80.4	83.4	78.0	265.6	286.7	248.4	404	181	223

Table 33. Accumulative Experience and Rate: Marital Conception
For Ever-Married Females
By Age at Marriage

BY AGE	EVER-MARRIED FEMALES											
	Age at marriage				Age at marriage				Age at marriage			
	16–20	21–25	26–30	31–35	16–20	21–25	26–30	31–35	16–20	21–25	26–30	31–35
	Per cent of females with conception experience				Conceptions per 100 females				Number of females			
20	30.8				40.7				513			
25	75.1	44.4			160.2	61.7			377	865		
30	84.2	77.1	43.9		239.1	174.8	68.9		279	642	328	
35	88.1	84.7	72.3	37.8	276.7	243.7	162.4	51.2	193	471	242	82
40	88.9	84.6	76.0	54.5	310.3	281.4	207.2	109.1	126	306	167	55
45	90.9	86.4	76.8		318.2	317.0	218.9		77	176	95	

Table 34. Accumulative Experience and Rate: Marital Conception
For Ever-Married Females
By Educational Level

BY AGE	EVER-MARRIED FEMALES											
	Educational level 0-8 9-12 13-16 17+				Educational level 0-8 9-12 13-16 17+				Educational level 0-8 9-12 13-16 17+			
	Per cent of females with conception experience				*Conceptions per 100 females*				*Number of females*			
	0-8	9-12	13-16	17+	0-8	9-12	13-16	17+	0-8	9-12	13-16	17+
20		40.5	21.8	23.5		57.9	27.6	27.9		195	225	68
25	67.7	62.8	54.6	39.5	163.1	115.1	87.3	58.2	65	352	527	306
30	80.3	71.2	72.1	64.2	246.5	171.8	169.1	126.0	71	326	488	369
35	82.6	80.6	79.4	74.6	291.3	227.8	218.2	181.4	69	237	379	307
40	82.8	81.8	80.2	75.7	325.9	261.6	246.1	218.6	58	159	232	226
45	*82.9*	83.5	80.0	77.4	*363.4*	283.5	264.6	218.5	*41*	109	130	124

Table 35. Accumulative Experience and Rate: Marital Conception
For Ever-Married Females
By Decade of Birth

BY AGE	EVER-MARRIED FEMALES				
	Decade of birth				
	Before 1890	1890–1899	1900–1909	1910–1919	1920–1929
	Per cent of females with conception experience				
20		34.7	41.5	27.6	26.7
25	*66.7*	62.7	56.6	46.4	61.0
30	77.6	78.3	68.4	66.0	
35	79.7	82.5	76.8	76.5	
40	81.1	83.0	75.9		
45	81.8	82.6	73.3		
	Conceptions per 100 females				
20		40.8	53.4	38.0	36.6
25	*168.8*	110.1	90.7	74.5	116.1
30	234.3	197.4	147.8	145.2	
35	304.1	242.0	194.1	189.9	
40	331.1	265.9	214.0		
45	327.3	271.4	194.2		
	Number of females				
20		49	118	163	172
25	*48*	169	389	526	118
30	67	230	538	409	
35	74	257	542	119	
40	74	264	336		
45	77	241	86		

Table 36. Accumulative Experience and Rate: Marital Conception
For Ever-Married Females
By Religious Devoutness

BY AGE	EVER-MARRIED FEMALES			
	Religious devoutness			Jewish
	Protestant			
	Devout	Moderate	Inactive	Inactive
	Per cent of females with conception experience			
20	32.6	31.6	34.8	18.9
25	55.7	53.1	49.4	56.0
30	76.7	67.7	62.4	76.1
35	80.7	78.5	72.3	85.4
40	82.6	79.6	71.5	83.7
45	86.3	79.3	72.6	83.3
	Conceptions per 100 females			
20	40.4	46.3	50.4	20.8
25	99.6	92.6	88.6	86.2
30	177.1	155.6	136.2	171.6
35	227.3	213.2	185.5	233.8
40	259.9	240.8	212.4	270.2
45	273.5	269.0	221.7	286.4
	Number of females			
20	89	95	141	106
25	264	256	332	218
30	275	266	348	197
35	238	205	282	151
40	167	147	186	104
45	102	87	106	66

Table 37. **Accumulative Experience: Marital Conception**

For Ever-Married Females

By Age at Marriage and Decade of Birth

BY AGE	EVER-MARRIED FEMALES							
	Decade of birth				Decade of birth			
	1890–1899	1900–1909	1910–1919	1920–1929	1890–1899	1900–1909	1910–1919	1920–1929
	Age at Marriage 16–20							
	Per cent of females with conception experience				*Number of females*			
20	*34.7*	40.4	26.9	25.4	*49*	114	160	169
25	*83.7*	79.8	65.6	*82.6*	*49*	114	151	*46*
30	89.8	85.1	79.8		*49*	114	94	
35	*89.8*	90.5			*49*	105		
40	*89.8*	90.0			*49*	60		
45	*00.5*				*42*			
	Age at Marriage 21–25							
25	54.2	46.5	38.2	46.5	120	271	372	71
30	90.0	75.2	71.1		120	270	218	
35	91.7	80.5	85.9		120	256	64	
40	91.6	78.1			119	155		
45	90.3	*73.8*			103	*42*		
	Age at Marriage 26–35							
30	45.9	43.3	40.6		61	150	96	
35	65.9	63.5			88	178		
40	70.5	71.3			88	108		
45	74.1				85			

Table 38. Age-Specific Conception Rate: Marital Conception
For Ever-Married Females
By Marital Status at Interview

AGE-PERIOD	EVER-MARRIED FEMALES					
	Marital status at interview			Marital status at interview		
	Ever married	Married once, still married	Ever S.D.W.	Ever married	Married once, still married	Ever S.D.W.
	Conceptions per 100 marital years			*Number of marital years*		
16–20	22.2	15.8	27.7	1,012	467	545
21–25	23.7	22.4	26.3	4,296	2,822	1,474
26–30	24.3	25.0	22.5	5,051	3,636	1,415
31–35	15.7	15.9	15.3	4,040	3,043	997
36–40	7.7	7.8	7.7	2,736	2,098	638
41–45	2.1	2.1	2.1	1,543	1,166	377
46–50	0.2	0.2	*0.5*	822	633	*189*

Table 39. Age-Specific Conception Rate: Marital Conception
For Ever-Married Females
By Age at Marriage

AGE-PERIOD	EVER-MARRIED FEMALES							
	Age at marriage				Age at marriage			
	16–20	21–25	26–30	31–35	16–20	21–25	26–30	31–35
	Conceptions per 100 marital years				*Number of marital years*			
16–20	21.5				979			
21–25	29.3	20.7			1,520	2,759		
26–30	20.6	26.5	21.3		877	3,031	1,130	
31–35	7.6	14.1	21.5	17.1	526	2,006	1,217	286
36–40	4.7	5.5	9.3	14.9	319	1,281	778	281
41–45		0.8	2.2			727	405	

Table 40. Age-Specific Conception Rate: Marital Conception
For Ever-Married Females
By Educational Level

AGE-PERIOD	EVER-MARRIED FEMALES							
	Educational level				Educational level			
	0–8	9–12	13–16	17+	0–8	9–12	13–16	17+
	Conceptions per 100 marital years				*Number of marital years*			
16–20		28.5	14.8			410	405	
21–25	*34.7*	26.3	24.1	17.4	*225*	1,178	1,917	976
26–30	28.8	21.5	26.1	23.3	267	1,234	2,114	1,436
31–35	*15.1*	13.9	15.9	17.0	*225*	925	1,623	1,267
36–40		6.7	6.5	10.2		613	1,039	900
41–45		1.6	2.5	2.1		382	554	470

Table 41. Age-Specific Conception Rate: Marital Conception
For Ever-Married Females
By Decade of Birth

AGE-PERIOD	EVER-MARRIED FEMALES							
	Decade of birth				Decade of birth			
	1890–1899	1900–1909	1910–1919	1920–1929	1890–1899	1900–1909	1910–1919	1920–1929
	Conceptions per 100 marital years				*Number of marital years*			
16–20		*27.4*	20.3	20.0		*226*	301	350
21–25	29.9	22.4	19.8	25.4	549	1,221	1,639	731
26–30	29.5	20.6	24.3		891	1,973	1,841	
31–35	14.9	13.6	19.4		986	1,974	795	
36–40	7.2	7.8			962	1,419		
41–45	2.4	1.3			845	445		

Table 42. Age-Specific Conception Rate: Marital Conception
For Ever-Married Females
By Religious Devoutness

AGE-PERIOD	EVER-MARRIED FEMALES							
	Religious devoutness				Religious devoutness			
	Protestant			Jewish	Protestant			Jewish
	Devout	Moderate	Inactive	Inactive	Devout	Moderate	Inactive	Inactive
	Conceptions per 100 marital years				*Number of marital years*			
16–20		27.4				248		
21–25	26.5	24.0	22.7	22.4	978	859	1,055	821
26–30	24.7	23.1	22.0	25.3	1,186	1,081	1,273	826
31–35	17.0	15.7	16.1	14.0	994	875	1,051	600
36–40	8.6	7.0	10.0	3.6	706	586	718	387
41–45	2.3	2.1	1.7	*3.3*	426	341	351	*240*

Table 43. Accumulative Experience and Rate: Pregnancies Terminated in Marriage

For Ever–Married Females
By Marital Status at Interview

BY AGE	EVER-MARRIED FEMALES					
	Marital status at interview			Marital status at interview		
	Ever married	Married once, still married	Ever S.D.W.	Ever married	Married once, still married	Ever S.D.W.
	Live Birth					
	Per cent of females with experience			*Outcome per 100 females*		
20	23.7	22.0	25.1	27.2	24.6	29.2
25	43.8	45.8	41.0	60.9	63.6	57.3
30	60.8	66.8	53.2	105.2	119.7	86.8
35	70.2	76.6	62.7	138.9	157.3	117.5
40	72.1	77.4	67.0	156.6	173.5	139.8
45	73.8	80.1	68.6	165.6	180.7	153.4
	Spontaneous Abortion					
20	5.0	3.0	6.5	5.4	3.0	7.2
25	11.4	9.9	13.4	14.6	12.5	17.4
30	17.1	16.7	17.7	26.6	25.9	27.4
35	21.6	22.1	21.0	35.7	36.1	35.2
40	25.6	27.1	24.2	46.4	48.5	44.2
45	27.7	31.5	24.7	51.7	58.6	46.2
	Induced Abortion					
20	9.9	6.9	12.4	13.4	8.2	17.5
25	13.2	8.0	20.1	19.6	10.9	31.2
30	17.5	12.6	23.6	31.6	21.9	43.8
35	22.0	17.8	26.9	41.5	32.6	52.0
40	23.4	20.2	26.5	47.0	42.9	51.0
45	21.5	17.7	24.7	50.2	49.2	51.1
	Number of Females					
20	523	232	291	523	232	291
25	1,250	714	536	1,250	714	536
30	1,254	699	555	1,254	699	555
35	992	534	458	992	534	458
40	675	336	339	675	336	339
45	404	181	223	404	181	223

Table 44. Accumulative Experience and Rate: Pregnancies Terminated in Marriage

For Ever-Married Females

By Age at Marriage

BY AGE	EVER-MARRIED FEMALES							
	Age at marriage				Age at marriage			
	16–20	21–25	26–30	31–35	16–20	21–25	26–30	31–35
	Live Birth							
	Per cent of females with experience				*Outcome per 100 females*			
20	22.8				25.5			
25	62.6	35.3			102.4	42.3		
30	72.8	68.1	35.7		141.9	118.8	46.0	
35	77.2	77.9	62.0	31.7	165.8	161.6	107.4	37.8
40	78.6	79.1	68.3	45.5	177.8	180.4	138.9	72.7
45	75.3	83.5	70.5		177.9	196.6	149.5	
	Spontaneous Aportion							
20	5.1				5.5			
25	17.2	9.0			22.8	11.1		
30	21.9	17.9	11.9		38.4	27.3	15.6	
35	24.4	22.5	22.3	8.5	36.8	39.1	37.6	9.8
40	28.6	27.1	25.7	14.5	50.0	49.7	49.1	20.0
45	27.3	29.5	30.5		48.1	58.5	55.8	
	Induced Abortion							
20	9.7				13.3			
25	22.5	9.0			39.5	10.9		
30	28.0	18.2	7.0		60.2	30.8	8.5	
35	33.2	24.6	13.6	4.9	74.1	46.3	18.2	4.9
40	35.7	25.8	15.6	14.5	83.3	54.6	21.0	18.2
45	37.7	24.4	11.6		92.2	65.3	13.7	
	Number of Females							
20	513				513			
25	377	865			377	865		
30	279	642	328		279	642	328	
35	193	471	242	82	193	471	242	82
40	126	306	167	55	126	306	167	55
45	77	176	95		77	176	95	

Table 45. Accumulative Experience and Rate: Pregnancies Terminated in Marriage

For Ever-Married Females

By Educational Level

BY AGE	EVER-MARRIED FEMALES							
	Educational level				Educational level			
	0–8	9–12	13–16	17+	0–8	9–12	13–16	17+
	Live Birth							
	Per cent of females with experience				*Outcome per 100 females*			
20		33.8	14.2	8.8		39.5	15.1	8.8
25	64.6	54.3	43.5	27.8	118.5	78.7	56.4	35.9
30	74.6	62.0	63.7	53.1	160.6	107.1	112.3	83.5
35	76.8	71.7	70.7	66.8	188.4	143.9	140.9	121.5
40	77.6	73.0	72.8	69.5	201.7	161.0	153.4	145.1
45	80.5	75.2	73.1	71.0	202.4	179.8	160.0	146.8
	Spontaneous Abortion							
20		5.6	5.3	2.9		6.7	5.3	2.9
25	15.4	15.1	11.0	7.2	18.5	19.0	13.9	9.8
30	18.3	22.7	15.4	14.4	28.2	34.0	24.4	22.5
35	21.7	28.3	18.5	20.2	36.2	44.7	34.0	30.6
40	24.1	33.3	24.1	22.1	41.4	60.4	46.6	37.6
45	31.7	35.8	24.6	22.6	53.7	66.1	50.0	40.3
	Induced Abortion							
20		12.3	8.4	8.8		16.9	11.1	11.8
25	16.9	15.3	12.5	11.1	36.9	22.4	19.4	13.1
30	22.5	17.2	19.3	14.4	67.6	33.7	33.2	20.6
35	24.6	21.5	24.0	19.2	76.8	41.4	44.1	30.6
40	27.6	23.9	23.3	22.1	93.1	42.8	47.0	38.1
45	26.8	23.9	22.3	16.9	112.2	40.4	55.4	33.1
	Number of Females							
20		195	225	68		195	225	68
25	65	352	527	306	65	352	527	306
30	71	326	488	369	71	326	488	369
35	69	237	379	307	69	237	379	307
40	58	159	232	226	58	159	232	226
45	41	109	130	124	41	109	130	124

Table 46. Accumulative Experience and Rate: Pregnancies Terminated in Marriage

For Ever-Married Females

By Decade of Birth

BY AGE	EVER-MARRIED FEMALES									
	Decade of birth					Decade of birth			
	Before 1890	1890– 1899	1900– 1909	1910– 1919	1920– 1929	Before 1890	1890– 1899	1900– 1909	1910– 1919	1920– 1929
	Live Birth									
	Per cent of females with experience					*Outcome per 100 females*				
20		*28.6*	29.7	20.2	20.3		*30.6*	33.1	22.7	24.4
25	*54.2*	52.7	43.2	38.0	54.2	*91.7*	79.9	55.3	50.6	85.6
30	74.6	67.4	58.7	57.5		138.8	129.6	93.5	100.5	
35	77.0	74.7	67.3	68.9		186.5	160.7	124.9	126.1	
40	78.4	76.1	67.6			206.8	173.9	132.1		
45	77.9	75.9	64.0			203.9	173.9	108.1		
	Spontaneous Abortion									
20		*4.1*	6.8	3.7	5.8		*4.1*	8.5	3.7	5.8
25	*25.0*	13 0	9.8	9.5	17.8	*39.6*	16.6	11.6	12.0	22.9
30	29.9	23.5	13.9	14.9		55.2	35.2	20.1	24.2	
35	33.8	24.5	18.3	22.7		78.4	37.7	29.3	33.6	
40	35.1	26.9	22.3			83.8	43.9	39.6		
45	36.4	27.8	19.8			83.1	46.5	38.4		
	Induced Abortion									
20		*4.1*	12.7	11.0	8.1		*6.1*	13.6	16.6	11.1
25	*12.5*	12.4	18.5	10.3	10.2	*37.5*	17.8	26.2	14.8	14.4
30	11.9	17.0	22.1	12.5		40.3	35.7	36.1	22.3	
35	12.2	19.8	25.5	16.8		39.2	46.7	41.7	31.1	
40	13.5	20.5	27.7			40.5	51.5	44.6		
45	14.3	21.2	29.1			40.3	53.9	48.8		
	Number of Females									
20		*49*	118	163	172		*49*	118	163	172
25	*48*	169	389	526	118	*48*	169	389	526	118
30	67	230	538	409		67	230	538	409	
35	74	257	542	119		74	257	542	119	
40	74	264	336			74	264	336		
45	77	241	86			77	241	86		

Table 47. Accumulative Experience and Rate: Pregnancies Terminated in Marriage

For Ever-Married Females

By Religious Devoutness

BY AGE	EVER-MARRIED FEMALES							
	Religious devoutness				Religious devoutness			
	Protestant			Jewish	Protestant			Jewish
	Devout	Moderate	Inactive	Inactive	Devout	Moderate	Inactive	Inactive
	Live Birth							
	Per cent of females with experience				*Outcome per 100 females*			
20	30.3	29.5	23.4	7.5	34.8	32.6	24.8	8.5
25	49.6	44.1	35.5	44.0	72.7	63.7	49.7	56.0
30	69.5	59.0	51.4	64.0	130.2	104.9	81.0	105.6
35	73.1	71.2	63.5	72.2	156.7	146.3	112.4	142.4
40	74.9	73.5	64.5	76.9	179.6	164.0	125.8	164.4
45	79.4	74.7	64.2	74.2	194.1	182.8	125.5	163.6
	Spontaneous Abortion							
20	3.4	4.2	7.8	2.8	3.4	5.3	8.5	2.8
25	12.9	11.7	12.3	7.3	17.4	14.1	16.3	8.7
30	20.7	15.4	16.7	14.2	29.8	21.4	24.4	23.4
35	26.1	18.5	20.6	20.5	48.3	29.3	30.9	35.1
40	31.1	23.8	22.6	21.2	59.9	38.1	40.3	40.4
45	34.3	26.4	24.5	21.2	61.8	47.1	43.4	42.4
	Induced Abortion							
20	3.4	9.5	15.6	9.4	4.5	15.8	20.6	11.3
25	8.3	12.9	16.3	17.4	11.7	19.5	26.2	23.4
30	12.0	16.2	18.4	26.4	18.2	32.7	32.8	43.7
35	14.3	17.1	24.8	35.8	23.1	41.0	44.3	57.0
40	15.0	17.0	27.4	36.5	21.6	42.9	48.9	66.4
45	12.7	12.6	29.2	39.4	18.6	41.4	55.7	81.8
	Number of Females							
20	89	95	141	106	89	95	141	106
25	264	256	332	218	264	256	332	218
30	275	266	348	197	275	266	348	197
35	238	205	282	151	238	205	282	151
40	167	147	186	104	167	147	186	104
45	102	87	106	66	102	87	106	66

Table 48. Age-Specific Rate: Pregnancies Terminated in Marriage
For Ever-Married Females

By Marital Status at Interview

By Age at Marriage

AGE-PERIOD	EVER-MARRIED FEMALES						
	Marital status at interview			Age at marriage			
	Ever married	Married once, still married	Ever S.D.W.	16–20	21–25	26–30	31–35
	Live Birth						
	Outcome per 100 marital years						
16–20	14.2	13.1	15.2	13.6			
21–25	15.7	16.1	15.0	19.3	13.7		
26–30	16.1	17.3	13.1	12.9	18.0	13.8	
31–35	11.0	11.3	9.9	4.9	10.2	14.5	11.9
36–40	5.1	5.0	5.6	2.5	3.6	7.2	7.8
41–45	0.9	0.8	1.3		4.1	0.7	
	Spontaneous Abortion						
16–20	2.8	1.5	3.9	2.8			
21–25	3.7	3.4	4.2	3.6	3.7		
26–30	4.0	4.0	4.0	3.6	3.8	5.0	
31–35	2.9	2.7	3.3	1.1	2.2	4.6	3.1
36–40	1.6	1.8	1.1	0.9	0.9	1.8	3.9
41–45	0.7	0.9	0.3		1.4	0.7	
	Induced Abortion						
16–20	6.6	4.1	8.8	6.6			
21–25	4.4	2.8	7.6	5.9	3.7		
26–30	3.5	3.0	4.9	3.4	3.9	2.7	
31–35	1.7	1.5	2.0	1.3	1.6	1.8	1.4
36–40	0.8	0.8	1.1	1.3	1.0	0	2.1
41–45	0.4	0.3	0.5		2.8	0.5	
	Number of Marital Years						
16–20	1,012	467	545	979			
21–25	4,296	2,822	1,474	1,520	2,759		
26–30	5,051	3,636	1,415	877	3,031	1,130	
31–35	4,040	3,043	997	526	2,006	1,217	286
36–40	2,736	2,098	638	319	1,281	778	281
41–45	1,543	1,166	377		727	405	

Table 49. Age-Specific Rate: Pregnancies Terminated in Marriage
For Ever-Married Females

By Educational Level

By Decade of Birth

AGE-PERIOD	EVER-MARRIED FEMALES								
	Educational level				Decade of birth				
	0–8	9–12	13–16	17+	Before 1890	1890–1899	1900–1909	1910–1919	1920–1929
	Live Birth								
	Outcome per 100 marital years								
16–20		19.3	8.1				16.8	12.3	13.1
21–25	23.6	18.0	15.8	10.9		21.9	13.9	13.8	16.4
26–30	17.6	13.3	17.7	16.0	18.5	18.1	13.7	17.2	
31–35	11.6	9.8	10.7	12.0	15.3	10.4	9.4	13.8	
36–40		4.4	3.8	7.3	5.3	4.6	5.2		
41–45		0.5	1.1	1.1	1.2	1.3	0		
	Spontaneous Abortion								
16–20		3.4	2.7				3.5	2.0	3.7
21–25	4.9	4.5	3.4	2.9		4.7	2.6	3.1	4.1
26–30	3.0	4.3	3.6	4.5	6.3	5.9	2.9	3.6	
31–35	1.3	2.9	3.0	3.0	7.5	1.5	2.6	3.6	
36–40		1.3	1.8	1.8	1.5	1.7	1.4		
41–45		0.8	0.4	1.1	0.8	0.7	0.9		
	Induced Abortion								
16–20		7.3	6.2				7.1	8.3	5.1
21–25	8.4	4.2	4.4	3.9		4.6	6.3	3.1	2.9
26–30	8.6	3.2	3.7	2.7	3.5	5.5	4.0	2.3	
31–35	2.2	1.2	1.7	1.8	0.7	3.0	1.6	0.5	
36–40		1.0	0.8	0.7	0.4	1.0	0.8		
41–45		0.3	0.9	0	0.4	0.4	0.4		
	Number of Marital Years								
16–20		410	405				226	301	350
21–25	225	1,178	1,917	976		549	1,221	1,639	731
26–30	267	1,234	2,114	1,436	254	891	1,973	1,841	
31–35	225	925	1,623	1,267	281	986	1,974	795	
36–40		613	1,039	900	266	962	1,419		
41–45		382	554	470	252	845	445		

Table 50. Age-Specific Rate: Pregnancies Terminated in Marriage

For Ever-Married Females

By Religious Devoutness

AGE-PERIOD	EVER-MARRIED FEMALES			
	Religious devoutness			Jewish Inactive
	Protestant			
	Devout	Moderate	Inactive	
	Live Birth			
	Outcome per 100 marital years			
16–20			*12.9*	
21–25	18.5	16.6	12.7	14.7
26–30	18.7	15.6	14.1	15.6
31–35	11.8	11.3	10.9	9.3
36–40	5.9	5.3	6.1	2.6
41–45	1.4	0.9	1.1	*0.4*
	Spontaneous Abortion			
16–20			*4.4*	
21–25	5.1	3.8	3.6	1.8
26–30	3.7	3.4	3.9	4.1
31–35	4.3	1.9	2.9	2.3
36–40	2.4	0.7	2.2	0
41–45	0.9	0.3	0.3	*2.1*
	Induced Abortion			
16–20			*11.3*	
21–25	2.8	3.8	6.4	5.7
26–30	1.6	3.5	3.2	4.8
31–35	0.5	2.1	2.1	2.3
36–40	0.3	1.0	1.0	1.0
41–45	0	0.6	0.3	*0.8*
	Number of Marital Years			
16–20			*248*	
21–25	978	859	1,055	821
26–30	1,186	1,081	1,273	826
31–35	994	875	1,051	600
36–40	706	586	718	387
41–45	426	341	351	*240*

Table 51. Outcome Ratio

For Pregnancies Terminated in Marriage by Females
Aged 36 and Older at Interview and Married by
Age 30

By Number of Pregnancies and Marital Status at
Interview

NUMBER OF PREGNANCIES TERMINATED IN MARRIAGE	NUMBER OF FEMALES	PREGNANCIES TERMINATED IN MARRIAGE			
		Type of marital outcome			Total terminated pregnancies
		Live birth	Spontaneous abortion	Induced abortion	
		Ever Married			
		Per cent			*Number*
0	151				
1	137	65.0	16.1	19.0	137
2	222	83.1	7.0	9.9	444
3	162	70.0	14.0	16.0	486
4	119	64.9	19.5	15.5	476
5	55	58.5	22.5	18.9	275
6+	64	42.7	22.9	34.4	520
		Married Once, Still Married			
0	57				
1	63	74.6	12.7	12.7	63
2	130	91.9	4.6	3.5	260
3	95	76.1	11.9	11.9	285
4–5	106	66.1	20.7	13.3	460
6+	28	41.5	27.4	31.2	234
		Ever Separated, Divorced, Widowed			
0	94				
1	74	56.8	18.9	24.3	74
2	92	70.7	10.3	19.0	184
3	67	61.2	16.9	21.9	201
4–5	68	57.0	20.6	22.3	291
6+	36	43.7	19.2	37.1	286

Table 52. Age-Specific Outcome Ratio

      For Pregnancies Terminated in Marriage

      By Marital Status at Interview

MARITAL STATUS AT INTERVIEW	AGE-PERIOD	PREGNANCIES TERMINATED IN MARRIAGE			
		Type of marital outcome			Total terminated pregnancies
		Live birth	Spontaneous abortion	Induced abortion	
		Per cent			*Number*
Ever married	All ages	65.7	17.3	17.0	3,645
	16–20	59.6	12.0	28.4	250
	21–25	64.8	15.8	19.4	1,079
	26–30	67.0	17.4	15.6	1,289
	31–35	69.3	18.3	12.4	720
	36–40	63.5	22.9	13.6	258
	41–50	*36.9*	*28.3*	*34.8*	*46*
Married once, still married	All ages	71.0	16.8	12.2	2,254
	16–20	70.2	8.0	21.8	87
	21–25	72.2	15.2	12.6	627
	26–30	71.3	16.4	12.3	884
	31–35	72.6	17.5	9.9	474
	36–40	66.2	23.6	10.2	157
Ever separated, divorced, widowed	All ages	57.0	18.1	24.9	1,391
	16–20	54.0	14.1	31.9	163
	21–25	54.6	16.6	28.8	452
	26–30	57.5	19.8	22.7	405
	31–35	63.0	19.9	17.1	246
	36–40	59.4	21.8	18.8	101

Table 53. Age-Specific Outcome Ratio
For Pregnancies Terminated in Marriage
By Age at Marriage

| AGE AT MARRIAGE | AGE-PERIOD | PREGNANCIES TERMINATED IN MARRIAGE | | | |
| | | Type of marital outcome | | | Total terminated pregnancies |
		Live birth	Spontaneous abortion	Induced abortion	
		Per cent			*Number*
16–20	All ages	61.1	15.6	23.3	1,078
	16–20	58.5	12.3	29.2	236
	21–25	65.1	13.3	21.6	487
	26–30	59.1	21.1	19.8	242
	31–35	60.5	14.5	25.0	76
21–25	All ages	67.8	16.0	16.2	1,841
	21–25	64.4	17.9	17.7	588
	26–30	70.2	14.7	15.1	802
	31–35	71.7	15.5	12.8	335
	36–40	62.3	17.3	20.4	98
26–30	All ages	67.3	23.0	9.7	588
	26–30	64.2	23.0	12.8	243
	31–35	68.4	23.1	8.5	260
	36–40	77.6	21.1	1.3	76
31–35	All ages	62.8	26.6	10.6	94

Table 54. Age-Specific Outcome Ratio
For Pregnancies Terminated in Marriage
By Educational Level

EDUCATIONAL LEVEL	AGE-PERIOD	PREGNANCIES TERMINATED IN MARRIAGE			
		Type of marital outcome			Total terminated pregnancies
		Live birth	Spontaneous abortion	Induced abortion	
		Per cent			*Number*
0-8	All ages	65.9	12.0	22.1	258
	21-25	63.6	12.9	23.5	85
	26-30	59.1	12.0	28.9	83
9-12	All ages	64.4	19.3	16.3	1,002
	16-20	63.3	11.5	25.2	131
	21-25	66.7	17.1	16.2	345
	26-30	61.9	22.1	16.0	294
	31-35	68.1	20.9	11.0	163
	36-40	63.1	24.6	12.3	57
13-16	All ages	65.8	16.5	17.7	1,481
	16-20	47.2	16.7	36.1	72
	21-25	65.3	15.2	19.5	473
	26-30	69.4	15.1	15.5	563
	31-35	69.1	18.5	12.4	275
	36-40	54.5	27.8	17.7	79
17+	All ages	66.7	17.9	15.4	904
	21-25	60.8	15.9	23.3	176
	26-30	69.1	18.6	12.3	349
	31-35	69.4	17.4	13.2	242
	36-40	71.0	18.7	10.3	107

139

Table 55. Age-Specific Outcome Ratio

For Pregnancies Terminated in Marriage

By Decade of Birth

DECADE OF BIRTH	AGE-PERIOD	PREGNANCIES TERMINATED IN MARRIAGE			
		Type of marital outcome			Total terminated pregnancies
		Live birth	Spontaneous abortion	Induced abortion	
		Per cent			*Number*
Before 1890	All ages	61.6	26.4	12.0	242
	21–25	51.5	27.1	21.4	70
	26–30	64.5	23.7	11.8	76
	31–35	66.2	30.9	2.9	68
1890–1899	All ages	64.0	16.8	19.2	740
	21–25	69.4	15.0	15.6	173
	26–30	60.8	19.8	19.4	268
	31–35	68.0	9.5	22.5	169
	36–40	58.8	22.4	18.8	85
1900–1909	All ages	63.4	16.2	20.4	1,265
	16–20	60.3	14.3	25.4	63
	21–25	59.2	11.8	29.0	297
	26–30	64.7	14.6	20.7	445
	31–35	67.7	19.7	12.6	309
	36–40	64.7	22.8	12.5	136
1910–1919	All ages	69.8	17.1	13.1	1,078
	16–20	52.8	8.6	38.6	70
	21–25	67.5	16.7	15.8	348
	26–30	72.6	17.2	10.2	470
	31–35	74.5	19.7	5.8	173
1920–1929	All ages	68.3	17.5	14.2	302
	16–20	60.2	15.7	24.1	83
	21–25	70.6	17.1	12.3	187

140

Table 56. Age-Specific Outcome Ratio

For Pregnancies Terminated in Marriage

By Religious Devoutness

RELIGIOUS DEVOUTNESS	AGE-PERIOD	PREGNANCIES TERMINATED IN MARRIAGE			
		Type of marital outcome			Total terminated pregnancies
		Live birth	Spontaneous abortion	Induced abortion	
		Per cent			*Number*
Protestant devout	All ages	72.0	20.2	7.8	872
	21–25	69.8	19.6	10.6	265
	26–30	76.4	15.5	8.1	296
	31–35	68.8	26.4	4.8	189
	36–40	66.6	29.2	4.2	72
Protestant moderate	All ages	68.7	14.0	17.3	729
	16–20	61.1	11.1	27.8	54
	21–25	66.8	15.2	18.0	217
	26–30	68.9	14.6	16.5	261
	31–35	73.2	12.7	14.1	142
	36–40	*72.9*	*12.5*	*14.6*	*48*
Protestant inactive	All ages	60.2	18.6	21.2	936
	16–20	45.4	15.6	39.0	77
	21–25	55.3	17.4	27.3	264
	26–30	64.6	19.3	16.1	305
	31–35	67.2	18.2	14.6	198
	36–40	62.0	22.8	15.2	79
Jewish inactive	All ages	61.3	14.7	24.0	587
	21–25	64.3	8.8	26.9	193
	26–30	63.7	16.3	20.0	215
	31–35	65.1	17.9	17.0	112

Table 57. Marital Status Comparisons: Percentages of Conceptions and Types of Outcome

For White Non-Prison Females Aged 36 and Older at Interview

By Educational Level

WHITE NON-PRISON FEMALES AGED 36 AND OLDER AT INTERVIEW

Marital status at event	Conception	Type of outcome			Total terminated pregnancies
		Live birth	Spontaneous abortion	Induced abortion	
Total Females					
	Per cent		*Per cent*		*Per cent*
Single	7.3	0.4	2.0	22.6	6.5
Married	89.1	99.3	96.0	65.4	89.9
Previously married	3.6	0.3	2.0	12.0	3.6
Total	100.0($N=2729$)	100.0($N=1571$)	100.0($N=444$)	100.0($N=708$)	100.0($N=2723$)
Educational Level 0–8					
Single	6.2	1.4	*0*	9.0	3.3
Married	91.3	97.9	*96.7*	85.0	94.2
Previously married	2.5	0.7	*3.3*	6.0	2.5
Total	100.0($N=241$)	100.0($N=144$)	100.0($N=30$)	100.0($N=67$)	100.0($N=241$)
Educational Level 9–12					
Single	6.1	0.5	1.6	20.7	5.3
Married	91.6	99.2	96.8	71.3	92.4
Previously married	2.3	0.3	1.6	8.0	2.3
Total	100.0($N=661$)	100.0($N=382$)	100.0($N=129$)	100.0($N=150$)	100.0($N=661$)
Educational Level 13–16					
Single	6.1	0.5	0.6	19.3	5.7
Married	90.2	99.3	98.1	67.8	90.5
Previously married	3.7	0.2	1.3	12.9	3.8
Total	100.0($N=1027$)	100.0($N=589$)	100.0($N=156$)	100.0($N=280$)	100.0($N=1025$)
Educational Level 17+					
Single	10.1	0	4.7	32.7	9.4
Married	85.1	99.6	92.2	51.7	85.7
Previously married	4.8	0.4	3.1	15.6	4.9
Total	100 0($N=800$)	100.0($N=456$)	100.0($N=129$)	100.0($N=211$)	100.0($N=796$)

Chapter 5

THE PREVIOUSLY MARRIED WOMAN

Despite the fact that the proportion of women who have been separated, divorced, or widowed has risen greatly in the twentieth century, virtually nothing has been known of their reproductive behavior during the time following the end of marriage and before remarriage. Much of this lack of knowledge is due to a reluctance to face what many would consider an insolvable moral problem. One can find hundreds of articles in newspapers and magazines and hundreds of chapters in marriage manuals directed at the woman who has yet to marry, but one has to search diligently to find discussions of the sexual problems of the previously married woman. In this respect, our brief chapter should be a needed contribution.

A considerable body of folklore pertaining to sex surrounds women who are separated from their husbands, divorced, or widowed (S.D.W.). The folklore is not without some foundation in fact. A woman who has known in marriage the satisfactions of coitus is not apt to abandon coitus when her marriage ceases to exist. In our previous study (1953:559) we found that in any five-year age-period before age fifty, some 47 to 72 per cent of the previously married women had coitus. In this present study we applied an educational level breakdown to the S.D.W. females and found that approximately three quarters of the high school educated, college educated, and postgraduate women at some time had postmarital coitus (76 per cent, 73 per cent, and 72 per cent, respectively). In brief, the continuation of coitus after the end of marriage is the rule rather than the exception.[1]

Our 754 white non-prison S.D.W. females had contracted 1,179 marriages (including their first marriages). Eighty of these were common-law marriages, entered into by 59 women, most of whom were high school educated, though some were college educated, and a few were grade school educated or postgraduates.

In the present sample 573 women had been separated or divorced,

---

[1] Terman 1938:418-419 found that a high proportion of divorced women who remarried had post-marital coitus, "Roughly four out of five of the divorced wives had premarital intercourse with the present spouse, and about four out of ten with others." Terman's sample, like ours, was predominantly (76 per cent) of females with college or postgraduate education.

but never widowed; 148 women had been widowed, but never separated or divorced; and 33 women had experienced separation or divorce as well as widowhood. Widows were naturally more numerous among women of forty or more: among women aged forty-six and over, 38 per cent had been widowed but never separated or divorced.

We found that 56 per cent of the S.D.W. women had had only one legal marriage, 33 per cent had had two legal marriages, 3 per cent had had three or more legal marriages, and 8 per cent had had common-law marriages or a combination of legal and common-law marriages. In connection with this, it is interesting that slightly over half (55 per cent) of our sample of S.D.W. women had remarried[2] prior to interview.

The median S.D.W. female married at age 21.8, whereas the female who married once and was still married at interview married at age 23.4. The S.D.W. women of lesser education married at younger ages than did those with more education: the median grade school educated female married at 19.9, the high school educated at 20.7, the college educated at 21.6, and the postgraduates at 23.6 years of age.

The median S.D.W. female's first marriage ended when she was 28.3 years old, the average duration of the marriage being 6.5 years. The average first marriage of the grade school educated lasted almost ten years, of the high school and college educated slightly over six years, and of the postgraduates about seven years.

PREGNANCY

Experience. Of our 754 S.D.W. women, 549 (nearly three quarters) had post-marital coitus; of these, 105 became pregnant in the post-marital period. Thus some 14 per cent of our total sample and 19 per cent of the sample of those with post-marital coitus conceived (Table 58). When we compare these figures with the pre-marital picture, it is evident that whatever knowledge of contraception these S.D.W. women obtained while married was to a considerable degree offset by their greater (as compared to pre-marital) frequency of coitus. Some of the women attributed their pregnancies to carelessness; it is not uncommon for wives occasionally to "take a chance" when contraceptives are not readily available, and this attitude seems to have carried over into the post-marital lives of some of them.

Examining the percentage of women who conceived as a result of post-marital coitus, we found that educational attainment was no

[2] Bernard 1956:51 notes that remarriage is commoner at younger ages and is becoming more so.

factor: the percentages ranged from 17 to 21 per cent for the different educational groups, a meaningless difference in view of the lack of trend and the relatively small number of women involved.

Table 58. Accumulative Experience and Rate: Post-Marital Conception

For Total Post-Marital Females and Post-Marital Females with Coitus

By Educational Level

TOTAL POST-MARITAL FEMALES					FEMALES WITH POST-MARITAL COITUS				
	Educational level					Educational level			
Total	0–8	9–12	13–16	17+	Total	0–8	9–12	13–16	17+
Per cent of females with conception experience									
13.9	10.0	16.1	12.3	14.7	19.1	*17.9*	21.1	16.7	20.3
Conceptions per 100 females									
21.2	12.0	20.3	20.6	25.7	29.1	*21.4*	26.7	28.1	35.5
Per cent with coitus					*Years of coitus per 100 females*				
72.8	56.0	76.3	73.3	72.3	474	*639*	454	426	536
Number of females									
754	50	236	277	191	549	*28*	180	203	138

Table 59. Age-Specific Frequency Per Week: Post-Marital Coitus

For Females with Post-Marital Coitus

By Experience in Post-Marital Conception

AGE-PERIOD	FEMALES WITH POST-MARITAL COITUS					
	Females without post-marital conception			Females with post-marital conception		
	Mean frequency per week	Median frequency per week	Number of females	Mean frequency per week	Median frequency per week	Number of females
21–25	1.4	0.8	122	*1.6*	*1.0*	*43*
26–30	1.2	0.5	168	*1.8*	*0.8*	*57*
31–35	1.1	0.4	158	*1.8*	*1.3*	*62*
36–40	1.2	0.5	125	*1.6*	*1.0*	*41*
41–45	0.9	0.4	89	*1.1*	*0.7*	*27*

As one might anticipate, the women who conceived as a result of post-marital coitus proved to have had coitus with greater frequency than the women who had coitus but did not conceive.

Rate. Table 58 indicates that of the total sample of S.D.W.'s there were 21 post-marital conceptions for every hundred females. Among only those with post-marital coitus there were 29 conceptions for every one hundred females.

The 105 women who became pregnant were responsible for 160 pregnancies. Some 73 per cent conceived once, 17 per cent twice, 4 per cent thrice, 2 per cent four times, 3 per cent five times, and one woman provided an astonishing record of 12 post-marital conceptions. One will recall that 81 per cent of those who conceived in pre-marital coitus did so but once (Chapter 3). Excluding most menopausal and post-menopausal women by confining our attention to women under forty-six, we calculate that the S.D.W. women who had post-marital coitus had a post-marital conception rate of 6.2 per hundred coital years. It would be interesting to compare this rate with an equivalent measurement for single women. However, we have no over-all rate calculated for single women under forty-six; consequently a less direct comparison must be made. Since we know that the median S.D.W. woman's first marriage ended when she was twenty-eight, we may compare her post-marital conception rate with the pre-marital age-specific conception rate of single women aged twenty-six to thirty, which is 5.7 per hundred coital years (Table 20). For single women aged thirty-one to thirty-five this rate is much lower, about 3 per hundred coital years. The differences between the pre-marital and post-marital rates derive from the greater frequency of coitus of the post-marital group. The pre-marital group had coitus on an average (median) of once every three weeks between ages twenty and forty-five, and less often before twenty; the post-marital group have an average (median) of from once in two weeks to nearly once per week (1953:334, 559).

Dividing the total S.D.W. sample according to educational achievement, we find that the high school educated had 20 post-marital conceptions per hundred women, the college educated 21, and the postgraduates 26 (Table 58). The grade school educated women of the sample had many fewer conceptions since a substantially smaller proportion had post-marital coitus. However, it must be stated that this sample of grade school educated is not only small but suffers from a serious bias, which is discussed in Chapter 7.

Among the S.D.W. women who had post-marital coitus, the grade school educated had a conception rate of 21 for every one hundred women, the high school educated 27, the college educated 28, and the postgraduates 36. The high post-marital conception rate among postgraduate women is also evident in the fact that 43 per cent became pregnant twice or more as against 18 per cent of the high school educated and 23 per cent of the college educated.

This discovery was contrary to any expectation: why should the best educated be so conception prone? The answer is simply that the postgraduates were exposed to the possibility of a post-marital conception for a longer period than were the less educated. The median postgraduate was aged 42.2 at reporting, whereas the median high school educated woman was 37.1, and the median college educated woman was 37.8 years old. The postgraduates averaged (mean) 11.4 years of post-marital life before age forty-five, of which 9.8 years had involved post-marital coitus. The college educated had 7.9 years, of which 7.1 were with coitus, and the high school educated had 6.5 post-marital years, of which 6.1 were with coitus.

In addition, there is evidence that the postgraduate women who conceived had post-marital coitus with greater frequency than did the lesser educated. For example, in Table 59 we saw that all the S.D.W. women with post-marital pregnancies had an average (mean) frequency of coitus, from ages twenty-one to forty, of between 1.6 and 1.8 per week. The postgraduate S.D.W. women who conceived had coital frequencies of 1.6 to 2.7 during the same age span.

OUTCOME OF PREGNANCY

While our sample contains 160 post-marital conceptions, only 157 of these had ended at the time of reporting. We excluded an additional 22 pregnancies that ended in post-marital life but that were conceived in marriage (20) or before marriage (2). It is interesting to note that of these 22 pregnancies 14 ended in birth, 6 in induced abortion, and 2 in spontaneous abortion.

Outcome ratio. Of the 157 terminated post-marital conceptions, 4 per cent resulted in live birth, 10 per cent in spontaneous abortion, 79 per cent in induced abortion, and 7 per cent were carried into a subsequent marriage. Comparing these figures with those relating to pre-marital outcome ratios (Table 60), we see that the proportions of live birth and induced abortion are about the same, but that the S.D.W. women, being generally older, are more prone to abort spontaneously—about twice as often as the single women. Likewise, the number of women who marry to escape their predicament is smaller among the S.D.W. than among the single, 7 per cent versus 15 per cent, and this, too, is partly a function of increased age.

As far as education is concerned, one finds that the proportion of pregnancies ended by induced abortion is least among the women who did not go to college. A larger proportion of their conceptions end in live birth, spontaneous abortion, and in subsequent marriage (Table

60). The post-marital ratios for the college educated and postgraduates are very similar to their pre-marital ratios, aside from the proportion of pregnancies carried into marriage. Among those of less than college education, there is less similarity between the post-marital and pre-marital ratios.

Table 60. Outcome Ratio

For Pre-Marital and Post-Marital Conceptions

By Educational Level

MARITAL STATUS AT CONCEPTION AND EDUCATIONAL LEVEL	PRE-MARITAL AND POST-MARITAL CONCEPTIONS				
	Type of outcome			Outcome in marriage	Total terminated pregnancies
	Live birth	Spontaneous abortion	Induced abortion		
	Per cent			*Per cent*	*Number*
All educational levels					
Pre-marital	4.8	4.5	75.8	14.9	417
Post-marital	3.8	10.2	79.0	7.0	157
Educational level 9–12					
Pre-marital	10.1	3.7	63.3	22.9	109
Post-marital	6.7	17.8	64.4	11.1	45
Educational level 13–16					
Pre-marital	2.4	4.3	81.7	11.6	164
Post-marital	3.5	5.3	85.9	5.3	57
Educational level 17+					
Pre-marital	1.6	6.2	82.9	9.3	129
Post-marital	0	8.2	85.7	6.1	49

It is also evident that the degree of education is related to reproductive behavior not only before marriage and in marriage, but also after the end of marriage.

The previously married woman is in many respects in a more awkward situation than the never-married girl. She has become accustomed to coitus and has shed many of her inhibitions; she finds it much more difficult to abstain from coitus than does the less experienced girl. Tradition labels her as being sexually acceptant, if not actually aggressive, and males react accordingly. One might say that a male hopes to have coitus with a never-married girl, but expects to have coitus with a divorcée or widow.

As a natural sequel to this situation, the previously married woman has a higher frequency of coitus than the never-married woman, but—despite her presumably better knowledge of sexuality and contraception—about the same incidence of pregnancy.

Unfortunately society makes no special provisions for the divorcée or widow who becomes pregnant. Moreover, she has, compared with the never-married woman, less opportunity and possibly less desire to solve the problem through marriage. In consequence social pressure forces her to the abortionist as inexorably as it forces the single girl.

Table 61. Accumulative Rate: Pre-Marital Conception

For Females with Pre-Marital Coitus

By Educational Level and Marital Status at Interview

BY AGE	FEMALES WITH PRE-MARITAL COITUS					
	Educational level 9–12		Educational level 13–16		Educational level 17+	
	Married once, still married	Ever S.D.W.	Married once, still married	Ever S.D.W.	Married once, still married	Ever S.D.W.
	Conceptions per 100 coital years					
20	8.3	12.5	6.5	10.5	3.9	9.7
25	9.6	10.8	6.8	9.1	5.7	7.7
30	9.3	10.5	6.8	9.3	6.9	9.6
	Number of coital years					
20	230	208	431	209	230	103
25	418	325	806	383	557	209
30	485	373	943	450	737	271

CHARACTERISTICS OF THE S.D.W. WOMAN

It is of considerable interest to ascertain if and how women who have been separated, divorced, or widowed differ from women who are still married to their first husbands, and to see if anything in premarital or marital life foreshadows the subsequent marital dissolution. It should be noted that the majority of our sample of S.D.W. women consists of the separated and divorced: those who were widowed but never separated or divorced comprise 20 per cent of the sample.

Since our S.D.W. sample differs from our married-once, still married sample in having a larger proportion of high school educated (31 versus 21 per cent) and fewer college educated (though about the same proportion of postgraduates), an educational level breakdown has always been made.

In pre-marital life we find that the S.D.W. women, in comparison to the married once, had higher rates of pre-marital conception during their teens and, to a lesser extent, during their twenties.[3] This is indicated in Table 61. Within marriage also, especially at younger ages,

[3] Christensen and Meissner 1953:643 in a study of pre-marital pregnancy as a factor in divorce state, "Premarital pregnancy has been found to be associated with disproportionately high divorce rates."

the women who were later separated or divorced apparently had higher marital conception rates than did the married once.

On the basis of Tables 61 and 62 one can conjecture that the factors that resulted in the S.D.W. females' having relatively high conception rates in early life, both before and in marriage, were also operative in post-marital life.

Table 62. Age-Specific Rate: Marital Conception

For Ever-Married Females

By Educational Level and Marital Status at Interview

AGE-PERIOD	EVER-MARRIED FEMALES					
	Educational level 9–12		Educational level 13–16		Educational level 17+	
	Married once, still married	Ever S.D.W.*	Married once, still married	Ever S.D.W.*	Married once, still married	Ever S.D.W.*
	Conceptions per 100 marital years					
16–20	*22.7*	*33.2*	*9.6*	*21.0*		
21–25	24.6	29.4	23.3	26.0	15.2	21.3
26–30	21.7	20.9	26.1	25.8	25.2	18.6
31–35	12.8	16.6	15.9	15.8	18.1	13.5
36–40	5.6	*9.0*	6.5	*6.8*	10.7	*8.3*
	Number of marital years					
16–20	*181*	*229*	*219*	*186*		
21–25	749	429	1,348	569	624	352
26–30	842	392	1,618	496	1,023	413
31–35	642	283	1,294	329	955	312
36–40	425	*188*	820	*219*	720	*180*

* For first marriages only.

One gains thus far the impression that as a group these S.D.W. women were sexually active and consequently, particularly at younger ages, rather conception prone. This impression, reinforced by our knowledge that a large proportion of them had post-marital coitus and rather high post-marital conception rates, made us suspect that within the S.D.W. sample there existed a group of women who might prove distinctive in their sexual and reproductive behavior. Since we have demonstrated that the women who conceived post-maritally had coitus with greater frequency than those who had coitus but did not conceive, we selected the former for more intensive study.

The 105 women who conceived as a result of post-marital coitus constitute a distinct group in other respects as well. Only three of them were widowed. Their pre-marital sexual life had been different from that of the average woman. Roughly half our total sample of ever-married women had had pre-marital coitus, but for our post-maritally pregnant group the proportion was higher: of the high school educated, 71 per cent; of the college educated, 62 per cent; and of the postgraduates, an astonishing 82 per cent. Consequently a high per cent (20) had also become pregnant before marriage.

These women also were more experienced in induced abortion. Whereas about 8 per cent of our ever-married women had had an induced abortion before marriage, and roughly one fifth during marriage, 40 per cent of the post-maritally pregnant group of high school education had had an induced abortion in or before marriage, 65 per cent of the college educated, and 46 per cent of the postgraduate.

Occupationally these women were exceptional. We devised an occupational category consisting of professional employment (e.g., physicians, psychologists, college teachers, artists, and so forth) and employment of a managerial or at least highly responsible nature (e.g., store manager, advertisement director, editorial worker, and buyer). Of our sample of post-maritally pregnant women, 34 per cent of the high school educated fell within this occupational category, 65 per cent of the college educated, and 86 per cent of the postgraduates, these percentages being larger than those given by census.[4]

In terms of personality these women were also exceptional. On each of our case histories the interviewer has made brief notes giving his impression of the subject's personality. Examining these notes, we found that between 47 and 58 per cent (varying with educational level) of the post-maritally pregnant women were described as assured, independent, aggressive, or in some way suggesting a high level of energy.

Their dynamism accounts for the fact that many of them went into business and professional occupations where, necessarily, they often faced male competition. Their particular qualities made them, even before marriage, rather independent of social mores. If they felt inclined toward coitus they had it, in or out of marriage. One also senses that these women would not be very tolerant of a husband's defects or play a submissive role, attitudes that may have played a part in the separation or divorce.

We suspect that in a more dilute fashion these same characteristics

---

[4] The 1950 U.S. Census provides data showing that of employed females of college education, 49 per cent may be classed as "professional, technical, and kindred workers" and about 5 per cent as "managers, officials, and proprietors" (excluding farm). This gives a total of 54 per cent for both groups which, when combined, are roughly equivalent to the occupational category we employ here. See U.S. Census, 1950, Special Reports, *Occupational Characteristics*, 1956:108-115, Table 10.

could be found among many of the women who had post-marital coitus but did not conceive: the characteristics enumerated do not, after all, guarantee a post-marital conception.

While obviously only a portion of the separated or divorced women are similar to those just described, that portion is sufficiently large to justify the apprehension that the average woman feels about the divorcée as a sexual competitor.

Chapter 6

THE NEGRO WOMAN

Our Negro sample is not large and consequently inferences drawn from analyses of it should be regarded with appropriate caution. However, the fact that our findings agree in general with vital statistics and with other studies makes us feel that they are valid insofar as trends are concerned and reasonably valid in terms of percentages and rates.

Our sample of Negro non-prison females consists of 572 individuals. Like the white sample, it is predominantly made up of young, urban women of above average education. Ninety-one per cent were urban as adults; 53 per cent were aged twenty-five or younger; and the median female had a twelfth grade education. Examining educational level in more detail, we find 23 per cent were grade school educated, 36 per cent high school, and 40 per cent had entered college. Census data show that of urban Negro females aged fourteen and over, 58 per cent were of grammar school education, 35 per cent high school, and 7 per cent college.[1] Of our sample, slightly more than half (55 per cent) had married. Both the median grade school educated and high school educated woman married at eighteen, whereas the median college educated woman married at nearly twenty-three. Of those who married, 63 per cent were subsequently separated, divorced, or widowed by the time they were interviewed.[2] The Negro sample is primarily (90 per cent) Protestant, the remainder being Catholic.

Since we have done virtually no interviewing of Negroes in southern states, the sample may be described as being one of northern Negroes

---

[1] U.S. Census, 1950, Special Reports, *Nonwhite Population by Race*, 1953:27.

[2] From U.S. Census, 1950, Special Reports, *Fertility*, 1955:66-81, Tables 20-21, one can calculate the percentage of ever-married white females who had been separated, divorced, or widowed (S.D.W.), according to educational level. Tables 22-23 provide the same data for Negro females. Considering only urban women of completed fertility (i.e., women aged forty-five to forty-nine at enumeration), one finds that separation, divorce, or widowhood is much more prevalent among Negroes than among whites. For example, of ever-married Negro women with eight grades of schooling, about 61 per cent were S.D.W. as opposed to 31 per cent for the whites; among the college graduates roughly 44 per cent of the Negroes and 24 per cent of the whites had been separated, divorced, or widowed.

in the sense that the individuals were born in or migrated to the northern states. Actually some of them had spent a considerable part of their lives in the South. Including Maryland, Kentucky, West Virginia, and the District of Columbia among southern states, we find that 48 per cent of our Negro non-prison females had lived for at least one year in the South (55 per cent of the grade school educated, 38 per cent of the high school educated, and 52 per cent of the college educated).

Negroes in the lower socio-economic level have a distinctive pattern of sexual attitudes and behavior. This pattern is in part the result of slavery, wherein reproduction was often encouraged and families broken up by sale. And in part it is the result of the fact that in the years since slavery, Negroes have been a socio-economically depressed and rather cohesive group set apart from the rest of society. Any cohesive group that is segregated is certain to develop distinctive attitudes and behavior patterns. It is true that this Negro pattern is similar in many respects to that of whites in the lower socio-economic level; yet it is distinct. Insofar as reproductive behavior is concerned, the lower social level Negro pattern may be simply described: coitus is regarded as an inevitable, natural, and desirable activity to be enjoyed both in and out of marriage, contraception is little known and considered at best a nuisance and at worst dangerous or unnatural; and pregnancy is accepted as an inevitable part of life; whether it occurs in or out of wedlock is a secondary issue. The result of this philosophy is a high conception rate, a high live birth rate, a high spontaneous abortion rate (exacerbated by poverty and disease), and a minimal incidence of induced abortion.

The upper socio-economic level Negroes have different attitudes and behavior, similar to those of the middle and upper socio-economic level whites. This similarity is largely due to vertical social mobility. It has been suggested that the different patterns among the Negroes themselves may stem from the strong distinction made in the days of slavery between the house servant and the field hand. The house servants had a higher social status, were more familiar with the sexual attitudes of whites, and adopted some of these attitudes. Following the Civil War, the descendants of the house servants were more likely than the descendants of the field hands to be in, or reach, the upper socio-economic level.

The vertical social mobility of the Negro has been largely a recent historical development, and we have numerous case histories of individuals who rose from lower social level origins to upper social level status. (By social level we mean social level in terms of society as a whole, and not the intra-Negro social hierarchy.) In cases of vertical mobility we find the individuals who move upward retain, to varying degrees, the sexual and reproductive patterns of the lower social level; this is true of both Negroes and whites. This fact, rather than any inherent racial difference, is at the core of the differences in reproductive behavior seen between Negroes and whites.

Since socio-economic level is the crux of the phenomena to be examined, we have divided our Negro women into categories of educational attainment, which is our measure of socio-economic level. However, the correlation between educational attainment and socio-economic level is weaker among Negroes than among whites. To use a simple illustration, one can say that most of our high school educated white females come from the middle socio-economic level, but a considerable proportion of our high school educated Negro females come from the lower socio-economic level. Similarly, it is commoner among Negroes than among whites to find a college student whose parents have only grammar school educations.[3]

It is imperative that an educational level breakdown be employed, and since our Negro sample is small we have been forced to limit our other breakdown factors to marital status and age.

THE SINGLE NEGRO WOMAN

Since in our volume *Sexual Behavior in the Human Female* we presented no Negro data, it is necessary at this point to note the percentages of women with experience in pre-marital coitus and the number of coital years involved. In the light of our preliminary comments concerning social level and vertical social mobility, it should come as no surprise to learn that pre-marital coitus is quite prevalent among Negro women of less than college education, and more prevalent among college educated Negro women than among college educated whites.

By age fifteen, 62 per cent of the grade school educated had had pre-marital coitus, and by age twenty, 82 per cent. Among the high school educated the percentage by age fifteen is 48 per cent and by age twenty, 82 per cent. Of the Negro women who went to college or on into graduate work, only 8 per cent had had pre-marital coitus by age fifteen, 49 per cent by age twenty, and 71 per cent by age twenty-five (Table 63). The fact that these levels of experience in

[3] Frazier 1957:81-84 pointed out the low socio-economic backgrounds from which many Negro college students have been drawn. See also Brenman 1943.

pre-marital coitus are higher than those of white females of equivalent age is in part accounted for by the earlier age at marriage of the Negro women. The same relationship between educational level and coital experience was seen among white women up to age twenty.

Our calculation for the number of years in which pre-marital coitus occurred show that the average Negro girl of less than college educa-

Table 63. Accumulative Experience and Rate: Pre-Marital Conception

For Negro Females: Total Females and Females with Pre-Marital Coitus

By Educational Level

BY AGE	TOTAL NEGRO FEMALES			NEGRO FEMALES WITH PRE-MARITAL COITUS		
	Educational level			Educational level		
	0–8	9–12	13+	0–8	9–12	13+
	Per cent of females with conception experience					
15	22.8	9.5	0.4	36.7	19.8	
20	38.3	34.8	8.7	46.6	42.6	17.9
25	41.9	40.6	19.8	52.0	50.0	28.0
30	41.0	38.0	21.1	52.5	47.5	27.9
	Conceptions per 100 females					
15	26.8	9.5	0.4	43.0	19.8	
20	42.1	39.1	11.6	51.1	47.9	23.8
25	46.2	47.8	28.3	57.3	58.9	40.0
30	43.6	48.0	31.6	55.7	60.0	41.9
	Per cent with coitus			*Years of coitus per 100 females*		
15	62.2	48.2	7.8	242	228	
20	81.5	81.7	48.8	351	324	340
25	80.6	81.2	70.8	395	441	487
30	78.2	80.0	75.4	410	580	586
	Number of females					
15	127	199	230	79	96	
20	107	115	172	88	94	84
25	93	69	106	75	56	75
30	78	50	57	61	40	43

tion who has had pre-marital coitus, had about two and a third years of coital experience by age fifteen, three and a half years by age twenty, and about four years by age twenty-five. These periods of time are very similar to those derived from our white sample except that the Negroes are "ahead" five years: for example, the Negroes at age twenty and the whites at age twenty-five have accumulated the same number of coital years.

PREGNANCY

Accumulative experience. Our sample of grade school educated
women, including those without coital experience, indicates that
roughly one fifth had a pre-marital pregnancy by age fifteen and ultimately 41 per cent by age thirty. If only women with pre-marital coitus
are considered, we see that 37 per cent have a pre-marital pregnancy
by age fifteen, 47 per cent by age twenty, and then 52 to 53 per cent

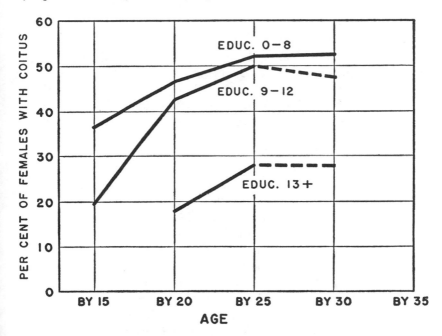

Figure 15. Accumulative Experience in Pre-Marital Conception for Negro Females
with Pre-Marital Coitus by Educational Level.
Data from Table 63.

thereafter (Table 63, Figure 15). A similar "leveling off" was noted
among white women, though it began at older ages.

The total high school educated sample provides an accumulative
experience percentage of about 10 by age fifteen and rises to a 38 to
41 per cent level. Of the females with pre-marital coitus, 20 per cent
had been pregnant by age fifteen, 43 per cent by age twenty, and
about 50 per cent by age twenty-five.

The college educated represent a definite departure from the reproductive picture described above. Less than half of 1 per cent of the

total college sample had conceived by age fifteen, 9 per cent had been pregnant by twenty, and 20 to 21 per cent by ages twenty-five and thirty. The figure for females with pre-marital coitus is 18 per cent by age twenty and 28 per cent thereafter.

Educational level relates to pre-marital conception experience among Negroes much as it does to the experience among whites, the lesser educated showing a higher proportion of women who became pregnant before marriage.[4] It is noteworthy, however, that the Negro grade school and high school educated are similar by age twenty and beyond. The effects of vertical social mobility are not sharply evident until one compares the college educated with those of lesser education.

Accumulative rate. Among the grade school educated Negroes with pre-marital coitus there were, by age fifteen, 43 pre-marital conceptions per hundred females; this rate increases somewhat and stabilizes at about 56 per hundred. Among the high school educated the accumulative rate of pre-marital conception is at first less, being 20 by age fifteen, but subsequently the rate is similar to that of the grade school educated. Those who went into college display lower rates: 24 per hundred by age twenty (as opposed to 51 and 48 per hundred among the less educated by the same age), and eventually the rate reaches its maximum of about 40 (Table 63).

The rates for all women regardless of coital experience are, of course, lower, being usually about four fifths of the rates for the sample consisting solely of women with pre-marital coitus.

It is our impression that the conception rates of the Negroes with pre-marital coitus exceed those of the whites primarily because of an absence of, or inadequacy of, contraception. Among Negroes of the lower socio-economic level there is an aversion to all forms of contraception except for the douche, and the douche is not only relatively ineffective but is often too long delayed.[5]

OUTCOME OF PREGNANCY

We have at our disposal for study 198 pre-marital conceptions of which 151 terminated while the females were unmarried. The others were carried into subsequent marriage. Six additional women were pregnant at time of interview.

---

[4] The same relationship was found in Pearl 1939:182. Of his sample of 5,633 fertile Negro women he reported 37 per cent pre-marital pregnancy experience for those with an elementary school education, 35 per cent for the high school group, and 18 per cent for the college or university educated Negro females.

[5] The relative omission of contraception among Negroes, aside from the douche, is cited by Tietze and Lewit 1953:564. Lack of knowledge of contraceptives among a group of unmarried Negro mothers was noted by Hertz and Little 1944:77.

Accumulative rate. On examining the outcome of pre-marital pregnancy, one sees that the grade school educated Negro females with pre-marital coitus have an accumulative rate of live births varying

Table 64. Accumulative Rate: Pre-Marital Outcome

For Negro Females: Total Females and Females with Pre-Marital Coitus

By Educational Level

BY AGE	TOTAL NEGRO FEMALES			NEGRO FEMALES WITH PRE-MARITAL COITUS		
	Educational level			Educational level		
	0–8	9–12	13+	0–8	9–12	13+
	Live Birth					
	Outcome per 100 females					
15	8	6	0	13	11	
20	13	16	2	16	19	4
25	14	19	2	17	23	3
30	12	18	2	15	*23*	*2*
	Spontaneous Abortion					
15	11	0	0	18	0	
20	8	2	0	10	2	0
25	10	1	0	12	2	0
30	9	4	0	11	*5*	*0*
	Induced Abortion					
15	4	3	0	6	5	
20	7	10	9	9	12	18
25	8	12	24	9	14	33
30	9	12	26	11	*15*	*35*
	Outcome in Subsequent Marriage					
15	4	2	0	6	3	
20	13	12	1	16	15	2
25	15	16	3	19	20	4
30	14	14	4	18	*18*	*5*
	Number of Females					
15	127	199	230	79	96	
20	107	115	172	88	94	84
25	93	69	106	75	56	75
30	78	50	57	61	*40*	*43*

from 13 to 17 per hundred females (up to age thirty). The high school educated begin with a rate of 11 by age fifteen and reach a rate of 23. The college educated have markedly lower rates, ranging from 2 to 4 per hundred (Table 64). Our total Negro sample, including those

with and without pre-marital coitus, provides an accumulative rate of
10 live births per hundred females by age twenty-five.[6]

Spontaneous abortion is commoner among the grade school group
(10 to 18 per hundred females) than among the high school educated
(2 to 5 per hundred), and our women of college education had had
very few (actually only two) spontaneous abortions.

Induced abortion rate is much higher among the better educated.
For example, by age thirty the grade school educated had had 11

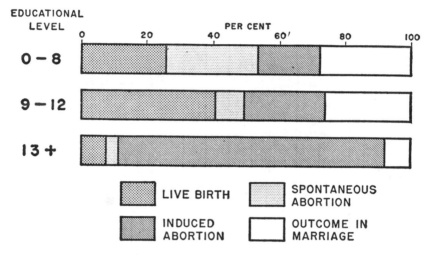

Figure 16. Outcome of Pre-Marital Conception for Negro Females by Educational
Level.

Data from Table 65.

abortions per hundred women with pre-marital coitus, the high school
educated, 15, and the college educated, 35. This sequence is in keeping with our finding that among white non-prison women the better
educated, when pregnant, resort to induced abortion more than do
the less educated.

The grade school and high school Negro females with pre-marital
coitus resolved pre-marital pregnancies by marriage at about the same
rates (by age thirty both rates are 18 per hundred), but the college
educated used this solution less often. Again this is the same situation
obtaining among the white females.

---

[6] U.S. Vital Statistics, Special Reports, 1950 (33): 74 showed a rate of 5.6 illegitimate births per hundred unmarried nonwhite females for the year 1947.
Williams and Thorner 1956:222 found a rate of 10 per hundred unmarried
Negro females for the state of Florida in 1950. The 259 never-married females
in the present sample reported 20 births, a rate of 7.7 per hundred women.

Outcome ratio. Turning our attention now to outcome ratio (Table 65, Figure 16), the proportions of pre-marital conceptions resolved in pre-marital live birth, spontaneous abortion, induced abortion, or in subsequent marriage, it is seen that the college educated ended only 8 per cent of their conceptions in live birth, as opposed to 41 per cent for the high school group and 26 per cent for those with grade school education. The fact that the college educated had the smallest proportion of live births agrees with our findings among white females; but the fact that the high school educated Negroes exceed the grade

Table 65. Outcome Ratio

For Negro Females: Pre-Marital and Marital Conceptions

By Educational Level

EDUCATIONAL LEVEL	NEGRO FEMALES: PRE-MARITAL AND MARITAL CONCEPTIONS				
	Type of outcome			Outcome in marriage	Total conceptions
	Live birth	Spontaneous abortion	Induced abortion		
	Pre-Marital Conceptions				
	Per cent			Per cent	Number
0–8	25.9	27.6	18.9	27.6	58
9–12	40.8	8.6	24.7	25.9	81
13+	7.5	3.8	81.2	7.5	53
	Marital Conceptions				
0–8	63.4	26.6	10.0		290
9–12	60.9	31.6	7.5		187
13+	56.9	23.5	19.6		102

school educated in this respect is puzzling and cannot be wholly dismissed on the basis of small sample size. Since it is clear that the prevalence of spontaneous abortion is the chief reason why the grade school educated do not have a high percentage of live births, one is tempted to seek some explanation involving nutrition and general health. However, the lower spontaneous abortion ratios derived not only from our white prison females but from the married Negro females and the Negro prison females of grade school education show any such explanation to be dubious. Nevertheless, vital statistics do exist which indicate that Negro women suffer a much higher proportion of late fetal deaths than do white women (see footnote 11).

Spontaneous abortion accounts for 28 per cent of the pre-marital conceptions of the grade school educated, 9 per cent of those of the high school educated, and 4 per cent of the pregnancies of the college educated.

Analysis of induced abortion presents the picture one could have predicted from accumulative rates: the better educated have a higher proportion of their conceptions thus terminated. The Negro college educated women aborted 81 per cent of their pregnancies (essentially the same percentage as for white college women), the high school educated women 25 per cent, and the grade school 19 per cent. These last two figures are much lower than among comparable categories of white women, as far as we can determine from our small sample of grade school educated white females.

The proportion of pre-marital pregnancies resolved in marriage varies inversely with educational achievement, ranging from 28 per cent for the grade school group to 8 per cent for the college group. This, too, agrees with our findings for white women.

In summary we may say that the single Negro women, in comparison with whites of the same education, have a higher percentage of pre-marital coitus and higher rates of pre-marital conception among those having coitus.[7] As far as the outcome of their pregnancies is concerned, the Negro and white single women of college education are similar, but among single women of lesser education the Negroes are far more likely to have live births and less likely to resort to induced abortion.[8] Educational level seems, in general, to correlate with reproductive behavior in Negroes as it does in whites.

---

[7] Pearl 1939:181 found 36 per cent of his total Negro sample of 5,633 women had pre-maritally conceived, in contrast to 9 per cent in his larger white sample.

Beebe 1942:61-62 also found that pre-marital conception was commoner among Negroes than among whites. The Logan County, W. Va., group he reported on showed 37 per cent experience for Negroes as against 15 for white women.

[8] Peckham 1936:112 stated, "In our experience [Johns Hopkins Hospital], it is extremely rare for a colored woman to induce an abortion upon herself, or to have such a procedure done by midwife or doctor."

Hertz and Little 1944:77-78 noted that their subjects (unmarried Negro mothers) were ignorant of or opposed to induced abortion and added that "a large number of Negroes, predominantly from the lower class, accept illegitimacy more or less as a matter of course." Drake and Cayton 1945:592-595 also discussed the negative attitude toward abortion and the relative acceptance of illegitimate birth.

U.S. Vital Statistics, Special Reports, 1955 (42):256 estimated on the basis of states reporting on illegitimacy, 1938-1953, that 16 to 19 per cent of the registered births of nonwhite women were illegitimate. In the present sample, 66 non-marital births out of a total of 422 provides a percentage of 16.

Young 1954:120-122 warned that while this acceptance of illegitimacy may be true of some Negro groups, the more status-striving Negroes have adopted the upper social level condemnation of illegitimacy.

THE MARRIED NEGRO WOMAN

In our Negro sample with marital experience, we have 313 ever-married women whose reproductive histories can be studied. Here, where the factor of coitus is held more constant, one would expect lesser differences between Negroes and whites, and this expectation is partially realized.

PREGNANCY

Accumulative rate. As with white women, the married Negro wives of grade school education have the greatest rates of conception in marriage and the college educated have the smallest (Table 66). For example, by age twenty-five the grade school wives have had 182 conceptions per hundred females, the high school educated 144, and the college educated 92. Judging from very small samples (by age thirty-five only 27 high school educated and 24 college educated women), these educational level differences do not lessen at older ages but become greater.

The grade school and high school educated Negro wives of our sample are more fecund than equivalent white wives. However, the college educated Negro wives prove ultimately to have had fewer marital conceptions than their white counterparts. By age thirty these Negroes appear (on the basis of 36 cases) to have had about 130 conceptions per hundred wives, whereas by the same age the white rate is 169.

OUTCOME OF PREGNANCY

Accumulative rate. In view of the higher marital conception rate it is not surprising to find the Negro live birth rate exceeds that of the whites.[9] Among the grade school educated, the rates of the two ethnic groups are roughly the same up to age thirty, but by age thirty-five the Negroes achieve an accumulative rate of 235 live births per hundred wives (Table 66), whereas the whites in our sample have a rate of only 188. Among the high school educated the live birth rates are lower than those of the grade school educated, as they were among our white women, but exceed the white rates at any age. For instance,

[9] The U.S. Census, 1950, Special Reports, *Fertility*, 1955:66-81, reveals that while more Negro than white wives are childless, those Negro women who bear children do so at a rate sufficiently high to make the Negro birth rate exceed that of the whites. The problem of Negro fertility is discussed by Pearl 1939:113, Beebe 1941:194, Kiser 1942:38-40, Grabill 1955:89-90, and Mayer and Klapprodt 1955:152-154.

by age thirty the Negro wives had 141 births per hundred women as compared to 107 for the whites. Among the college educated, however, there is reason to believe that the whites have more live births than do the Negroes. Despite the small sample, we feel that the finding is probably valid;[10] the college educated Negroes have, unfortunately, considerable difficulty in establishing themselves in positions in society commensurate with their educations, and as a result children are more of an economic handicap to them than to the whites. The decision to

Table 66. Accumulative Rate: Marital Conception and Outcome

For Ever-Married Negro Females

By Educational Level

BY AGE		EVER-MARRIED NEGRO FEMALES			
	Conception	Type of outcome			Total females
		Live birth	Spontaneous abortion	Induced abortion	
		Educational Level 0–8			
		Rate per 100 females			Number
20	126.5	74.7	45.8	24.1	83
25	181.8	111.4	58.0	29.5	88
30	244.2	163.6	63.6	32.5	77
35	326.7	235.0	72.0	37.0	60
		Educational Level 9–12			
20	85.1	59.5	29.7	10.8	74
25	143.6	101.8	45.5	10.9	55
30	204.3	141.3	54.3	19.6	46
		Educational Level 13+			
25	92.3	48.1	25.0	25.0	52

have few children so that these few may be given material and educational advantages is probably more of a factor among college educated Negroes than among college educated whites.

One large and inexplicable difference between the Negroes and whites lies in the rates of spontaneous abortion, the Negro rates being roughly double those of the whites by any age.[11] The fact that

---

[10] The 1950 U.S. Census volume on fertility cited previously shows that among urban college educated females, many more Negroes than whites are childless, and that the Negro birth rate in this educational group is less than that of the whites. The decreasing fertility among Negro women with increasing education is also clear in the census tables. This trend was also noted by Kiser 1942:247 and Frazier 1948:330-331.

[11] The New York City Department of Health records show that for 1952-1954 spontaneous abortion was about twice as common in nonwhites as in whites. See Erhardt and Jacobziner 1956:831.

among the Negro wives the rates decrease with educational level suggests some health factor may be involved, but if so, this is not evident among the white females. However, it is known that syphilis, a factor in spontaneous abortion, is more prevalent among Negroes than among whites,[12] and one would expect its incidence to be greatest among the less educated. It is also feasible to postulate that, owing to economic reasons, the Negroes, as a group, live in less healthful conditions than do whites, and that therefore one might expect a higher spontaneous abortion rate. This supposition receives some indirect support from the fact that our white prison females, who are also an economically

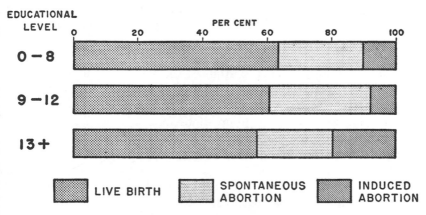

Figure 17. Outcome of Marital Pregnancy for Negro Females by Educational Level.
Data from Table 65.

depressed group, likewise display high spontaneous abortion rates in marriage.

Induced abortion rates present a different and more complex picture. Among the grade school and high school educated women, the Negro wives have lower rates of induced abortion than do whites, despite the fact that the Negro wives have higher conception rates. Among the college educated the reverse seems true: the Negro rates surpass those of the whites.

Outcome ratio. A study of outcome ratio reveals that educational level makes relatively little difference in the proportion of marital pregnancies that end in live birth: the figures range from 57 for the college educated to 63 per cent for the grade school educated Negro wives

[12] According to the *Journal of Venereal Disease Information* 1948, Vol. 29, p. 29, U.S. Public Health figures for 1947 show a rate that is 15 times higher for all stages of syphilis among Negro women than among whites.

(Table 65, Figure 17). Among white wives the proportions ranged from 64 to 67 per cent (Table 54).

The proportions accounted for by spontaneous abortion follow the pattern we have seen in accumulative rate; the Negroes have a much greater proportion of their pregnancies thus aborted than do whites.[13] However, the difference lessens with increased education: while the grade school educated Negroes aborted 27 per cent of their pregnancies spontaneously and the whites only 12 per cent, among the college educated the equivalent figures are 24 per cent versus 17 per cent.

Likewise, the proportions of pregnancies ending in induced abortion parallel the accumulative rates. The grade school and high school educated Negro wives had about half as great a percentage of induced abortions as did the white wives of the same education (8 per cent versus 16 per cent among the high school educated).[14] The college educated Negroes, however, had about the same percentage of abortions as did the college educated whites (20 per cent versus 18).

One is left with the impression that the Negro wives of less than college education are as a group quite fertile, unusually subject to spontaneous abortion, and rather opposed to induced abortion. The college educated Negroes, on the other hand, appear to have emulated the reproductive behavior of the college educated whites, and matched them in induced abortions. This fact, coupled with the prevalence of spontaneous abortion that also exists among college educated Negroes, resulted in depressing the number and proportion of live births below the level of the white females.

SUMMARY

The differences between Negro and white women stem primarily from differences in cultural and socio-economic background. Some of these differences may be the heritage of the peculiar sexual and reproductive behavior associated with slavery. The grade school and high school educated Negro women, for the most part, belong to the lower socio-economic level where social sanctions against pre-marital coitus and illegitimacy are weak, and where contraception is inadequate.

---

[13] Strandskov and Einhorn 1948 found a greater prevalence of stillbirth among the "colored" in comparison with the whites, in their survey of data.

Stix 1941:185 reported outcome ratio of 16 per cent spontaneous abortion and Beebe 1942:116 showed 14 per cent among Negro women in their samples. See also footnote 11.

[14] Pearl 1937:1389 and 1939:222-230 noted less induced abortion among Negro than among white wives. A similar finding is reported in Stix 1941:185 and Beebe 1942:116.

Consequently the percentages of women who have had pre-marital coitus, pregnancy, and live birth are high in comparison with the white women. Owing to a relative scarcity of induced abortion and to adverse health factors, pre-marital spontaneous abortion is also prevalent among the Negroes. One also finds that the Negro wives have relatively high rates of conception, live birth, and spontaneous abortion.

The single college educated Negro woman presents a different reproductive pattern. A recent product of vertical social mobility, she retains vestiges of the lower socio-economic sexual pattern, which accounts for her exceeding the college educated white woman in pre-marital coital experience and pregnancy. However, she aborts spontaneously and deliberately the same percentage of her pre-marital conceptions as does the white woman, and presumably for the same reasons.

The married college educated Negro woman, often striving for status in a rather adverse social and economic environment, tends as a result to be less fertile than the white wife. Equaling the white wife in percentage of pregnancies ended by induced abortion, the Negro wife has a larger proportion of spontaneous abortions; hence the percentage of her pregnancies resulting in live birth is lower than that for the white woman.

Chapter 7

THE PRISON WOMAN: THREE STUDIES

Between 1941 and 1946 the members of our research organization carried on interviews in three women's correctional institutions. These institutions were places to which women were legally committed and kept in custody; therefore they fulfill the dictionary's definition of prisons and will be referred to as such, despite the fact that two of them did not include the word "prison" in their official titles.

It has always been our policy to refrain from publishing our findings on any single identifiable organization, just as we have refrained from publishing data on an identifiable individual. We regret that, for this reason, we cannot name the superintendents and staff members whose co-operation made our work possible. Although they must remain anonymous, we wish to express our appreciation for their efforts on our behalf. Acknowledgment must also be gratefully expressed to the inmates who contributed their sexual histories. No small amount of courage and trust is involved when an inmate confides information that, if it came to official ears, could result in delay of parole and the imposition of additional restrictions.

From the three prisons 1,250 individual case histories were obtained; these represent nearly a 100 per cent coverage of the inmates in the institutions at the times we were working in them. Of the 1,250 women, 900 were white, 309 were Negroes, and the remainder were of other races.

While this prison study is based upon the inmates of only three institutions, in terms of numbers of inmates it is impressive. The U.S. Census reports that as of April 1, 1950, there were in the state and federal prisons and reformatories of this country, 3,975 white females of whom 3,775 were between ages fifteen and fifty-nine. Our sample of white females of the same age, accumulated over seven years, constitutes nearly one quarter of this figure. The census also provides the number of Negro females in prisons, reformatories, and training schools, and our Negro prison sample constitutes slightly over 6 per cent of this number.

To the best of our knowledge this study of prison women is unique. No other large-scale comprehensive study of the sexual behavior, past and current, of prison women exists. The admirable work of the Gluecks is the nearest approach, but they were concerned with a broad investigation of which sexual behavior was but a part and hence it did not receive detailed treatment. While this chapter is confined to the reproductive behavior of prison women, we hope to publish subsequently on their sexual behavior.

The three institutions differed considerably in nature and in the characteristics of their inmate populations; hence they receive separate treatment. However, the small number of Negro women in two of the institutions precludes their being separated, so it was necessary to analyze our Negro prison sample as a whole unit. A description of the characteristics of the inmates of two of the institutions (the third was an all-Negro institution) follows.

PRISON A

This institution in a midwestern state was populated chiefly by women convicted of misdemeanors; felons usually constituted only about 10 per cent of the annual commitments. However, 11 per cent of the women interviewed had had prior felony convictions. In the course of six years a total of 886 white and Negro women inmates were interviewed. This represents an almost complete census: of those inmates available (i.e., those not hospitalized, mentally capable of being interviewed, and able to speak English or Spanish) only five refused to be interviewed.

The white inmates of Prison A (698 in number) were largely small town or rural in background, and 14 per cent had been primarily rural as adults: 67 per cent had not gone beyond grammar school, 31 per cent had some high school education, and 2 per cent had attended college. Eighty-seven per cent had married, the median age at marriage being 17.6 years. Four out of every five of these ever-married women had also been separated, divorced, or widowed.[1] Some of the presumably permanent separations and the divorces stemmed, naturally, from imprisonment. Eighty-two per cent of the women were Protestant, the majority being inactive religiously and, with the exception of one Jewish woman, the remainder were Catholic. The average age was somewhat high, the median female being 29.8 years old.

These 698 white females provide us with data on 149 pre-marital conceptions, on 1,440 marital conceptions, and on 39 post-marital conceptions.

---

[1] Glueck and Glueck 1934:95 reported on their sample of 500 women paroled from the Massachusetts Reformatory, Framingham, Massachusetts. Nearly the same percentage (76 per cent) of the marriages of their delinquent women were broken up.

PRISON B

This institution derived its population chiefly from a large eastern metropolis, accepting misdemeanants, delinquents, and a few first-time felons. It was designed for females ranging in age from the late teens to the late twenties; older females were almost never accepted. The median inmate was aged 19.5 years.

As in the case of Prison A, our sample from this prison was nearly the total available inmate population: 273 contributed their histories and one female refused. Of the 273 women, 202 were white females whose characteristics are given below.

The white inmates were almost wholly urban; only 7 per cent had been primarily rural as adults. Forty-four per cent had grammar school educations and 56 per cent had entered or completed high school. Thirty-two per cent had married, and about three out of four of these women had had their first marriage terminated by separation, divorce, or death, despite the youthfulness of the group. The median female married when 17.8 years old. Fifty-five per cent were Protestant, 41 per cent were Catholic, and the remainder were Jewish.

The Prison B females had had 93 pre-marital conceptions, 71 marital conceptions, and 17 post-marital conceptions.

One aspect of Prison B deserves specific mention: one of the criteria used by the courts in determining whether a girl was delinquent was whether or not she had had pre-marital coitus. The impression was widespread among the inmates and persons associated with the prison and the courts that there was an unofficial policy excluding virgins from Prison B. While this is probably an exaggeration, it is given some substance by the fact that 91 per cent of the Prison B females had had pre-marital coitus by age twenty, and an unexpected number of single females were pregnant at commitment. The inmates jokingly maintained that there was but one virgin in the institution, and that she owed her virginity to having always been exclusively homosexual.

PRISON C

This institution situated in an eastern state served as a training school for Negro girls committed to its custody as delinquents. There were 50 inmates, ranging in age from adolescence to eighteen, and all of them contributed their sexual histories to our research. Twenty-seven girls were aged eleven to fifteen, and 23 were aged sixteen to eighteen. Of the latter, 22 of the 23 had had pre-marital coitus with 14 resultant pregnancies. None of the Prison C girls had married. About half of the girls were in grammar school grades, and half in high school grades.

THE WHITE SINGLE PRISON WOMAN

The characteristics that distinguish females who are convicted by the courts from females who are never tried or convicted are poorly known, and any enumeration of them must be general. One can note that poverty, poor education, mental retardation, alcoholism, and so forth are to be found more commonly among women convicted of offenses. Of their sexual and reproductive behavior very little is known. One could hypothesize that women convicted of asocial or antisocial behavior would be, as a group, less inclined to follow the regulations of society, including sexual regulations. This present study will, in addition to providing much needed descriptive data, test this hypothesis insofar as reproductive behavior is concerned.

PREGNANCY

Before taking up the subject of pre-marital conception, mention must be made of the percentage of women who had had pre-marital coitus. This amounted to nearly half of the Prison B inmates by age fifteen and nine tenths of them by age twenty. In this respect Prison B cannot be compared to either of our other samples since, as we have pointed out, there were selective factors that account for the unusually high incidence of pre-marital coitus among the Prison B women.

Prison A provides a problem: by age fifteen, 22 per cent of its inmates had had pre-marital coitus, and 45 per cent by age twenty; but thereafter the percentages successively decrease. This decrease with age is, as we have previously demonstrated (Chapter 3), partly due to the fact that proportionately fewer women born in earlier decades engaged in coitus before marriage, the percentage of those who did rising with each successive birth decade. The decrease in percentages begins, in our Prison A sample, after age twenty because we do not have for older ages the women born between 1920 and 1929. By age twenty 66 per cent of these 1920–1929 women had had pre-marital coitus;[2] calculations for age twenty-five must be based on other and older women of whom considerably fewer had coital experience (by age twenty-five the women born between 1910 and 1919 had the largest percentage with coitus, and this percentage was 50 rather than

---

[2] Glueck and Glueck 1934:88-90 found 74 per cent of their delinquent girls had had pre-marital coitus, and that 57 per cent had such experience prior to age 19. Tappan 1947:153 reports that of 150 cases before the New York Wayward Minor Court in 1942, 104 were accused of sexual delinquency. In a more popularly written book, Sullivan 1956, concerning Massachusetts Reformatory, 20 of the 36 cases used as illustrations are mentioned as having had pre-marital coitus and such experience seems, from the text, likely to have been had by an additional six.

66). Thus, as one can see, our accumulative figures were predestined to decrease with age. In our non-prison sample the decrease does not begin until long after age twenty because we continued to interview women of the 1920–1929 birth decade throughout the years and hence

Table 67. Accumulative Experience and Rate: Pre-Marital Conception

For Prison Females: Total Females and Females with
Pre-Marital Coitus

By Race and Institution

BY AGE	TOTAL PRISON FEMALES			PRISON FEMALES WITH PRE-MARITAL COITUS		
	Race and institution			Race and institution		
	White females Prison A	White females Prison B	Negro females	White females Prison A	White females Prison B	Negro females
	Per cent of females with conception experience					
15	4.6	8.9	18.8	20.5	18.4	31.7
20	15.3	33.9	40.8	34.2	37.3	52.5
25	13.0		35.8	32.2		51.8
30	11.6		27.6	31.9		*45.7*
35	9.9			30.7		
	Conceptions per 100 females					
15	4.6	11.9	20.2	20.5	24.5	34.1
20	16.4	33.9	47.5	36.9	37.3	61.2
25	13.2		40.8	32.8		59.0
30	12.6		35.5	31.9		*58.7*
35	9.9			30.7		
	Per cent with coitus			*Years of coitus per 100 females*		
15	22.3	48.5	59.2	156	217	233
20	41.6	91.1	77.7	232	286	335
25	40.4		69.2	279		377
30	36.3		60.5	314		
35	32.2			365		
	Number of females					
15	698	202	282	156	98	167
20	590	56	179	263	51	139
25	431		120	174		83
30	311		76	113		*46*
35	233			75		

had them available for calculations involving older ages; but interviewing in Prison A ceased by 1946, and consequently most of the 1920–1929 prison females were "lost" to us beyond age twenty.

Accumulative experience. The Prison A women, as a total, reported 5 per cent of their number as having had a pre-marital conception by

age fifteen. By age twenty this figure reached 15 per cent and thereafter declined (Table 67). Among only those Prison A women who
had had pre-marital coitus the equivalent percentages are naturally
greater, being 21 per cent by age fifteen and 34 per cent by age twenty.

Prison B women present a different picture. Of the total group, 9
per cent had experienced a pre-marital conception by age fifteen and
34 per cent by age twenty. Among those with coitus the equivalent
percentages are 18 and 37 per cent.[3]

Compared to non-prison women, these are high percentages. Of
the total sample of non-prison women who married by age twenty (a
group similar in this respect to the prison sample), only 9 per cent
experienced pre-marital conception; and of those with pre-marital
coitus, 18 per cent had had a pregnancy before marriage (Table 16).
Our high school educated non-prison sample of women with coitus had
22 per cent with pre-marital conception experience by age twenty, but
even this is far below the prison female percentages.

Accumulative rate. As one would anticipate, the number of pre-
marital conceptions per hundred females among Prison B inmates is
roughly twice that of the Prison A inmates (Table 67). By age twenty,
for example, the Prison B females had 34 conceptions per one hundred
females as opposed to 16 for the Prison A inmates. However, if the
sample is confined only to those who had pre-marital coitus, the accumulative rates of conception are essentially identical for both prison
groups: 21 per cent and 24 per cent by age fifteen, and 37 per cent
for both groups by age twenty. These rates exceed those of the non-
prison females of the same age. However, one cannot conclude from
these figures that the amount of coitus and the contraceptive practices
of the women of Prison A were the same as those of the women of
Prison B. By age fifteen the average girl of Prison B had had slightly
over two years of pre-marital coitus, while the girl of Prison A had
had one and a half; by age twenty the girl of Prison B had accumulated an average of almost three coital years, while the girl of Prison
A had roughly two and a third.

However, in their early years the females in both prisons had more
coital years than the non-prison females. At first this may not be ap-

---

[3] On the other hand, Glueck and Glueck 1934:92 report a higher figure for their
sample of delinquent females, of whom 54 per cent had experienced a pre-
marital pregnancy. Of 150 cases before the New York Wayward Minor Court
in 1942, Tappan 1947:153, notes 7 were unmarried mothers and nineteen
were pregnant. In Mrs. Sullivan's book (1956) concerning the Massachusetts
Reformatory, she uses for illustration 36 cases of whom 12 were described as
having been pre-maritally pregnant. This is obviously a minimal figure since
data were not given for the remaining 24.

parent: by age twenty our non-prison females had accumulated between 225 and 251 years of coitus per hundred females (Table 17), and the prison figures of 232 and 286 do not appear dissimilar. However, since our average prison woman married before eighteen, comparison should be made with non-prison women who married young. In doing so, we see that the non-prison women with pre-marital coitus who married by age twenty, accumulated only 163 years of pre-marital coitus per hundred females (Table 16), a number markedly lower than that of our prison women. This explains why the prison girls with pre-marital coitus had a rate of 37 conceptions by age twenty while the non-prison girls who also married young had a rate of only twenty-one.

The small decreases in pre-marital conception rates at ages beyond twenty, among women with pre-marital coitus, may be fortuitous or related to decade of birth. However, these rates are reasonably similar to the rates shown by our high school educated and college educated women of the same ages. One is left with the impression that the difference in the pre-marital conception rate of prison and non-prison women is pronounced only in their teens and is associated with an early age at marriage.

Among non-prison women we found that the more education a woman had, the less likely she was to have become pregnant before marriage. To determine whether this inverse relation between education and pre-marital conception exists among prison women we combined Prison A and Prison B samples and then classified them by educational level. By age fifteen the grade school educated had had 25 conceptions per hundred females while the high school educated had had 17; by age twenty the figures are 39 as against 34; and by age twenty-five, 36 as against 31. In brief, pre-marital conception is commoner among the less educated prison women, as it was among the less educated non-prison women.

OUTCOME OF PREGNANCY

The most interesting and indeed startling differences between prison and non-prison women are to be seen when the outcome of pre-marital pregnancy is studied.

Outcome ratio. Among the Prison A women, 39 per cent of the pre-marital pregnancies ended in live birth, 14 per cent in spontaneous abortion, 10 per cent in induced abortion, and 37 per cent were carried into a marriage (Table 68). Among the Prison B women, 42 per cent ended in live birth, 18 per cent in spontaneous abortion, 23 per cent in induced abortion, and 17 per cent were resolved in subsequent marriage. While these figures describe the situation that existed, no allowance has been made for the fact that four fifths of the Prison A women were married as opposed to only one third of the Prison B women. Therefore we must examine outcome ratio in other ways as well.

If one studies only those conceptions terminated prior to marriage it is evident that Prisons A and B are alike in the proportions of spontaneous abortion (23 and 21 per cent), but that the Prison A women were more inclined to live birth (62 versus 51 per cent), and less in-

Table 68. Outcome Ratio

For Prison Females: Pre-Marital and
Marital Conceptions

By Race and Institution

RACE AND INSTITUTION	PRISON FEMALES: PRE-MARITAL AND MARITAL CONCEPTIONS				
	Type of outcome			Outcome in marriage	Total conceptions
	Live birth	Spontaneous abortion	Induced abortion		
	Pre-Marital Conceptions				
White females	*Per cent*			*Per cent*	*Number*
Prison A	38.7	14.1	9.9	37.3	142
White females					
Prison B	42.2	17.8	23.3	16.7	90
Negro females	51.7	20.0	5.5	22.8	145
	Marital Conceptions				
White females					
Prison A	74.2	23.8	2.0		1,475
White females					
Prison B	76.9	23.1	0		78
Negro females	57.4	40.0	2.6		265

clined toward induced abortion (16 versus 28 per cent). The tendency of the Prison B females toward induced abortion at the expense of live birth probably is in part explained by the fact that Prison B had a higher proportion of high school educated inmates: 56 per cent in contrast to 32 per cent for Prison A. Also, the Prison B females were metropolitan, whereas the Prison A inmates were largely rural or small town in background, and we know that illegal abortions are more readily secured in large cities.

A side calculation showed that if one confines the ratio study to ever-married women, Prison A and B inmates proved identical in the proportions of live birth, nearly identical in the proportions of conceptions carried into marriage, and differed only in terms of abortion, the Prison B women having more induced and fewer spontaneous. Combining the ever-married women of Prisons A and B, we find that 31 per cent of their pre-marital pregnancies ended in live birth, 10 per cent in spontaneous abortion, 9 per cent in induced abortion, and 50 per cent terminated in subsequent marriage.

Regardless of which of the several ways of examining outcome ratio is employed, it is clear that the prison women differ dramatically from our sample of non-prison women, having had a vastly larger proportion of live births, a considerably larger proportion of spontaneous abortions, and a much smaller proportion of induced abortions. While in our total sample the prison women ended 39 to 42 per cent of their pre-marital pregnancies with a pre-marital birth,[4] our non-prison high school educated women ended only 10 per cent in this way; and they had proportionately more live births than any other non-prison group (Table 28). Spontaneous abortion accounted for some 14 to 18 per cent of the prison women's pregnancies, whereas among non-prison women the percentages usually lie at a 3 to 5 per cent level and never exceed 8. The induced abortion figures of 10 and 23 per cent shown by the prison women are dwarfed by those of the non-prison: the lowest non-prison per cent is 43 and is found among those who married by age twenty. It is unfortunate that we do not have an adequate non-prison grade school educated sample for comparative purposes; however, it may be of some interest that of the 17 pre-marital conceptions among non-prison grade school educated women, only 6 (35 per cent) were deliberately aborted.

Turning now to the proportion of pregnancies carried into subsequent marriage, we find that the 17 per cent figure of the Prison B women is not particularly different from the percentages of various non-prison groups. One cannot compare in this respect the prison women with the non-prison women who married by age twenty, since not all the prison women had married. However, such a comparison is possible when one deals with the ever-married prison women. We have seen (Chapter 3) that, by age twenty, the non-prison women had carried 51 per cent of their pre-marital conceptions into marriage; the equivalent per cent for the Prison A women is 51 and for the Prison B women 47. It would appear that the prison females were

---

[4] While direct comparison cannot be made, it is worth noting that Glueck and Glueck 1934:92 report that 54 per cent of their sample had experienced pre-marital pregnancy and 35 per cent had experienced an "illegitimate birth." These figures would suggest that an outcome ratio of the Glueck sample would show live births accounting for well over the 40 per cent we find in our sample.

equally able to, and equally desired to, solve the problem by marrying.[5]

One may ask why the prison women differ radically from the non-prison women in their pre-marital reproductive behavior. Since equally striking differences will be disclosed in discussion of the married women, we shall postpone our discussion of this question.

THE WHITE MARRIED PRISON WOMAN

Inasmuch as there were but 64 ever-married women in our Prison B sample, we have based our study of married prison women solely on the 607 ever-married women of Prison A, mentioning the Prison B wives only at specific points.

PREGNANCY

One might assume that since imprisonment necessarily interrupts marital coitus (at least in this country), the prison wives would have fewer marital conceptions than the non-prison. This assumption proves false.

Accumulative rate. The Prison A wives averaged by age fifteen some 42 marital conceptions per 100 females; by age twenty, 137; by age twenty-five, 218; and eventually by age forty-five, 379 conceptions (Table 69).[6] These rates are considerably higher than the rates for the non-prison wives by any equivalent age. They exceed the rates of the non-prison grade school educated, and also the rates of the non-prison wives who married young. In later life the prison versus non-prison differences lessen but are never obliterated; actually the discrepancy in later life would be even greater were it not for the fact that the high proportion of S.D.W. women reduces the conception rates of the prison sample.

As one would anticipate, the conception rates of the grade school educated wives of Prison A are greater than those of the high school educated. For example, by age twenty the grade school rate is 141 while the high school rate is 128; by age thirty-five the rates are, respectively, 336 versus 294 (the latter figure is based on only 34 women).

---

[5] Glueck and Glueck 1934:94 found that roughly one third of the marriages of their delinquent women had been "forced." However, some of these "forced" marriages involved pre-marital coitus that did not result in pregnancy.

[6] On the other hand, Glueck and Glueck 1934:94 found that from the 301 marriages contracted by 254 of their delinquent women only 155 children resulted —a definitely low live birth rate.

OUTCOME OF PREGNANCY

In describing the manner in which the pregnancies of the married prison women ended, we are once again faced with marked differences between the prison and non-prison wives.

Accumulative rate. The Prison A married women appear as early as age fifteen with a live birth rate of 37 births per hundred females (Table 69). This rate rapidly increases to 161 by age twenty-five and

Table 69. Accumulative Rate: Marital Conception and Outcome

For Ever-Married Prison Females

By Race

BY AGE	EVER-MARRIED PRISON FEMALES									
	White females, Prison A					Negro females				
	Con-cep-tion	Type of outcome			Total females	Con-cep-tion	Type of outcome			Total females
		Live birth	Spon-taneous abortion	Induced abortion			Live birth	Spon-taneous abortion	Induced abortion	
	Rate per 100 females				*Number*	*Rate per 100 females*				*Number*
15	42	37	13	0	145	28	38	9	0	53
20	137	100	39	5	463	102	70	47	3	132
25	218	161	57	6	396	128	86	51	5	110
30	262	192	65	8	300	179	110	76	4	72
35	323	236	78	8	227					
40	353	262	79	10	143					
45	379	278	88	13	80					

finally to 278 by age forty-five. These rates dwarf those of the non-prison wives; the nearest approach is the live birth rate of the non-prison grade school educated. Even in this comparison the differences are sizable: by age twenty-five the prison rate is 161 while the non-prison rate is 119, by age thirty-five the figures are 236 as against 188, and by age forty-five, 278 as against 202.

The situation is similar for spontaneous abortion, the prison wives having rates markedly greater than any non-prison group. By age twenty the prison women had a rate of 39 spontaneous abortions per hundred females; by age thirty, a rate of 65; and by age forty, a rate of 79. Our non-prison sample of grade school educated wives provides rates of 28 by age thirty, and of 41 by age forty. The non-prison wives who married by age twenty display a rate of 6 by that age, of 38 by age thirty, and of 50 by age forty. These two non-prison groups are the most comparable to our prison women, yet fall far below them in prevalence of spontaneous abortion.

Also, the induced abortion rates for the prison women are extraordinarily low in comparison to the rates of the non-prison women; differences of ten diameters occur. The prison women had a rate of 5 induced abortions per hundred females by age twenty, which gradually increased to 10 by age forty. In contrast, the non-prison grade school educated had a rate of 93 by age forty—the highest rate of any educational level. The non-prison women who married young likewise have the highest rate by age forty (83) of any age-at-marriage group. In brief, judging from the point of view of educational attainment and age at marriage, our prison sample should have had a high rate of induced abortion, but the reverse is true.

Outcome ratio. The married women of Prison A ended 74 per cent of their marital conceptions in birth, 24 per cent in spontaneous abortion, and 2 per cent in induced abortion. The small number of married Prison B wives provided similar proportions.

The same ratio trend that we saw in the non-prison women when they were grouped by education obtains among prison women: the less educated have proportionately more live births and fewer induced abortions.

No non-prison groups in our sample have induced abortion ratios at all similar to those of the prison wives. For example, the non-prison grade school educated ended 22 per cent of their pregnancies artificially—11 times the percentage that the prison females showed.

DISCUSSION OF DIFFERENCES

Thus far we have presented descriptive and comparative data without attempting to explain the marked differences. At this point we shall present a hypothesis that should serve as at least a partial explanation.

Our basic contention is that in terms of social background, economic status, and mores, women who sooner or later are sent to prison are, as a group, different from non-prison women.

Our educational level breakdown is inadequate to separate the prison from the non-prison women. The grade school educated group contains at one end of its social gamut persons who are ordinary citizens. The majority of these women or their husbands are occupationally semiskilled or skilled. Some are fairly prosperous, some are poor: they belong primarily to the middle or lower middle class. In their behavior, sexual and reproductive, they are not unlike the high school educated who, for the most part, may be classed in the middle and upper middle socio-economic levels. It is these grade school educated who constitute most of our non-prison grade school educated sample.

In this connection we must add that our grade school sample was accumulated in such a way as to make it more likely for us to obtain this
upper stratum of the grade school educated. For example, persons of
this upper stratum are more likely than persons of the lowest stratum
(described in the following paragraph) to belong to accessible groups.
Furthermore, there is another selective mechanism that may be described by a simple illustration: let us say that a person of the upper
socio-economic level wishes to assist the research by persuading his
spouse, relatives, and friends to contribute their case histories. Among
the persuaded individuals will be some of grade school education, but
these will almost necessarily prove to be from the upper stratum of
the grade school educated.

At the lower end of the scale of the grade school educated are the
impoverished, the underprivileged, the untrained, and the rejects of
society. These are the women who constitute a large part of our prison
sample. It is difficult to obtain an adequate sample from this lowest
stratum: the individuals do not belong to organized groups whose
co-operation could be obtained through lectures. They must be
reached on an individual basis, which is time-consuming and expensive. If one is fortunate, one can facilitate the accumulation of case
histories through use of a "contact," a person of sufficient status and
enthusiasm to bring his friends and acquaintances to the interviewer.
Here, however, one must be alert to selective factors.

To some degree the same division into lower and upper strata can
be applied to the high school educated. Classed as high school educated there could be both the daughter of a prosperous and respect-
able storekeeper, who was graduated with honors from high school,
and the daughter of the town drunk and a prostitute mother, who was
placed in the ninth grade only because the law required her to be in
school until a given age. This dichotomy existing within the high
school group explains why we find marked differences between our
prison and non-prison high school educated women.

What follows is a description of the attitudes toward sex and reproduction generally held by those in the lowest socio-economic level; it
is based upon our case histories and upon our personal impressions
during interviews.

Coitus is looked upon as natural and inevitable, and as one of the
chief pleasures available. Virginity is encouraged verbally but not
expected. Pre-marital coitus, especially between persons contemplating
marriage, is common and pre-marital pregnancy is also a frequent
precursor of marriage. If the marriage does not occur, this is considered
a misfortune, but the unwed mother is not stigmatized; disapproval is

apt to be directed at the male who escaped the marriage. Since there is relatively little social disapproval of illegitimacy, the women do not have such a strong reason to seek an abortion. Also, for these people the cost of an abortion is often prohibitive, and many of them have a general distrust and fear of physicians. A pregnant woman may attempt self-abortion and, when repeated efforts fail, she may overcome her misgivings and scrape together enough money for an operative abortion, only to find that her pregnancy is too far advanced for the professional abortionist.

Among the married women there is a general feeling that women are intended to bear children and that repeated pregnancies are to be expected and accepted with resignation. Other wives take a certain pride in their fertility, regardless of consequences. These attitudes, coupled with the economic considerations mentioned above, account for the rarity of induced abortion. The women of this stratum are those who have given rise to the popular conception of the poor wife in rags surrounded by numerous children.

As a rule induced abortion is strongly connected with status-striving. Abortion is practiced to preserve reputation, to provide much for a few children rather than little for many children, to maintain or raise a level of living, and the like. These motives are weak or even absent in the people of the lowest social stratum, and one often has the impression that they are passive, resigned, and prone to follow the path of least effort. After all, obtaining an illegal abortion requires considerable courage and initiative as well as money.

The high incidence of spontaneous abortion indicated by our prison sample stems from various sources. First of all, a low rate of induced abortion is conducive to an increased rate of spontaneous abortion, since induced abortions would terminate some pregnancies that would otherwise abort spontaneously. Secondly, there is the possibility that poorly educated women may think any delay in their menses means a pregnancy, and consider a resumption of menstruation proof of a spontaneous abortion. Thirdly, and more important, there is the health factor. At the lowest social stratum the cumulative effect of syphilis, malnutrition, and poor living and working conditions could markedly increase the spontaneous abortion rate.

To many, the low induced abortion rates and the high spontaneous abortion rates would suggest that the prison women may have reported their induced abortions as spontaneous, for fear of jeopardizing their chances for parole. We doubt if such deception has been a significant factor. The prison women who reported no induced abortions frequently reported other behavior that would be more damning from the point of view of officialdom. Furthermore, it is noteworthy that the grade school educated non-prison Negro women, who, as a group, are similar to the prison women in being socially and economically depressed, displayed spontaneous abortion figures comparable to those of the white prison women.

SUMMARY

The importance of this group of white prison women does not lie in their having been convicted and incarcerated, but in the fact that they give us a better idea of the lowest socio-economic level for which we have otherwise an inadequate sample.

Both before marriage and in marriage the prison women, in comparison with non-prison women, show higher conception rates, more live births and spontaneous abortions, and markedly fewer induced abortions. We believe these are social level differences and have nothing to do with criminality or imprisonment; this belief is strengthened by noting that within the sample of prison women the same educational level differences exist that we saw among non-prison women, the less educated having the greater number of conceptions and live births.

From these prison data, from our grade school educated non-prison females, from our impressions from field work, and from data derived from male case histories, we can arrive at a general idea about fertility among people of urban lower socio-economic level. Two substrata may be differentiated: a lower stratum that furnishes most of our prison sample, and an upper stratum, which furnishes most of our non-prison sample. In the lower stratum, pre-marital coitus is common at younger ages and conception is correspondingly frequent, especially since adequate contraception is seldom employed. The group mores are tolerant regarding pre-marital pregnancy, which is looked upon as a prelude to marriage; effective induced abortion is prohibitively expensive for many; and an element of procrastination and irresponsibility leads others to delay too long. All these factors combine to produce a high pre-marital live birth rate and to minimize induced abortion. With induced abortion low, and in an economically depressed group, it is no surprise to find spontaneous abortion common. In marriage the same picture obtains: high rates of conception, of live birth, and of spontaneous abortion, with induced abortion being rather uncommon. It requires a considerable amount of courage for a wife to seek and to obtain an induced abortion: friends and relatives may know of the pregnancy, she and her husband may have ambivalent feelings, abortion is contrary to religious teachings, abortion is expensive, abortion is illegal and, of course, a varying amount of physical pain and danger is involved. In many ways it is easier for the pregnant wife to conform to social pressures and bear her unwanted child. In this lower substratum, large families are not looked upon with disapproval and the men and women involved are not especially status-striving.

Turning to the other group, the upper stratum of the grade school educated, one finds more of its members concerned with improving their status socially, economically, and intellectually. It is an unfortunate truth that children interfere with such improvement; children do require expenditure of time, effort, and money. In consequence, as one progresses up the social scale there is an increasing use of contraception and also an increasing resort to induced abortion in cases where contraception fails.

THE NEGRO SINGLE PRISON WOMAN

Our Negro prison sample consists of 188 females from Prison A, ranging in age from eighteen to sixty, 71 females from Prison B, ranging in age from eighteen to thirty, and 50 girls from Prison C, ranging from adolescence to eighteen: a total of 309. Since the small number of those from Prisons B and C preclude separate treatment, we have combined all our Negro prison females.

Sixty-one per cent of the Negro prison women had not gone beyond grade school, 37 per cent were high school educated, and 2 per cent had entered college. The median female had 8.5 years of schooling. Fifty-seven per cent of the women had married and, as was also true of our white prison sample, the majority of the first marriages had terminated—87 per cent, to be exact. The median age at marriage was 17.6 years. The sample is highly urban; only 2 per cent of the women were classed as having been primarily rural as adults. However, some of these urban females had come from rural areas. The women were primarily Protestant (88 per cent) with most of the remainder being Catholic. The median female was aged 23.2 at the time of reporting. Forty-eight per cent of the Negro prison females had lived one year or more in the south. Those of grade school education were, using this definition, more "southern" (55 per cent) than those of more education (38 per cent).

PREGNANCY

The Negro prison females do not particularly differ from the Negro non-prison females of grade school education in the percentage of young girls who had pre-marital coitus. For example, by age fifteen, 59 per cent of the prison girls had had pre-marital coitus and by the same age some 62 per cent of the non-prison girls were no longer virgin.

After twenty, by which age 78 per cent had had pre-marital coitus (as opposed to 82 per cent for the non-prison women), the figures decrease, as in the case of the white women of Prison A and probably for the same reason.

Accumulative experience. By age fifteen, 19 per cent of the Negro prison girls had been pre-maritally pregnant, and by age twenty, 41 per cent. Taking for a denominator only those with coitus, 32 per cent were pregnant by fifteen and 53 per cent by age twenty (Table 67). The reader may recall that the non-prison grade school educated Negro females showed nearly the same percentage (47 per cent).

Following age twenty, the percentages decrease in keeping with the decrease in the percentage with pre-marital coital experience. This decrease, though less marked, is also seen in the sample of females with coitus, but here it seems the result of sample size vagary.

Accumulative rate. The rates of pre-marital conception per hundred females of the prison sample (Table 67) are not dissimilar to those of the non-prison women of grade school education. The prison rate, for all prison females, is 20 by age fifteen, and 48 by age twenty; the equivalent figures for the non-prison grammar school group are 27 and 42. If we confine the sample to women who had pre-marital coitus, the rates are 34 by age fifteen and 61 by age twenty for the prison group, and 43 by age fifteen and 51 by age twenty for the non-prison grade school educated.

OUTCOME OF PREGNANCY

With only 145 terminated pre-marital conceptions available, we decided to limit the analysis of these to outcome ratios and dispense with rates.

Outcome ratio. The Negro prison women had 52 per cent of their pre-marital pregnancies end in live birth, 20 per cent in spontaneous abortion, 6 per cent in induced abortion, and 23 per cent were carried into subsequent marriage (Table 68). Despite the similarity between the prison women and the grade school educated non-prison women in terms of conception, some marked differences appear when comparison is made in terms of outcome ratio. The non-prison grade school educated had only half as great a proportion of their pregnancies end in pre-marital birth (26 per cent versus the prison 52 per cent), and three times as great a proportion end in induced abortion (19 per cent versus the prison 6 per cent). The proportions ending in spontaneous abortion and in marriage were roughly the same in both groups.

Just as we saw in our comparison of prison and non-prison white females, the Negro prison women have a larger proportion of live births and a smaller proportion of induced abortions than do non-prison Negro females. Among the whites the prison group also had more spontaneous abortions, but this is not the case among the Negroes.

THE NEGRO MARRIED PRISON WOMAN

Of our total sample of 309 Negro prison women, 176 had married. These women accounted for 265 pregnancies terminated in marriage, of which 237 were conceived in marriage.

PREGNANCY

Accumulative rate. Whereas the white prison women proved to be more fertile than their non-prison counterparts, the Negro prison women are relatively infertile. Table 69 shows that by age twenty there were only 102 marital conceptions per hundred wives, 128 by age twenty-five, and 179 by age thirty. These conception rates are distinctly lower than those of the grade school educated non-prison women, Negro or white, and also lower than the rates of the white prison women. This infertility of our Negro prison sample will be discussed later.

OUTCOME OF PREGNANCY

Outcome ratio. The Negro prison women had 57 per cent of their pregnancies end in live birth, 40 per cent in spontaneous abortion, and 3 per cent in induced abortion (Table 68). The proportion of 57 per cent live births is rather low as opposed to 63 per cent for the grade school educated non-prison Negro wives, and to 66 per cent for the grade school educated non-prison white wives. The proportion of induced abortion is close to that of our white prison women (2 per cent), but is lower than the proportions found among non-prison grade school educated women (10 per cent for Negroes, 12 per cent for whites). In terms of spontaneous abortion, the Negro prison females are unique. The grade school educated, non-prison Negro and white, and the white prison females have spontaneous abortion ratios of from 22 to 27 per cent, but the Negro prison figure of 40 per cent represents a loss that is comparable to the pregnancy loss sustained by diabetics prior to modern therapy.

DISCUSSION OF DIFFERENCES

This examination of the Negro prison females leaves us with a number of questions that must be discussed.

1. Why are the Negro prison and grade school educated non-prison women so similar in pre-marital conception experience and rate when there was a marked difference in this respect between the white prison and grade school educated non-prison women?

2. Why do the married Negro prison women have fewer marital conceptions than the married non-prison women of equivalent education (both Negro and white) and the white prison wives?

3. Why is such a high proportion of the marital pregnancies of Negro prison women spontaneously aborted?

When we take up these questions in order, the answer to the first appears to be that the non-prison grade school educated whites derived from a social stratum above that of our prison grade school educated whites; hence their behavior differs. But our Negro non-prison grade school educated women and prison women came from more nearly the same social stratum, hence their similarity in pre-marital behavior. To put it succinctly, most of our non-prison grade school educated Negro females were interviewed in a slum environment, whereas most of our non-prison grade school educated white females were interviewed in connection with organizations and other groups belonging to the middle or upper socio-economic levels.

Questions two and three may be answered together. The low marital conception rate and the high ratio of spontaneous abortion among Negro prison women seems largely the result of several factors, the most important of which is venereal disease. The low marital conception rate was not, we determined, due to any lack of exposure: the number of marital years, the frequency of coitus, and contraceptive practices are very similar among Negro and white prison women. Both groups depended very heavily upon the douche and 30 per cent of each group did not practice contraception with any consistency. This similarity in contraceptive practice is all the more interesting because 27 per cent of the Negro prison women said that at the time of marriage they did not want to have any' children, whereas only 15 per cent of the white prison women held this attitude.

Regarding venereal disease, we found 58 per cent of the Negro prison women had had syphilis; in many cases this was verified medically on admission to prison. The white prison women had an equivalent figure of 32 per cent.[7] Since syphilis is known to cause spontaneous abortion and stillbirth, the high incidence of syphilis among the Negro

---

[7] According to the *Journal of Venereal Disease Information* 1948, Vol. 29, p. 29, U.S. Public Health figures for 1947 show a rate that is 15 times higher for all stages of syphilis among Negro women than among white. See also Nelson and Crain 1938:168, 176

prison women is undoubtedly a major factor in their infertility. This conclusion does not conflict with the pre-marital reproductive behavior of these women; as a group they married so young (median 17.6 years of age) that the consequences of pre-marital syphilis could not be expected to show themselves until after marriage, and some of the syphilis was contracted after marriage.

Our data as to gonorrhea, known to be an important cause of sterility, are not, we feel, especially trustworthy. Gonorrhea is not so easily recognized by women as by men, and uneducated women are particularly apt not to recognize the disease and to dismiss symptoms as being "the whites" (leucorrhea) or some other genital irritation.[8] Prison medical records can be expected to record only those cases which were active at time of admission. At any rate, 36 per cent of our white prison women reported having had (or were found to have) gonorrhea, as opposed to only 18 per cent of the Negro prison women. While it has been suggested that Negroes are less susceptible to gonorrhea than are white females,[9] we feel that this 18 per cent figure reflects inability to recognize the disease. Negroes of the lower socio-economic level even more than whites are apt to be confused and vague regarding venereal disease, often denying syphilis or gonorrhea but confessing to have had "bad blood."

Another factor that may be involved in the low conception rate of the Negro prison females is the large number who had engaged in prostitution. Prostitutes are surprisingly infertile and not all their infertility can be attributed to venereal disease or contraception; some other and as yet unknown factor may be involved. Fifty-six per cent of the Negro prison women admitted to or had been convicted for prostitution. The equivalent percentage for white prison women was 21 per cent, a figure that apparently did not adversely affect their fertility to any marked degree, but one which, if more than doubled, could be expected to exert some appreciable influence.

SUMMARY

The women composing our Negro prison sample came from essentially the same environment as the grade school educated of our

---

[8] Nelson and Crain 1938:106 note "These early signs and symptoms of gonorrhea are usually quite mild . . . Married women, especially brides, pay little attention to them. . . ." On page 170 they also state that in venereal disease surveys "It is probable, of course, that gonorrhea is missed in the female in a higher proportion of cases that in the male." On page 199, "Infection with gonorrhea is usually obvious to the male patient, less commonly to the female. . . ." Johnwick 1952:15 states, ". . . more than half of the women infected with gonorrhea do not recognize their own disease. . . ."

[9] Nelson and Crain 1938:168, 177.

Negro non-prison sample; hence the differences in reproductive be-havior between these two groups are small in comparison to the differences observed between white prison and white non-prison women.

About the same percentages of prison and grade school educated non-prison women had pre-marital coitus—over three quarters by age twenty. Also, the percentages of women who had pre-marital conceptions, and the frequencies with which they had these conceptions, were similar among the prison and grade school educated non-prison women. However, there are definite differences in how these pre-marital conceptions ended. The prison women had a much higher proportion of live births than did the non-prison women, and fewer of their pregnancies ended in induced abortion.

The prison wives were characterized by low conception rates and by the extraordinarily high proportion of their pregnancies that spontaneously aborted. These two phenomena explain, at least in part, why the Negro prison wives had so few induced abortions. The relative infertility of the married prison women and their proneness to abort spontaneously seem largely the result of the prevalence of syphilis and of prostitution, both being much more frequent among the prison women than among non-prison women of the same socio-economic status.

The Negro prison women married young (the median females being aged between seventeen and eighteen at marriage) and consequently many of them had not contracted syphilis by the time of marriage, or had not by that time suffered its effects, and many of them had not had extensive experience in prostitution. Therefore the adverse effects of syphilis and prostitution on reproduction are not evident in the pre-marital years, but are clearly seen in years of married life.

Chapter 8

INDUCED ABORTION

THE BACKGROUND

Unwanted pregnancy has been a problem of mankind since, probably, the appearance of the first mammals meriting the term "human." The human animal is so constituted that abstention from coitus is not generally a practical solution, and until recent times effective contraceptive methods were largely unknown. The inevitable unwanted pregnancies have often been dealt with by induced abortion and infanticide. These two methods of reproductive control are universally known and practiced to some degree in all societies.[1]

On the other hand, Murdock points out that ". . . society as a whole has so heavy a stake in the maintenance of its numbers, as a source of strength and security, [that] abortion, infanticide, and neglect, unless confined within safe limits, threaten the entire community and arouse its members to apply severe social sanctions to the recalcitrant parents."[2] Different societies have different ideas as to what constitutes "safe limits"; among some abortion is approved or at least tolerated, among others it is considered a serious offense and is strongly condemned, and in still other societies it is almost mandatory that certain pregnancies be aborted.

Anthropological data on the prevalence of induced abortion are inadequate, as Devereux noted in his comprehensive volume on the subject,[3] usually consisting of loose impressionistic statements. Nevertheless, one can safely state that there is a great range among human societies in the degree to which induced abortion is practiced. This range runs the gamut from the improbable statement that the Mataco of South America abort all first conceptions[4] to the equally improbable statement that the Naskapi of North America abort none.[5]

---

[1] Ford 1952:765.

[2] Murdock 1949:9.

[3] Devereux 1955. Another comprehensive anthropological work on primitive abortion, with an extensive bibliography, is Berkusky, 1913. This work deserves mention since it has been largely unknown.

[4] Metraux in Steward 1940:319-320, "It is reported that even married Mataco women provoke a miscarriage at their first pregnancy to facilitate the delivery of the next child."

[5] Lips 1947:415 flatly stated, "Birth control and abortion are not practiced."

References to abortion appear in some of the earliest writing. Certain passages of the ancient Egyptian Ebers Papyrus may be construed as formulas for inducing abortion[6] and the Middle Assyrian laws stipulate punishment for abortion.[7]

The attitude toward induced abortion held by a society does not seem to correlate with the society's technological status; one cannot postulate that the "primitives" tended to condone abortion while "civilized" peoples condemned it. Induced abortion seems to have been tolerated in Egyptian and Roman civilizations,[8] and in Greece, Aristotle felt it mandatory in certain circumstances.[9] The attitude toward abortion takes on a particular intensity when abortion becomes a matter of religious rather than purely secular concern.

The penalties for induced abortion among disapproving societies range from scolding to the death penalty.[10] In a few societies, including our own, a person who assists a woman in aborting is also held punishable.[11]

The reasons for induced abortion are, and have been, legion in human history. Usually the motive is powerful and compelling, as in instances where poverty or ill health is involved, or where a birth would result in serious social complications. In other instances the motive is, to western minds, trivial: for example, some women on the island of Lesu abort because pregnancy interferes with dancing, which is one of the chief pleasures of life.[12]

[6] Ebbell 1937:109-110 translated these passages of the Ebers Papyrus. It is not clear whether the formulas were intended to hasten labor or to cause abortion. Subsequent sections deal with the prevention of spontaneous abortion.

[7] Pritchard 1950:185. The Middle Assyrian law stipulated that a woman who aborts herself shall be impaled on stakes.

[8] Hertzler 1956:242 noted that abortion and infanticide were "publicly recognized and socially condoned" in Rome and Greece.

[9] Aristotle, *The Politics*, Book VII:xiv expressed his view, ". . . there must be a limit fixed to the procreation of offspring, and if any people have a child as a result of intercourse in contravention of these regulations, abortion must be practiced on it before it has developed sensation and life. . . . "

[10] Devereux 1955:62 noted that the woman who aborts herself is merely scolded on the island of Truk, but would be subject to the death penalty among the Jakun. As previously mentioned, the Middle Assyrian laws prescribe the death penalty, which was also in existence among the Kabyle (Aptekar 1931:134), the Inca (Guaman Poma 1943:11-12, 130), and the Visigoths (Carr-Saunders 1922:269).

[11] The punishment of those assisting a female to abort is mentioned for the ancient Germans (Devereux 1955:56) and the Inca (Guaman Poma 1943:11-12, 130). The present-day laws of Germany, Peru, and Switzerland also provide for such a penalty. See Schönke 1951:508; Mac-Lean 1942:349; and Panchaud 1951:77. The states of Alabama, Delaware, Florida, Massachusetts, Rhode Island, and Vermont included punishment for a person who aided, assisted, or abetted in an abortion according to Taussig 1936:455-471.

[12] Powdermaker 1933:243 lists dancing as a motivation for abortion.

Primitive societies have employed various methods to cause abortion; these may be grouped roughly into four major categories:

1. Abortion through external treatment. This is common, and includes massaging, pounding, and compressing the abdomen. Violent physical exertion such as jumping and lifting heavy weights is often employed. The application of substances or of heat to the abdomen is less common.

2. Abortion through insertion of objects into the vagina or uterus. Sharp instruments have been used to injure the embryo or puncture the membrane, an effective but dangerous procedure. In other cases irritant substances are placed in the vagina or in the os of the cervix.

3. Abortion through oral ingestion. Drinking or eating some substance to cause abortion is a very common method and one which, if it fails, may be followed by other methods. The majority of substances taken are ineffective and may be more magical than practical. However, in some societies certain substances do seem to be definite abortifacients.

4. Abortion through magic. It is rather uncommon for females to use methods that they consider purely magical.[13] It is interesting to note that the pregnant woman who desires a child observes various taboos, often numerous and annoying, in order to prevent spontaneous abortion or stillbirth, yet this same woman must be aware that women who have deliberately broken such taboos in order to provoke abortion have been singularly unsuccessful.

In our culture there has been much concern over the physical danger of abortion, particularly when self-induced or performed by someone not a physician. It is undeniable that invasion of the uterus with clumsily handled or nonsterile instruments can result in perforation, hemorrhage, and/or infection that may result in serious illness or death. It is surprising, therefore, to find historical and anthropological literature almost devoid of references to such serious sequelae. The very fact that a substantial number of societies have accepted or condoned abortion may well indicate that the physical consequences are not ordinarily severe. On the other hand, one must also realize that women of pre-literate cultures may better withstand trauma than women of our own culture or, possibly, accept the consequences with relatively less concern. Hrdlička, in speaking of abortion among an Indian group (presumably the Pima), stated, "There was found nowhere much fear of serious bodily consequences, which suggests that

---

[13] For example, Devereux 1955:364-371 in a trait list finds magico-religious methods of abortion in only 30 of 482 groups (6 per cent).

these may be more limited than under similar circumstances among white women."[14]

Up to this point we have been speaking in broad terms of ancient civilizations and pre-literate societies. In our own culture we find an ambivalent attitude in regard to illegal abortions.[15] There are laws against such practices in all 48 of our states. Penalties for the crime of inducing an illegal abortion range from one year (Kansas) to as much as 20 years in prison (Mississippi). In 15 states the woman who solicits or consents to the abortion is also guilty, but usually with a lesser penalty. In 18 states the woman must actually be pregnant, whereas in most of the remaining 30 states an attempted abortion is punishable even though she was in actuality not pregnant. Some states differentiate the stages of pregnancy: if the child in utero has "quickened," i.e., if the mother has felt life, the penalty for an abortion is greater.[16]

It would seem that all the states have been consistent in condemning the practice of induced abortion (except for therapeutic abortions) even though they have not been consistent in the degree of penalty attached to it. It is also true that the churches, and particularly the Catholic Church, have been most severe in their condemnation of induced abortion.

However, on the other side of the coin, we find that defense lawyers know that their best way to win an abortion case is to secure a jury rather than a court trial. Police and other officials often allow known abortionists to practice since it is felt that there is a need for their services.[17] In 1944 only 116 persons were convicted for illegal abortions in the twenty-four states of the union reporting on this.[18] This amounts to one abortion conviction for every 625,000 persons in the population in that year. This, again, is a demonstration of society's unwillingness to penalize the abortion specialist. In our own sample we find that the great percentage of the women who had an illegal abortion stated that it had been the best solution to their immediate problem. This widespread difference between our overt culture as expressed in our laws and public pronouncements and our covert culture as expressed in what people actually do and secretly think is as true with abortion as with most types of sexual behavior.

Methods of abortion receive scant attention in medical schools in this

---

[14] This quotation from Hrdlička is given by Aptekar 1931:147.
[15] For elaborations on this point see Amen in Taylor 1944:134-135; Ellis 1951:92-94; Sontheimer 1955.
[16] Sherwin 1949:61-64.
[17] Amen in Taylor 1944:135; Sontheimer 1955.
[18] U.S. Census 1945-1946, *Judicial Criminal Statistics, 1944.*

country; the student is told of the indications for therapeutic abortion, is warned of the social and legal problems, and is taught how to dilate and curette. This method is almost the only one used by American physicians.[19] Actually, owing to our mores and laws, the study of abortifacients is a scrupulously avoided field, though much money and energy have been devoted to research in contraception. The difficulty involved in testing the abortifacient with humans, and the fear that it might escape from the jurisdiction of physicians and be surreptitiously produced and widely used, all combine to deter the would-be investigator. Nevertheless, it is already evident that it would not be difficult to develop effective and safe abortifacients, including some to be taken orally. The fact that such a development has not been made is basically a moral matter.

METHODS OF ILLEGAL ABORTION

The females in our sample who had had illegally induced abortions were questioned about the methods used in the abortion. Further information was obtained by asking the same questions of the males in our sample who were responsible for pregnancies that ended in induced abortions.

As indicated in Table 70, almost all (91 per cent) of the illegally induced abortions of our white non-prison sample were operative.[20] By operative abortion we are here referring to any interruption of the life of the embryo, at any age prior to live birth, by insertion of any instrument or drug or other substance into the uterus or the os of the cervix. Medical opinion is that drugs used for inducing abortions if taken orally are of little value unless the female tends to miscarry easily.[21] Hence a report that 7 to 14 per cent of the induced abortions

---

[19] The late Dr. Robert L. Dickinson, famed gynecologist, was well aware that official medical circles showed wide gaps in knowledge of abortion techniques. During a discussion at the 1942 Abortion Conference, sponsored by the National Committee on Maternal Health, he pointed out that "although abortion is the only operation done on an invisible field, with hemorrhage difficult to control, training for necessary skill is handicapped or prevented," adding that "although [abortion is] sometimes needed to save life, research on methods, or on simple or non-surgical means of induction is neglected or absent." See Taylor 1944:50.

[20] Other studies of induced illegal abortion showing the large majority of cases reporting the use of operative procedure include: Watkins 1933:162; Stewart 1935:873; Parish 1935:1108; Peckham 1936:212; Brunner and Newton 1939: 88; Simons 1939:843; Brunner 1941:174. These surveys show percentages of operative type of abortion ranging from 66 to 90 per cent, with the lower figures reported from hospitalized abortion case samples. The Brunner study based on over 1,000 medical case histories parallels the figure from the present data.

[21] See Taussig 1936:352-355 and Guttmacher in Fishbein and Burgess 1947:217.

were brought on as a result of taking drugs is probably misleading, since some of the women involved would have had a spontaneous abortion in any case. The somewhat higher percentage of abortion by drugs in the previously married women (14 per cent) may be due to her older age, since we know that older women tend to have more spontaneous abortions.

Table 70. Method of Illegal Abortion

Reported by White Non-Prison Females and Males

By Marital Status at Event

METHOD OF ABORTION	FEMALE REPORT				MALE REPORT
	Pre-marital	Marital	Post-marital	Total	
	Per cent				Per cent
Drug	6.9	9.7	14.4	9.2	7.5
Operative	93.1	90.3	86.6	90.8	92.4
Injury	0	0	0	0	0.1
Total	100.0	100.0	100.0	100.0	100.0
Number abortions, method known	335	566	127	1,028	745
Number abortions, method unknown	1	13	2	16	1

Rarely did females in our sample deliberately attempt to injure themselves to produce an abortion, by intentionally falling down stairs, for instance, or having someone hit the abdomen with fist or board. In our entire sample, only eight males reported that females whom they had impregnated used this technique with success, and only two females reported using this method.

Of the abortions by oral use of drugs reported by females, about half were self-induced[22] (presumably the drugs were purchased at a pharmacy without a prescription), and the other half were either by prescription or by drugs given to them by a physician. Of the illegal operative abortions, less than 1 per cent were self-induced. Almost all the remaining operative abortions were performed by a "physician." This point is discussed more fully later in the chapter.

Whereas over 90 per cent of the white non-prison females reported that their abortions were operative, only 72 per cent of the white prison females, 79 per cent of the Negro non-prison females, and 65

[22] This wider reliance on self-induction with the use of drugs as an abortion method is also reflected in the reports of Stix 1935:360 and Évans in Van Hoosen 1938:47, in which three fourths of all self-induced abortions were by means of drugs.

per cent of the Negro prison females (based on only 19 cases) reported that their illegally induced abortions were operative. The lower socio-economic groups, as reflected in these last three categories, tend to have more fear of doctors, to have less money, and to be more aware of and responsive to the folklore concerning drug-induced abortions.[23]

It is the general medical opinion that abortifacients are either ineffective or extremely dangerous to the health of the mother.[24] As mentioned previously, if induced abortions by use of herbs or natural drugs are reported, there is a likelihood that a spontaneous abortion would have resulted in any case. Hence, among groups using such abortifacients the reported induced abortion rate may be somewhat too high and the spontaneous abortion rate correspondingly low. We found that white women rarely reported the use of tansy tea, apiol, aloes, and ergot of rye. The use of quinine and castor oil was frequently tried but was seldom reported as being successful. In only about 9 per cent of all the cases was a drug reported as inducing an abortion, although such drugs were tried in many instances before the woman resorted to an operation.[25]

Among the Negro women of the lowest socio-economic group, however, we did secure a higher percentage reporting the use of such abortifacients as drinking water in which a rusty nail was soaked, tansy tea, ginger tea, horse-radish, turpentine, bitters and whiskey, and bluing. In each of these cases a successful abortion was reported. Drinking turpentine, tansy tea, and rusty nail water were the three most common techniques. Earlier we stated that in considering whether an abortion was regarded as spontaneous or induced we felt justified in agreeing with the woman's interpretation of the event even if the sub-

---

[23] Hamilton 1940:922 showed a third more of her Negro sample reporting the use of drugs than the white sample in her study of abortion cases in Bellevue Hospital. Lewis-Faning in the 1949 study of family limitation in Great Britain (p. 171) also reported that the higher social classes used drugs less often and more operative procedures in attempting abortions.

[24] See, for example, Taussig 1936:352-355; Guttmacher in Fishbein and Burgess 1947:216-217 (never effective in the case of a normal, well-implanted egg); Fisher in Rosen 1954:6-7; Hyman 1946(3):2651. But also see Adair in Taylor 1944:59 (no evidence that it is not possible in very early pregnancy).

[25] Drugs used in abortion attempts, some successful, some unsuccessful, as reported in American and European studies, include: Chance 1931:57, 60 (salts, pills, gin, black medicine); Watkins 1933:162 (quinine, turpentine, ergot); Kopp 1933:125 (quinine, aspirin); Evans in Van Hoosen 1938:47 (Beecham's pills, pennyroyal pills, castor oil, Epsom salts, ammonia, black draught); Ministry of Health 1939:41-42 (apiol, pennyroyal, quinine, female pills, mustard, dolly-blue solution, water in which nails or pennies have been soaked, beer, stout, gin—often with iron filings); Davis 1950:124 (ergot in hot port wine); Auken 1953:250 (quinine, rosemary, herb tea, abluent, litharge, lavender, camphor drops); Rolph 1955:98 (opium tablets).

stance taken was of dubious efficacy. However, the belief in the abortifacient quality of rusty nail water, ginger tea, and substances of a
similar nature is stretching credulity beyond reasonable limits even
though the subjects were quite sincere in their convictions. Thus, such
cases were classified as spontaneous.

THERAPEUTIC ABORTION

There were 68 legal abortions (including operations for ectopic
pregnancies) reported by 51 white non-prison women in our sample.
Out of our total of 1,067 induced abortions this represents a percentage
of 6.4. When we use live births as a base for calculation, these 68 legal
abortions are 2.8 per cent of the 2,434 live births. There were 19 cases
in which extra-uterine pregnancy was given as the reason for the
therapeutic abortion, 6 cases of tuberculosis, 5 cases of cardiovascular
difficulty, 3 cases with psychiatric reasons, 1 case of toxemia, 7 cases
reporting other pathology, and 27 cases where the reasons were unknown or not given.

Recently published ratios of the incidence of therapeutic abortion
to deliveries in various hospitals range from 1:76 at Bellevue Hospital,
1935–49, to 1:285 at Los Angeles County Hospital, 1931–1950.[26] The
present data calculate to the higher ratio of 1:50, excluding extra-
uterine pregnancies. The two factors that contribute to this discrepancy are the disproportionate number of upper educational level females among our histories and the all white sample. Various sources
show that therapeutic abortions are more frequent among upper social
and educational level groups. In New York City, for example, the
ratio of therapeutic abortions to live births as reported by the Department of Health for 1951–1953 for private hospitals was five times that
reported for the municipal ones. This same tendency is reflected in
the generally low therapeutic abortion rate among Negro women,
which Dr. Tietze in 1950 reported as being half of that for white
women in New York City. These facts are particularly interesting in
view of the statement often found in medical writing that unfavorable
social and economic factors may play an unconscious role in a decision to do a legal abortion.[27] It appears that they do, but not in the
direction implied.

The ratio of therapeutic abortion to conception among the married
females was 1:61; among the unmarried females the ratio was 1:73.

---

[26] See Wilson in Rosen 1954:190 and Russell 1951:435.

[27] For statements regarding the part played by unfavorable economic and social
conditions in a decision to perform a therapeutic abortion see: Studdiford
1950:733; Moore and Randall 1952:37; Guttmacher in Rosen 1954:21; Speert
and Guttmacher 1956:204. The contrary point of view is ably expressed by
Kleegman in Rosen 1954:256 and by Mandy in Rosen 1954:288.

Hence, whether a woman was married or not appeared to have little effect on her chances of securing a legal abortion.

The therapeutic abortion rate appears to have decreased markedly in recent years and indications that are acceptable for therapeutic abortion have shifted considerably. The current lists, while including newer items such as the Rh factor and rubella (German measles), are much less inclusive than formerly. For example, fewer women are being aborted on account of cardiac disease, while tuberculosis, vomiting of pregnancy, and diabetes now are only rarely used as indications for therapeutic abortion.[28] Reports show that for a period during the 1940's when other medical indications for inducing an abortion were decreasing, psychiatric indications were assuming a much greater relative importance, but this trend appears to have slowed down in recent years.[29]

AGENT INDUCING ILLEGAL ABORTION

For about a third of the male and female samples, information was secured concerning the agent who induced the abortion. Our male sample consists as before of males who were responsible for pregnancies ending in induced abortion. As indicated in Table 71, the data from white non-prison female histories are within a few percentage points of the data from our male histories. Self-induced abortions accounted for 8 to 10 per cent, abortions by "physician" for 84 to 87 per cent, and by others for 5 or 6 per cent.[30] The term "physician" in this

---

[28] See Guttmacher in Rosen 1954:17-20.

[29] See Hellman in Cecil 1951:341; Russell 1952; Moore and Randall 1952; Heffernan and Lynch 1953; Kummer 1953; Tietze 1954:19; Guttmacher in Rosen 1954; Planned Parenthood 1955 Abortion Conference, Calderone 1958.

[30] Reports on the type of agent who brought about the induced abortion vary widely in other investigations. The following inquiries based on general samples record a high incidence of professional help either from a doctor, professional abortionist, or midwife, similar to the present study: Stone and Hart 1932:17 (56 per cent); Kopp 1933:Appendix, Table 30 (75 per cent); Stix 1935:360 (94 per cent); Brunner 1941:174 (91 per cent); and Whelpton in Taylor 1944:21 (70 per cent).

On the other hand, more selective samples based on induced abortion cases receiving hospital treatment show self-induction as much more common. For example: Watkins 1933:162 (73 per cent); Simons 1939:842-843 (79 per cent); and Olson et al. 1943:677 (82 per cent). This difference might indicate the less skillful methods of the self-operation or self-administered drugs, which would result more often in hospitalization, or it might reflect a greater reluctance of abortion patients to involve a second person when they are questioned by hospital personnel.

Alexandrow 1947:115 reported more than half of 450 abortion court cases in Zurich, Switzerland, as performed by lay persons, the others by doctors.

Sutter 1950:94, in his detailed survey of 1,300 cases in Paris, reported an even division between self-induced abortions and those done with the aid of another person.

context is used very loosely, as many persons were undoubtedly reporting as physicians abortionists who were in reality not licensed to
practice medicine. The subjects were often unable to differentiate
licensed physicians from others because of the brief and often furtive
contact with the abortionist. However, there were many who were
reputable physicians, in good standing in their local medical associa-
tions, who performed abortions on their wives, other relatives, friends,
or other patients out of sympathy. It is our conclusion that almost
every general practitioner has been asked to perform an illegal abortion sometime in his practice. It is impossible to determine how many
have allowed their sympathy toward a patient, who did not want the
pregnancy, to overrule the medical and legal ethics of the situation.

Table 71. Agent Inducing Illegal Abortion
Reported by White Non-Prison Females and Males

AGENT	FEMALE REPORT			MALE REPORT
	Operative	Drug	Operative and drug	Operative and drug
	Per cent			Per cent
Herself	2.5	54.0	9.5	7.9
Physician	91.2	38.0	84.0	86.7
Other	6.3	8.0	6.5	5.4
Total	100.0	100.0	100.0	100.0
Number abortions, known agent	320	50	370	240
Number abortions, unknown agent	613	45	658	506

The agent who induced the abortion was reported in a total of 96
cases for the Negro females and white and Negro prison females. In
29 of these cases (30 per cent) the abortion was reported as being
self-induced. This is to be expected, since the largest percentage of
these abortions was by use of drugs and we noted above that the
prison and Negro women reported a greater use of drugs for abortion.

Although in the course of taking sex histories we have acquired as
subjects several practicing abortionists, and have secured supplemen-
tary data on their practice of abortion, we do not have a wide enough
sample to generalize about them as a group. In the limited number of
professional abortion specialists interviewed we have been impressed
with their technical ability and the low number of deaths and ill effects resulting from their operations.[31] We have also been impressed

---

[31] For similar evaluation of the more skilled professional abortionists see Rongy
1933:134-135; Dickinson's discussion in Taylor 1944:50; Amen Report acc.
Human Fertil. 1941:185; Guttmacher in Fishbein and Burgess 1947:216; and
Planned Parenthood 1955 Abortion Conference, Calderone 1958.

with their obvious concern, in most cases, over the plight of a woman with an unwanted pregnancy. One abortion specialist, for instance, who had considerable evidence to support his claim that he had performed 30,000 abortions without a single death in the course of his medical practice, attempted to hire a psychiatric social worker to counsel prospective abortion patients on the social and emotional aspects of their problem. This attempt met with failure because of his inability to find a trained person who was willing to become associated with him in his illegal practice. To be sure, the profit motive is also present, as the practice of inducing illegal abortion is a lucrative one, but the particular abortionists who consented to be interviewed had a much higher quality of surgical and medical technique than much of the literature would lead one to expect.[32]

It would be invaluable to secure the histories of a goodly sample of abortionists to acquire a better understanding of their procedures and problems. Very few of them keep records because of the legal danger of doing so, but an accumulation of such records would be of considerable importance to an understanding of this social and medical phenomenon.

PRICE OF ILLEGAL ABORTION

Illegally induced abortions may cost from nothing to several thousands of dollars, depending on who is performing them and who is paying the bills. As with other illegal services, there is no fixed price, even in a given locality; the cost usually varies directly with the degree to which the abortion law is enforced and inversely with the availability of abortionists. Some abortionists have a fixed minimum price but will attempt to charge as much more as the particular exigencies of the situation will allow. Most persons seeking an illegal abortion have compelling reasons for wanting it and are emotionally so upset over the unwanted pregnancy that price is of secondary consideration. Hence the practitioner is able to charge more under these circumstances than he might otherwise.

For our total sample of white non-prison females, 11 per cent of the illegally induced operative abortions were secured without cost (Table 72). If we divided the sample by marital status, we find that the single females were able to secure only 6 per cent of their abortions free, whereas the married and previously married females se-

---

[32] For typical horror stories of abortion mills see: Child 1931 (orig. 1922):155; Pugh 1935:650 ff.; Pemberton 1955 (orig. 1948):162. Bromley and Britten 1938:262-266 give a more balanced picture including both the less trying and the more sordid sides of actual abortion experiences as reported by college students.

cured 16 per cent of their abortions for nothing. Only 14 per cent of the 58 induced operative abortions secured without cost were self-induced. The rest were usually performed by husbands, other relatives, and friends. Because of the fairly large number of histories we have from women connected with the medical profession (such as nurses, technicians, and physicians' wives) we may have an unduly

Table 72. Price of Illegally Induced Operative Abortion

Reported by White Non-Prison Females

By Marital Status at Event

By Educational Level

PRICE	Total	Marital status			Educational level			
		Pre-marital	Marital	Pre-viously married	0–8	9–12	13–16	17+
	Per cent	*Per cent*			*Per cent.*			
None	11.3	5.5	16.3	15.5	*0*	7.6	14.2	10.8
$ 1–25	7.0	4.7	10.0	5.6	*11.8*	5.0	5.4	10.8
26–50	21.0	23.9	21.5	9.9	*35.2*	26.0	20.4	15.8
51–75	12.2	14.0	10.0	12.7	*29.4*	7.6	10.8	16.6
76–100	15.5	14.9	15.8	16.9	*11.8*	18.5	14.6	15.1
101–150	11.1	11.9	10.0	11.3	*5.9*	12.6	9.2	13.7
151–200	8.5	9.4	9.1	4.2	*5.9*	11.8	10.4	2.9
201–300	8.0	8.9	5.3	12.7	*0*	6.7	7.9	10.0
301–400	2.1	2.1	0.5	7.0	*0*	2.5	2.1	2.2
401–500	2.1	2.6	1.0	4.2	*0*	1.7	3.3	0.7
501+	1.2	2.1	0.5	0	*0*	0	1.7	1.4
Total known	100.0	100.0	100.0	100.0	100.0	100.0	100.0	100.0
Number known	515	235	209	71	*17*	119	240	139
Number unknown	418	77	302	39	48	122	145	103
Median*	$83	$84	$77	$98	*$56*	$87	$87	$79

*Median of those who paid.

large percentage of cases in which the abortion was secured without cost. For the rest of the tabulations made on price of abortion we have omitted the free abortions and included only those for which actual payment was made. We feel this gives a better picture of the true market price of illegal operative abortion.

The median amount paid for an illegal operative abortion was $84 for the single female, $77 for the married female, and $98 for the previously married female (Table 72).[33] The lower price for abortion

---

[33] Among other sources citing specific amounts charged for performing an illegal abortion are the following:

Wisconsin Legislative Committee 1914:137, 145-146 ($50 to $100 cited

Table 73. **Price of Illegally Induced Operative Abortion**
Reported by White Non-Prison Females
By Age at Outcome
By Year of Abortion

	FEMALE REPORT					
	Age at outcome			Year of abortion		
PRICE				Before		
	−20	21–30	31+	1930	1930's†	1940's†
	Per cent			Per cent		
None	6.4	10.7	20.4	11.4	10.9	11.9
$ 1–25	9.2	6.1	7.7	8.6	8.6	4.0
26–50	24.8	22.3	10.3	31.4	25.9	10.2
51–75	13.8	12.2	10.3	5.7	15.4	8.0
76–100	13.8	15.5	17.9	22.9	17.1	11.4
101–150	15.6	9.8	10.3	8.6	10.5	12.5
151–200	8.2	10.1	2.6	8.6	5.3	14.2
201–300	5.5	7.9	11.5	2.8	3.9	15.9
301–400	0	2.4	3.8	0	0.7	5.1
401–500	2.7	1.8	2.6	0	1.0	4.5
501+	0	1.2	2.6	0	0.7	2.3
Total known	100.0	100.0	100.0	100.0	100.0	100.0
Number known	109	328	78	35	304	176
Number unknown	69	247	102	119	239	60
Median*	$75	$83	$93	$76	$67	$143

Median of those who paid.
These dates can be only approximations because of the way the data were trans-
ferred to punched cards. Actually, a few abortions in the second group occurred
as early as 1921 and a few as late as 1944. However, the great majority occurred
in the 1930's. Likewise, in the third group, a few occurred as early as 1936.

several times as current price in Wisconsin cities in testimony at the White
Slave Traffic hearings).

Grotjahn 1921:52 (customary charge of $10 to a laborer's wife in New
York City according to this early German report).

Stix 1935:361 (from $2 to $200, with an average of $60 in New York
City).

Time, Oct. 19, 1936:71 (from $35, if woman is six weeks pregnant, to
$300, if pregnancy has advanced to seven months, charged by California
abortion chain).

Bromley and Britten 1938:262-267 (from $35 to $250 in six cases reported
by college students).

Time, July 28, 1941:60 (prices ranging from $60 to $500, charged by professional abortionist).

Time, March 6, 1944:60 ($100 in single case in New York City).

Tietze 1949:60 (from $300 to $500 charged by physicians in an eastern
city).

Rolph 1955:98 (£20 paid by a British prostitute for an abortion in
London).

paid by the married may reflect their less concern over the outcome of the pregnancy. The married woman may not want the child, but knows that at least she will not suffer social disapproval if she does have it. Hence she is in a somewhat better bargaining position with the abortionist when it comes to arranging for the cost of the abortion. The higher rate for abortion paid by the previously married woman is probably related to her somewhat older age as well as to her marital status.

The cost of induced abortions also varies with the education of the woman. Our few cases of grade school educated women indicated that they paid only about half as much for their abortions as did the better educated women. High school, college, and postgraduate educated women paid approximately the same amounts for their abortions (Table 72).

Females over thirty-one years of age tend to pay more for abortions than females who are younger. The median amounts are $93 versus $75 (Table 73). One may assume that older women have somewhat more money than younger women and therefore are able to pay more.

It must be remembered that the abortions reported by our sample of women occurred throughout the first half of this century. Inasmuch as we experienced a considerable variation in the purchasing power of the dollar during this period of time, it is of interest to determine whether the price of abortion also fluctuated proportionately. In classifying the abortion cost data in a time series we find that abortions secured up to 1929 averaged $76, abortions secured primarily in the depression years of the 1930's averaged $67, and abortions secured in the 1940's averaged $143 (Table 73).[34] This rise is consistent for all marital classifications. Although part of it may well be due to increased enforcement against abortion practices, it is also true that abortion, like all other services and commodities, is subject to inflation.

The males in our sample were asked the amounts that they contributed toward the cost of abortions of pregnancies for which they were responsible. The median amount paid by the male was $62, as compared with $83, which is the median price reported by the female. In some cases the male was unaware of the pregnancy, as we found from our female histories. In other cases he refused to pay even though he did know of it. The female or one of her relatives usually then paid

---

[34] The increasing cost of obtaining an illegal abortion was also pointed out by Timanus, who contrasted the costs in the "early days" ranging from $25 to $100, with the $150 and $200 charges in "later years," and by Kleegman, who stated that charges in New York City had risen from $300 to $1,000 or $1,500 per abortion. See Planned Parenthood 1955 Abortion Conference, Calderone 1958.

the bill. In a very few cases among the married women the husband himself was unaware of the abortion, although even in these cases he probably paid for it indirectly.

It has been possible to analyze abortion costs for three other groups of females: Negro, white prison, and Negro prison groups. These three classifications were withheld from our total sample because it was believed they were select groups that did not fairly represent the total population. It is of interest, however, to see how costs of illegal operative abortions compare among these three special groups. Although the median price of abortion was $83 for the white non-prison part of our sample (Table 72), it was only about $45 for the Negro non-prison sample and for the prison samples of whites and Negroes taken as a whole.[35] The prices reported for these three groups are based on a total of only 89 cases, however, and can be considered only a very rough approximation. The low price reflects the lower socio-economic constitution of these samples. Table 72 indicates that the white non-prison females who did not go beyond eighth grade paid an average of only $56 for their abortions.

CONSEQUENCES OF INDUCED ABORTION

The literature is replete with statements about the horrors of illegally induced abortions. Vivid word pictures are painted concerning the unsanitary conditions, possibilities of infection, subsequent sterility, guilt, shame, and even death that inevitably follow such a heinous act.[36] Usually the unfavorable sequelae of abortion are em-

---

[35] Timanus at the Planned Parenthood 1955 Conference on Abortion similarly described the variation in the charges for abortion to persons of different income levels, citing a range from $25 to $100 in "early days." See Calderone 1958.

[36] The following are some typical statements of the disastrous results likely to follow an illegally induced abortion:

Popenoe 1946:212, " . . . death-rate is many times that of normal childbirth, and it may result in lifelong infection, in sterility, or in a partial unsexing of the woman due to the disturbance of her endocrine glands."

Christensen 1950:155, ". . . both life and health are endangered. It is estimated that some ten thousand women in this country lose their lives each year through this practice. Many others suffer long periods of illness or have their health permanently impaired. . . . Often just the emotional upset surrounding this experience is sufficient to cause a nervous breakdown or to incline one toward frigidity."

Skidmore and Cannon 1951:316, "Abortion . . . is . . . unreliable, and dangerous. . . . Many a prospective mother loses her life in the crude, unsanitary, unsafe practice of illegal abortion with or without the aid of medical practitioners. If she escapes infection and death, she may suffer sterility or infertility."

Koos 1953:203, "Infection—possibly followed by sterility, chronic illness, or (in extreme cases) death—is likely to result because of the circumstances under which such operations are performed."

phasized as a means of frightening persons from having pre-marital intercourse, just as are the horrors of venereal diseases.

The extreme concern over the practice of illegal abortion during the past twenty-five years was apparently triggered by the 1930 League of Nations Report that pointed out the degree to which abortion contributed to maternal mortality rates. Since the over-all death rates from puerperal causes had been shrinking, it was natural that abortion, especially illegal abortion, should receive attention in the effort to further reduce maternal mortality. Figures cited in the 1930's and 1940's usually attribute 20 to 30 per cent of all maternal mortality to abortion, with illegal abortion bearing the brunt of the responsibility.[37]

Figures on the mortality of illegally induced abortions must, for obvious reasons, be secured from other studies.[38] We have interviewed no one who has died from an abortion! Nor have we interviewed any male whose partner died from an abortion. However, we do have in-

---

Drummond 1953:256, "The risk to health and life incident to the performance of an illegal abortion is regarded by physicians as far more grave than the commission of the crime itself. . . . Frequently also the women . . . are rendered absolutely sterile. . . . "

Bowman 1954:486, ". . . it is still a killer of considerable magnitude. . . . other results which over a longer period may affect the mother's health or her ability to bear children normally. Infertility is very common. . . . "

Gordon in Becker and Hill 1955:336, "The dangers of induced or 'criminal' abortion cannot be too strongly stated." The author follows this statement with the observation that "the enormous development of antibiotic therapy during the past decade . . . has eased somewhat the extreme anxiety concerning septic complications of abortions induced by instrumentation and has significantly brightened the outlook for victims of these misfortunes."

Pemberton 1955:162, "There is all likelihood of infection. . . . The chances thus taken add up to possible quick death right there, permanent invalidism, or complete sterility."

---

[37] See, for example, Holmes et al. 1929:1440; U.S. Dept. Labor, Children's Bureau 1934:103 (25 per cent for 15 states); Dunn in Taylor 1944:14 (a higher estimate of 30 to 35 per cent for all United States); Newberger 1946:378 (19 per cent in Illinois hospitals).

[38] An inspection of 16 studies of fatality rates in abortion cases admitted to hospitals shows a range from 0.35 per cent (Galloway and Paul 1939:251, Evanston, Ill. hospital, 15-year period, 1,114 cases) to 1.9 per cent (Simons 1939:845, Minneapolis General Hospital, 1896-1934, 1,000 cases). Since the more serious cases are the ones that are hospitalized, these death rates cannot, of course, be considered as applying to abortions in general. Tietze 1948 showed a steady decrease in deaths associated with abortions, 1927-1945, based on vital statistics data. Since this summary the figures have dropped considerably. For 1953 the total for the country was 294, and for 1954 it was reported as 287. See U.S. Vital Statistics, Special Reports, 1955: Vol. 42, No. 12, p. 275, and 1956: Vol. 44, No. 14, p. 321.

Mrs. Dorothy Thurtle, in a minority report of the 1939 British Ministry of Health Abortion Committee (see pp. 139 ff.), supported the view, based on British government figures, that abortion in poor circumstances showed no higher mortality than birth in good.

formation on the presence or absence of other unfavorable consequences in 43 per cent of our female sample as well as in an additional
38 per cent of the abortions of pregnancies for which the males reported being responsible.

Table 74. Unfavorable Consequences of Illegal Operative Abortion

Reported by White Non-Prison Females and Males

By Marital Status at Event

| UNFAVORABLE CONSEQUENCES | FEMALE REPORT | | | | MALE REPORT |
	Pre-marital	Marital	Post-marital	Total	Total
	Per cent				*Per cent*
None	67.7	81.8	78.4	74.2	86.6
Mild physical	4.1	2.0	2.7	3.2	3.2
Moderate physical	7.7	5.4	6.8	6.8	2.5
Severe physical	6.4	6.8	6.8	6.6	2.8
Psychological	13.6	4.1	5.4	9.0	4.2
Social	3.6	0	0	1.8	1.1
Legal	0	0	0	0	0
Total	103.1	100.1	100.1	101.6	100.4
Number abortions, consequences known	220	148	74	442	283
Number abortions, consequences unknown	92	363	36	491	406

It should be pointed out here that the "unknowns" total 62 per cent
of the cases because questions concerning sequelae of abortions were
not added until later in the research. Because of the way the histories
were taken the great percentage of these unknown cases would show
no unfavorable consequences. If the women (in the instances where
the question was not specifically asked) volunteered the information
that the consequences had been unfavorable, their answers were recorded. But they would be much less apt to mention the subject if
there were no unfavorable result. Hence we believe that if all women
had been routinely asked this question, the percentage of unfavorable
consequences would have been considerably lower than is indicated
in Table 74.

About three fourths of the white non-prison women on whom we
have data indicated that there were no unfavorable consequences of
the abortion.[39] Among single women about two thirds reported no

[39] Only a few other studies present data on complications in induced abortion on
   any wide sample, since most such material is drawn from medical descriptions
   of hospital cases, which would be nontypical.
   Stix 1935:362 showed complications in 14 per cent of 686 illegally induced

unfavorable results, whereas among married women 82 per cent so
reported.[40] Males reported an even higher percentage (87 per cent)
of the aborted women whom they made pregnant as having had no
unfavorable sequelae from the abortion.

About 16 per cent of the women reported an unfavorable physical
aftermath to abortion. Such sequelae were defined as follows: the
classification of mildly unfavorable was made if there was a history
of bleeding, cramps, temporary menstrual difficulties, or if it was
necessary to go to the hospital for a day or two; moderately unfavorable if there was a history of severer bleeding or cramping for a longer
period of time, some infection, more than temporary menstrual difficulty, and if it was necessary to go to the hospital for several days;
severely unfavorable if there was a history of septicemia, peritonitis,
other serious infections, a long hospital stay, invalidism, or a record
of almost dying. A slightly higher percentage of single women reported such unfavorable effects than married women. The smaller
percentage of mildly unfavorable physical effects as compared to the
moderate and severe ones may be the result of failure to report
the milder consequences as not being worth mentioning; or it may be
the result of classification.

The question has often been raised of the likelihood of subsequent

---

abortions reported by clients of a New York City birth control clinic. Complications were reported in only 9 per cent of those done by physicians, but in
76 per cent of the self-induced ones, and in 14 per cent of those induced by
midwives.

Evans in Van Hoosen 1938:58 showed 3.4 per cent with fever among 280
cases of abortion in a British sample.

Brunner and Newton 1939:89 showed immediate complications (fever,
bleeding) in 12 per cent of 1,216 induced abortions reported in 4,500 case
histories at the New York University College Clinic.

Brunner 1941:174 showed less than 10 per cent incidence of any type of
morbidity except bed confinement (36 per cent) in 475 induced abortions.

Dickinson in a discussion at the 1942 Abortion Conference pointed out that
considering the large number of induced abortion cases with no aftercare,
"the relative and extraordinary absence of after-troubles is most remarkable."
See Taylor 1944:50.

[40] That complications are more usual among single women was confirmed in Davis
1950:123, who in a hospital study showed 14 per cent severe complications
for single women, and only 6 per cent for married. He suggested that the
answer lay in the combination of several factors including "inexperience,
isolation, and desperate nature of their predicament." It is also evident that
a selective factor would be operating here since single females would be more
likely to delay hospitalization until their condition was more severe.

Østergaard 1949:3 also found more febrile cases among single women
hospitalized for abortion cases in Denmark.

Dr. Milton Helpern, chief medical examiner of New York City, in his discussion of the illegal abortion problem at the Planned Parenthood 1955
Abortion Conference pointed out that single women are peculiarly exposed
to bad abortion techniques. See Calderone 1958.

sterility following induced abortion.[41] An analysis was made of our data on this point by a special study of our white non-prison women who had been married for the full five years between ages twenty-six and thirty. This group was divided into those who had had an induced abortion prior to age twenty-six and those who had conceived but had not had an induced abortion before twenty-six. All women who had no conceptions up to age twenty-six were omitted from this calculation.

There were 389 females who had conceived before age twenty-six and who had been married continuously from twenty-six to thirty. Of these 389 females, 26.7 per cent (104) had had an induced abortion, and 73.3 per cent (285) had conceived but had had no induced abortion.

Not only was the percentage conceiving between twenty-six and thirty almost identical (74.0 versus 75.8 per cent), but also the rate at which they became pregnant was almost the same. The conception rate for those with prior induced abortions was 26.9 per hundred marital years, and the conception rate for those with no prior induced abortions was 24.5 per hundred marital years. This identity prevailed when live birth rates between ages twenty-six and thirty were also

---

[41] Concern over sterility subsequent to induced abortion is expressed in many sources. See, for example, Davis 1923:119; Rubin 1931:213-214; Child 1931: 154; Taussig 1936:274; and Taussig in Taylor 1944:40-42. Adair, joining in the discussion at the 1942 Abortion Conference, stated, "a good many of these abortion cases are subsequently sterile." (Taylor 1944:37). There has, however, been a lack of adequate data on the subject.

The study of Rubin 1931 is often cited as authority for the fact of high incidence of later sterility in induced abortion cases. Actually, this study is based entirely on a sample of sterile women, and his investigation was concerned with the relative frequency of tubal occlusion in various categories of his sterile cases. He concluded that sterility was more frequently due to tubal occlusion in sterile women who have had a previous induced abortion than it was in women whose sterility had been preceded by either a spontaneous abortion, a previous live birth, or no pregnancy (primary sterility). After citing this work, Meaker 1934-47 pointed out that it was remarkable how severe some inflammations of the post-abortal type may be without destroying tubal function.

Rosen 1954:178 in a detailed footnote differed with Manfred Guttmacher and Taussig on their interpretation of the significance of the early Russian findings on unfavorable after-effects (including sterility) of induced therapeutic abortion.

The following studies, based on women who had undergone therapeutic abortions, have reported on the extent of subsequent involuntary sterility: Vögel 1928:191-197 (U.S.S.R. data on over 2,500 cases, total fertility same as that of the control group); Svanberg 1949:1265 (2 per cent involuntary sterility among 174 Swedish cases); Ekblad 1955:235 (1 per cent involuntary sterility among 479 Swedish cases); Mehlan 1956a:876 ff. (1 to 2 per cent among 253 cases in East Germany). One of the problems of therapeutic abortion as it is practiced in Sweden and Japan is, in fact, a second unwanted pregnancy following a legalized abortion.

compared: a live birth rate of 15.6 for those with induced abortions as against 16.8 for those without induced abortions. Hence our data would indicate that having an induced abortion before twenty-six does not lower the ability to conceive or to have live birth in women between ages twenty-six and thirty.

Social consequences of an unfavorable nature were reported only by the single females, and here in little more than 3 per cent of the cases. Their difficulties consisted of such things as gossip about the abortion, family rejection, a loss of friends, having to leave school, and subsequent difficulty in marriage over the abortion. Although each of these is serious enough, the low percentage of women adversely affected is a testimonial to the secret nature of abortion. This is true both of our samples of white and Negro males and females and of our samples of prison males and females. Although court records are certainly available concerning fines and imprisonment for having secured or being an accessory to an illegally induced abortion, it is of some note to record that in our entire sample of 18,000 male and female histories we did not secure a single such case.

Much has been said concerning the psychological trauma resulting from having an induced abortion, and in recent years there seems to have been an increased concern about this possible after-effect. This was perhaps related to the increasing use of the psychiatric indication for therapeutic abortion in the 1940's; this in turn led to a weighing of the psychic ill effects of continuing the pregnancy against the psychologic trauma that might result from the therapeutic abortion itself.[42] As post-abortional medical techniques and care have improved, it appears that the emotional side effects are considered by many authorities to be the most injurious feature of an induced abortion. Some psychiatrists in fact have argued that women must inevitably be upset by terminating a life that they have started.[43] Abortion is considered murder in some systems of law and philosophy, yet less than 10 per cent of the females in the present sample reported psychological upset over their induced abortions.[44] In most cases this

---

[42] For example see Taussig 1936:276 and Rosen 1954:240 ff.

[43] Among the psychiatrically oriented writers such statements as the following are found:

Cenac 1939 acc. Taussig in Taylor 1944:45, "Should an abortion be produced, the woman is left psychically wounded. . . ."

Coghill 1941:686, "All of these women [clinic cases] . . . have guilt feelings in regard to abortions."

Deutsch 1945 (2):183, " . . . interruption of [unwanted pregnancies] must constitute a trauma regardless of reality."

[44] Among the authors who, with varying results, have investigated the problem of psychologic trauma following induced abortion are the following:

was given in general terms, e.g., they were emotionally upset or, in a smaller number of cases, they were depressed or had guilty feelings. A few said they were nervous for some time after the abortion. One regretted a subsequent sterility, one almost committed suicide, one reported that it affected her subsequent sexual relations adversely, another that she was "ruined mentally." Hence although in the great majority of cases there appears to be little psychological trauma,[45] a considerable amount of unfavorable reaction does show up in a few cases. As might be expected, women married at the time of abortion showed less of the psychological after-effects than the single fe-

---

Taussig 1936:376 cited a few case histories of known psychoses following induced abortion, but made no estimate as to the general incidence of such consequences.

Hamilton 1940:925 in a sample at Bellevue found 8 to 9 per cent of induced abortion patients expressing remorse or fright and 23 per cent expressing regret. The fact that these interviews were held largely within 24 hours of hospital admission must be taken into account.

Siegfried 1951 acc. Ekblad 1955:23 reported over half of 61 Swiss women who had been artificially aborted as showing slight remorse, guilt feelings, unpleasant memories, or conflict about the operation, while 13 per cent showed definitely unfavorable psychologic sequelae.

Sjövall 1953:84 described the phenomenon of increased guilt feelings following an induced abortion as he had observed it in his clinical work among Swedish women, particularly if they were already upset over marital problems. This suggests the type of case that might be likely to show psychological trauma.

Ekblad 1955 has provided the most comprehensive follow-up study of psychologic after-effects of induced abortion, based also on Swedish therapeutic cases. He reported 14 per cent experiencing mild self-reproach and 11 per cent serious self-reproach (see pp. 168-218). Since these cases had all been referred on psychiatric grounds, they would tend to include a less stable type of personality.

Dr. Bard Brekke at the Planned Parenthood 1955 Abortion Conference (Calderone 1958) reported a 2 per cent unfavorable psychologic reaction in 88 cases of therapeutic abortion studied in Norway. He contrasted this with the 1951 Swedish study by Malmfors, which reported over half of 84 cases as dissatisfied.

Mehlan 1956a:876 ff. reported 10 per cent of 243 women expressing regret following a legal induced abortion in East Germany. Eighty per cent of the abortions in the total sample had been granted on social indications.

---

[45] The present findings concur with the general viewpoint expressed by Mandy in Rosen 1954:291-292, who stated that he saw little evidence in his obstetrical experience to justify the exaggerated warnings of psychiatrists as to the frequency of serious depressions following induced abortions. "We have seen in our clinic," he wrote, "a number of patients who admitted to as many as 15 or 20 self-induced abortions without any evidence of guilt or serious depression consequent to these acts." Up to that time no attempt had been made, he pointed out, to gather data on the thousands of women who had one or more induced abortions without suffering any ill effects. Rosen and Lidz expressed the same general point of view at the Planned Parenthood 1955 Abortion Conference, see Calderone 1958.

males, with the previously married women falling between them.

Several other methods were used in attempting to weigh the traumatic effect of pre-marital induced abortion. It might be reasoned, for instance, that girls who have a pre-marital induced abortion might discontinue pre-marital intercourse because of fear of another pregnancy, if the experience of the abortion were as horrible as some of the descriptions in the literature might lead one to believe. When we examine our data we find that of 235 females who had a pre-marital induced abortion, 211, or 90 per cent, continued pre-marital intercourse after the abortion. However, 9 of these 211 females delayed pre-marital coitus for three or more years after the abortion. Only

Table 75. **Percentage of Marital Coitus Leading to Orgasm**

For White Non-Prison Females with Pre-
Marital Coitus

By Pre-Marital Abortion Experience

PER CENT MARITAL COITUS WITH ORGASM FIRST YEAR OF MARRIAGE	FEMALES WITH PRE-MARITAL COITUS	
	Without pre-marital abortion	With pre-marital abortion
	Per cent	
0	24.1	15.8
1– 29	10.9	12.3
30– 59	13.5	11.6
60– 89	11.2	13.7
90–100	40.3	46.6
Total	100.0	100.0
Number of females	936	146

8 females, or 3.4 per cent, stopped pre-marital coitus after the abortion. In 5 of these cases there had been a limited amount of intercourse before the abortion (four times or less), in one case there had been intercourse ten times, and in the other 2 cases the women married very shortly after the abortion. In the 16 cases (7 per cent) in which it was unknown whether intercourse had continued after the abortion, either a marriage took place or the history was taken within that year. Hence our data seem to indicate that having a pre-marital induced abortion had not deterred the female from continuing with pre-marital coitus in the great majority of cases.

Another approach to the question of the effect of a pre-marital induced abortion is to tabulate the percentage of orgasm in marital coitus experienced by women who had and did not have an abortion. Here again one might reason that the traumatic effect of an abortion before marriage would hinder the woman from responding as well in marital coitus, particularly in the early days of marriage. The following table compares percentages of orgasm in the first year of marital coitus for those who had had intercourse but no abortion before marriage with those who did have a pre-marital abortion.

From Table 75 we see that 24 per cent of the women who had coitus but no abortion before marriage had no orgasm in the first year of marital intercourse, whereas only 16 per cent of the women who had had a pre-marital abortion had no orgasm in the first year of marital intercourse. It also shows that a lower percentage of the females without pre-marital abortion (40 per cent) had orgasm always or almost always in the first year of marital coitus than did the females with an abortion before marriage (47 per cent). It is probable that females who had an induced abortion before marriage had a somewhat higher frequency of pre-marital coitus than those without such experience, but this factor could not be controlled in this comparison. Again it would seem that a pre-marital induced abortion did not affect adversely the sexual adjustment in marriage as measured by the rate of orgasm in the first year of marital intercourse.

A third measure of the traumatic effect of a pre-marital abortion can be obtained by ascertaining the percentage of pre-marital induced abortion among the females whose first marriages held together as against the percentage for those whose marriages broke up. Table 22 gives these percentages. It is found that for women aged thirty-six and older at report, 6.9 per cent of the ever-S.D.W. women had had a pre-marital abortion, whereas 8.2 per cent of the married-once, still married women had had such an abortion. There is no evidence in these data to suggest that a pre-marital induced abortion is sufficiently traumatic to the woman to lead to the breakup of a subsequent marriage.

SUMMARY

Although there are laws against non-therapeutic induced abortions in all 48 states of the Union, these laws have been only sporadically enforced, with much ambivalence in the minds of law enforcement officers and the public concerning their usefulness.

The greatest percentage (91 per cent) of the illegal operative abortions for our white non-prison sample were operative. Nearly 10 per cent were reported as the result of taking drugs, but it is felt that in reality even this low figure is misleadingly high, because in some of these instances the women would have had a spontaneous abortion in any case. Almost never was a deliberate physical injury reported as inducing an abortion. A smaller percentage (two thirds to three fourths) of white prison women and Negro non-prison and prison women reported their abortions were by operative techniques.

"Physicians" accounted for about 85 per cent of the abortions in our white non-prison sample, although in some of these cases the "physician" did not have a medical license. Although operative techniques were reported to have been used in over 90 per cent of our white non-prison sample, they were reported in only 72 per cent of the white prison sample, 79 per cent of Negro non-prison, and 65 per cent of the Negro prison females.

Therapeutic abortions comprised 6.4 per cent of all abortions in our sample, and amounted to 2.8 per cent of the number of live births. The marital status of the woman appeared to have little or no relation to her chances of securing a therapeutic abortion.

Prices for abortion ranged from nothing to several thousand dollars. Eleven per cent of the illegal operative abortions of the white non-prison sample were free. For those who did pay, the median amount paid was $84 for the single female and $77 for the married female. Older women tended to pay more for their abortions than did younger women. For those thirty-one years of age and older the median price was $93, whereas for those under thirty-one the median price was only $75.

Abortions, like many other services, are becoming more expensive. The median price paid was $76 for the abortions secured before 1929, $67 for the depression years of the 1930's, and $143 for abortions secured in the 1940's.

Abortion costs vary with education. Grade school educated females paid about half as much for their abortions as did the better educated groups.

There is a considerable quantity of material in the literature concerning the horrors of abortions and their deleterious consequences. Our own data show that in three fourths of the white non-prison cases there were no unfavorable sequelae of any sort reported. Among single women about two thirds reported no unfavorable results, whereas among married women 82 per cent reported none. Three per cent reported mild physical difficulties, 7 per cent moderate, and 7 per cent severe physical difficulties. Nine per cent reported unfavorable psychological sequelae. Nearly 4 per cent of the single females reported unfavorable social sequelae, but none were reported by the married women. There were no legal complications from securing illegal abortions reported by any of our female or male subjects.

An attempt was made to determine the amount of sterility resulting from illegal abortions. Women married for a full five years between ages twenty-six and thirty were divided into those who had an abortion before age twenty-six and those who had conceived but had no abortions before this age. The percentage who conceived and the rates of conception of these two groups between ages twenty-six and thirty were almost identical.

It was found that females in our sample who had a pre-marital induced abortion stopped pre-marital coitus in only 3.4 per cent of the cases. The data showed that orgasm in the first year of marriage for those who had a pre-marital induced abortion was about the same or a little higher than for those without that experience. It was also found that females with a pre-marital induced abortion became separated, divorced, or widowed slightly less often than those without such an abortion.

IN CONCLUSION

We have provided an analysis of the reproductive histories of the 7,074 women who gave us an account of their sex behavior and reproductive experiences. We have reported the extent of pre-marital pregnancy, pre-marital birth, and pre-marital abortion (spontaneous and induced) among the single women and among the married women during their pre-marital years. In all parts of the sample, but in varying degrees, it was found that the induced abortion of a pre-marital pregnancy was a fairly common event.

Similarly, the pregnancies, births, and abortions during the years of marriage have been presented in statistical form. Here we have found that a much smaller percentage of pregnancies was intentionally aborted. We found, however, that the great majority of all induced abortions stems from pregnancies in marriage. This is because many more married women become pregnant than do single women.

Among both the married and single females, we have explored the importance of age at the time of marriage, of the decade in which the woman was born, of her degree of religious devoutness, and of the extent of her education. All these factors were found to be linked to differences in the pattern of pregnancy and its outcome.

In examining the reproductive experiences of women in our sample who had once married but who, by the time of the interview, had been separated, divorced, or widowed, we found surprisingly high levels of conception outside of marriage, and these in turn led to pregnancy losses similar to those found in the as yet unmarried.

The sexual and reproductive histories provided by Negro females revealed reproductive behavior among single women that was unique in its low incidence of induced abortion in combination with high numbers of spontaneous abortions and births out of wedlock. Similar findings in regard to spontaneous and induced abortions held for the married Negro women. Educational differences were especially marked in this part of our sample.

Three prison samples, studied individually, provided a glimpse of pregnancy, birth, and abortion patterns in a lower socio-economic group, with findings consistent with the broader analysis of the general sample.

The agent who induced the abortion, the method used, and the price range were analyzed. In an attempt to study the adverse side effects of induced abortions on the female, we tabulated the reported physical and psychological after-effects, and also examined the possibility of subsequent sterility and of later sexual maladjustment in marriage as reflected in orgasm capacity. In our sample, ill effects after an induced abortion appear less frequently than had been previously assumed. From a statistical point of view, it can be said that our material gives no evidence of resulting sterility or damage to orgasm capacity.

The social implications of pregnancy, birth and abortion are dependent on a knowledge of the facts themselves, various aspects of which are set forth here for the first time, but a consideration of these broader questions must of necessity be left to others who are specialists in the various fields of the social sciences. We can do no better here than to restate the following words of Dr. Alfred Kinsey, which appeared in the concluding paragraph of *Sexual Behavior in the Human Male:* ". . . we have explored, and we have performed our function when we have published the record of what we have found. . . ."

Appendix

SOME NOTES ON ABORTION PROBLEMS IN OTHER COUNTRIES

While the fact that the legal status of induced abortion varies widely from country to country is of course well known to students of social history, the average person is not aware of these broad contrasts. Some detailed articles on the status of abortion in certain countries outside the United States have been published, but recent general surveys of such material are scarce.[1] For this reason it has seemed worthwhile to draw together from various sources information on the status of induced abortion abroad to provide a background before which our own data and that of other American studies could be placed.

Those countries having the most liberal laws and attitudes concerning abortion naturally provide a greater amount of data than countries such as ours whose laws and attitudes are more restrictive. Since Russia was the earliest experimenter in abortion reform, the sequence of events in that country will be described first.

ABORTION IN THE SOVIET UNION

The course of legalized abortion in the Soviet Union has been a checkered one, and because of two sharp reversals of policy by the government has drawn wide attention. Free legal abortion in government hospitals was inaugurated in the U.S.S.R. in 1920, two years after the Soviet revolution. At the time it was widely publicized as a social reform movement and as part of the general program to emancipate women and to give them equal rights with men by not asking them to bear unwanted children.[2] Another declared aim was to eliminate, or at any rate reduce, the many illegal, clandestine abortions admitted

---

[1] Taussig's 1936 authoritative volume on abortion covered earlier Russian and German material in detail, but chiefly with a medical approach. Tietze 1954, Rosen 1954, Williams 1957, and the Planned Parenthood 1955 Abortion Conference, Calderone 1958, all furnish foreign material but with varying emphasis.

[2] Field 1932:75.

215

to exist[3] and which, according to medical belief, were associated with a high incidence of illness and death.[4] In addition to these ostensible reasons, immediate economic conditions may have been a factor.[5] Smaller families would clearly be advantageous in the shift to an industrialized economy in which the woman was needed primarily in the factory rather than at home. The relative importance of these three underlying purposes is difficult to assess, even in the light of later events.

By the early 1930's the Russian medical literature began suddenly to set forth the undesirable side effects of even legally induced abortions (especially when repeated) upon the fecundity, libido, and general health of the women whose pregnancies had been interrupted.[6] In June 1936, the government shifted its policy in accord with these findings, and therapeutic abortion, except for strict medical indications, was outlawed again. This change of front gave rise to many questions. Most gynecologists in the western world had looked askance at the unorthodox Russian program, and their doubts about its soundness were pleasantly substantiated by this retreat of the Soviet social reformers. There has been some difference of opinion, however, about the reliability and validity of the Russian statistics on the severity of the sequelae of induced abortion.[7] This was understandable since the reports on the shrinking number of illegal abortions, low mortality, slight morbidity, and lack of serious after-effects had been enthusiastic and glowing in the 1920's.[8] There had also been repeated denials

---

[3] Weissenberg acc. Hirsch 1911, for example, reported two thirds of 100 abortions in his private practice at Elizabethgrad, Russia, as induced. See also the article on abortion in Volume 1 of the newly issued Soviet Medical Encyclopaedia, col. 25.

[4] A 50 per cent incidence of infection and 4 per cent mortality was cited in the official decree. See Schlesinger 1949:44.

[5] See the letter of the Soviet Ambassador to Great Britain in J. Obstet. & Gynaec. Brit. Emp. 1939:46:90.

[6] Wide sterility and libido damage, for example, were reported by Kakuschkin in 1934, who also claimed that a "hormone trauma" frequently resulted from interrupting the first pregnancy. (Hodann 1937a:220-223). Naiditch et al. in 1935 reported 26 per cent incidence of pelvic pathology following induced abortion according to J. Contracep. 1936:1:167. A detailed account of similar findings is presented by Taussig 1936:413-415 and Taussig in Taylor 1944: 40-44.

[7] Taussig in Taylor 1944:41; Haire 1947:9; Rosen 1954:178, footnote.

[8] Pasche-Oserski 1929:233 at the 1928 Sexual Reform Congress reported the reduction of criminal abortions by 61 per cent in the cities and 25 per cent in the rural areas in 1924, and a further reduction of 25 per cent in both areas the following year. Gens 1930:147 claimed less than 5 per cent illness after abortion, 1921-1923. Low death rates are cited, for example, by Haro 1934:365; Hodann 1937a:222; and Haire 1947:9. Haro cites a single death in 23,000 abortions and contrasts it with Taussig's figure for U.S. experience, which is 460 times as great. Hodann's figure is .06 deaths per 1,000 for a ten-year

that legal abortions had produced "any material decline" in the birth rate,[9] so that superficially it appeared that it was simply the previously illegal abortions that were now being performed openly in the well regulated government abortaria.[10] Education in birth control methods through public clinics had been promoted during the 16-year period that abortions were legal,[11] and a wide program of maternity aid had also been instituted, including maternity leaves from work, state help for large families, and a broad system of crèches, nursery schools, and kindergartens to aid in the care of children.[12] Thus it might be assumed that the authorities had decided that the time had come for the Russian citizen to put complete dependence on contraception for family limitation.

There are several accounts of visits to the Soviet abortaria by American doctors interested in investigating the Russian abortion problem.[13] They seemed impressed with the simplicity of the arrangements and the "gruesome" efficiency of the clinics, but reported that the doctors involved regarded the operations as a "necessary evil." Although the Soviet doctors were obliged to provide a woman with an abortion if she requested it,[14] they apparently tried to dissuade many of the applicants from carrying out their original intention.[15] This being the

---

period in Moscow. Gens 1930:146 stated flatly, "we do not observe any deaths after abortions performed in hospitals." Hodann 1937a and Haire 1947 both reported low complication rates and no effect on fertility that could be observed. It has been suggested that the practice of discharging the abortion patient from the abortarium a few days after the operation, with any later follow-up care falling upon the regular hospitals, was an important factor in the low incidence of deaths in the official abortarium records.

---

[9] Taussig 1936:362. See also *Soviet Medical Encyclopaedia,* article on abortion, Vol. 1, col. 25.

[10] According to Gens (see Taussig 1936:363) there had been about a 30 per cent increase in total abortions by 1926. This was probably concentrated in the cities and towns. The official abortion rates by 1928 showed abortion as more than equaling births in both Moscow and Leningrad, where between 55 and 60 per cent of all pregnancies were legally terminated. See Tietze 1954:18. The government abortion services were more available to city populations and more used by them, apparently, since decreases in illegal abortion also were less marked in rural districts. See Batkis and Gurwitsch 1929:45. Likewise, Peller 1931:848 showed lower rates of legal abortion for rural areas in the Ukraine based on the Tomilin and Schreider 1927 figures.

[11] Gens 1930:153-154; Field 1932:77; Taussig 1936:408.

[12] See article on abortion in Volume 1 of the *Soviet Medical Encyclopaedia,* col. 25.

[13] Taussig 1931; Taussig in Taylor 1944:53; Stone in the Planned Parenthood 1955 Abortion Conference, Calderone 1958. See also Field 1932:84,94.

[14] This was true providing the pregnancy was of less than three months' duration, and apparently after 1935 if it was not a first pregnancy.

[15] At the time of Mrs. Field's visit to Russia she reported that 20 per cent of all pregnant women were requesting an abortion, and that about half the applications were approved. Field 1932:82,90-92.

case, it may be well that the medical profession carried the day, and that the return to a narrowed program was largely the result of pressures from this source.[16]

On the other hand, there are definite suggestions in the available sources that economic and political motives demanded a cut in abortions so that a higher birth rate could produce a larger labor force and more manpower for a future possible war.[17] If this was the basic thinking, then the publicized medical findings provided a façade for more fundamental reasons that were not openly stated. These possible interpretations are interesting in the light of the newest developments. Nearly twenty years later, in November, 1955, Russia reversed her stand again, and for a second time instituted a broad program of permissive legalized abortion. It is too soon to know what the results of this step will be.[18] At the time of the public announcement official sources stated that the growth of the political conscience and cultural standards of the Russian woman made it possible to abolish the prohibition of abortion. Prevention of abortion could be insured, it was added, by extending the state measures for encouraging motherhood and by further educational work.[19] If this were true, one wonders why the law was changed at all. No mention was made of the improvement in the control of infection by antibiotics, or of the low incidence of complications in the legal abortion program in the Scandinavian countries, but one may suppose that these considerations had also played a role.

ABORTION IN JAPAN

The case of Japan is in some respects similar to the Russian experiment. Japan (and recently Communist China) are the only countries except Russia that have fully legalized abortion in modern times. Abortion has been legal in Japan since 1948. Over 19,000 doctors have been authorized to perform abortion operations, and abortion

---

[16] Extracts from the proceedings of the First Ukrainian Conference of Gynaecologists, Kiev, 1927, give a clear picture of the antagonism of the doctors to legalized abortion. See Schlesinger 1949:174-187. In a footnote the Congress is described as a demonstration against legalized abortion and Schlesinger pointed out that the criticism is more impressive when it is kept in mind that it came from doctors who evidently shared the basic assumptions of the Soviet system (p. 174, footnote 2).

[17] Hodann 1937a:221, footnote by Stella Browne; Haire 1947:9; Guttmacher in Rosen 1954:178; Stone in the Planned Parenthood 1955 Abortion Conference, Calderone 1958.

[18] The New York *Herald Tribune* of October 25, 1956, carried a news story from Russia reporting increased private abortions and the need for more extensive contraceptive education and services.

[19] *New York Times*, Nov. 23, 1955.

facilities have been established in over 800 health centers. Since the Shinto and Buddhist religions are ethically blank on the subject of induced abortion, and since infanticide had in past centuries been an accepted means of family limitation, it has not been difficult for legalized abortion to be readily adopted by the many who need a way to control family size.[20] Programs of sterilization and of more intensive education in contraception were later added with the hope that these would complement and gradually supplant the possibly too extensive use of abortion.[21]

That the abortion law has served as a curb on population increase can be inferred from the fact that the 1956 crude birth rate in Japan was down to 18.5 per thousand, a sharp drop from the 30 per thousand rate of 1937, and even from the 28 per thousand of 1950.[22] Recent government figures show over a million reported legal abortions annually,[23] and it has been estimated that there are an additional million unreported abortions, some by doctors who thus avoid heavy income tax payments, and others by unauthorized persons such as midwives or pharmacists. With 1,746,000 live births reported, the tentative two million abortion figure plus an unknown number of spontaneous abortions would represent well over a 50 per cent loss in all pregnancies.

While the abortion law in Japan is entitled the "Eugenic Protection Law," the immediate reasons given for the abortions are usually economic, medical, or personal, rather than strictly eugenic. One study reported over 80 per cent of a series of 1,382 first abortions requested for economic reasons, the remainder on the grounds of health.[24] A somewhat later survey showed the two reasons, "do not desire children" and "suffering from illness," as of equal weight and accounting for all but 10 per cent of 5,200 requested abortions. Since the decline in fertility in Japan is especially marked among wives over thirty-five, it appears that so far the impact of legalized abortion is largely on higher order births.[25]

It is difficult to get a clear picture of the findings in regard to complications from the various studies reporting abortion cases. One widely quoted study, based on 1,712 legally induced abortions, showed

[20] The low cost of Japanese abortions must also be taken into account. An abortion may be procured at less than the equivalent of $5.00, according to Pommerenke 1955:156, who also points out that the expense may be less than that of a year's supply of contraceptives.

[21] See Muramatsu 1955 and Koya 1957:22-23.

[22] See *U.N. Demographic Yearbook* for 1948 and *U.N. Monthly Bulletin of Statistics*, Oct., 1957, p. 8.

[23] Taeuber 1956:139.

[24] Koya 1954:288.

[25] Nakatsu 1955:234-235.

slight or severe complications in 47 per cent of the cases, with a somewhat higher incidence for second or third abortions.[26] The author comments that this is "much greater than was expected." Another more
recent study of over 5,000 cases authorized by the Mother and Child
Health Section of the Welfare Ministry reported only an 8 per cent
incidence of complications.[27] With such contrasts it is clear that either
criteria or samples vary widely. It may also be that the medical technique and sanitary controls are improving with experience.

The Japanese studies show an interest in the time interval between
an abortion and a subsequent pregnancy. Koya found that of 1,382
women who had had their first abortion, over 20 per cent were pregnant again in six months, and a total of almost 50 per cent within 18
months. Another survey in Kanagawa province showed that among
those who did not use contraception following an induced abortion, 53
per cent became pregnant within a year.[28] While such figures may be
reassuring when concern over subsequent sterility is at issue, they also
show starkly the temporary nature of abortion as a family limiting
device, and reveal the need for repeated operations if fertility is to be
controlled by this method alone.

Some opposition to the Japanese abortion law has been reported
from the start, an increase in opposition to abortion was reported in a
recent public opinion survey, and it is said that the results of the law
have disturbed even those who were originally in favor of it.[29] In
some of the Japanese discussions there seems to be almost a note of
apology to the West that the abortion program in Japan has met with
such docile co-operation by Japanese wives. "Abortion has become so
popular in our country that it is almost a fashion," was the opening
remark of one of the speakers at the Tokyo International Conference
on Planned Parenthood in 1955. The delegate, a doctor in the Public
Health Department, ended with a plea for revision and narrowing of
the abortion law.[30]

In reading the rather lurid description[31] of one nonauthorized abor-

---

[26] Koya 1954:292.

[27] Nakatsu 1955:235.

[28] See Koya 1954:291 and Koguchi 1955:233.

[29] For these various reports see Okasaki 1952:223; Kiser 1956; Burch 1955.

[30] See Koguchi 1955:231. Similar criticism is evident in even such an objective
treatment of the general abortion problem as is found in Williams 1957:236.
He writes only briefly of the Japanese program but refers to the "staggering
number" of abortions and cites the "unhealthy use of abortion as a form of
population control."

[31] This was the lowest grade of the three types of facilities visited by Dr. Pommerenke in Tokyo. No appointments by the patients were necessary, names of
the women were not recorded, the cost of the abortion was fixed by bargaining, and during the short interval while the instruments were bathed

tion clinic in a very poor district visited by an American doctor, one realizes that sheer legislation cannot provide an adequate solution to the abortion problem. Problems of methods, cost, hospital facilities, and public education must still be faced. But, according to Dr. Irene Taeuber, the harm that may be inherent in a legalized abortion in Japan must be balanced against the dangers of a home delivery by an untrained midwife. There is no evidence of an increase in mortality rates and, in fact, the deaths of women in childbearing ages have markedly declined.[32]

Thus it appears that there have been mixed results from the Japanese abortion program. While it has probably helped to reduce the long-range miseries of overpopulation on their already crowded islands, it has created other unsolved problems.

ABORTION IN SWEDEN

Sweden, a country that has led in many experiments in social reform, was in 1938 the first of the Scandinavian governments to legislate an abortion law with broad indications.[33] An official investigation in 1930 had led to the estimate that 10 to 20 per cent of the pregnancies were being illegally aborted.[34] Threat of punishment was held to have only a very slight deterrent effect, since the proportion of discoveries was so low. It was also felt that the stiffening of penalties would in part tend to prevent women who needed medical care following an illegal abortion from seeking it. Following largely the recommendations of the Commission on Abortion made public in 1935, which had by then been studied and discussed for several years, the 1938 law allowed induced abortion for medical, humanitarian, and eugenic reasons. Included with these was a combined medical-social indication, such as would apply to and provide for the "worn out mothers" category.[35]

The rate of legal abortions in the first years that the law was in force was lower than expected and represented less than 1 per cent of the live births by 1944.[36] In 1946, after considerable debate, the terms of

---

in an "'anti-septic' solution," one patient (in street clothes) "crawled off and another patient crawled onto the blood encrusted table." (Pommerenke 1955: 162).

[32] See Dr. Taeuber's remarks at the Planned Parenthood 1955 Abortion Conference, Calderone 1958.

[33] For a more detailed account of the Swedish abortion legislation and its background see Inghe 1947; Gille 1948; and Williams 1957:236-254. The comprehensive study by Ekblad 1955, which has been published in English, includes a full account of the events prior to the 1938 legislation and summarizes many earlier studies.

[34] Gille 1948:33.

[35] Ekblad 1955:10-15.

[36] Westman 1955:236.

the law were broadened to include what is variously described as "presumptive debility," "foreseen weakness," or "anticipated weakness." This term was intended to allow for such future contingencies in the mother's life as the strain of giving birth to and caring for the new child.[37] This modification of the law gave rise to much debate and sharp criticism.[38] Some authorities have argued that this is not "a true medical but, indeed, a true social indication more or less disguised as a medical one."[39] But in 1953, for example, we find that this new indication was used for only 11 per cent of the 4,915 approved abortions, while almost half of them were still granted on the basis of present debility or weakness. Thus this broadened indication apparently has not been applied in any wholesale manner. The total legal abortions rose to a peak of well over 5 per cent of all live births by 1951, but the number has stabilized at the lower figure of between 4 and 5 per cent in the years following.

A legal abortion in Sweden must be done prior to the 20th week of pregnancy save in exceptional circumstances. If the indications for the abortion are eugenic, the Special Committee dealing with abortions of the Royal Medical Board must give permission for the operation (exceptions are made for emergency cases). While abortion requests based on other indications can be passed upon by two doctors, one of whom must be a medical officer, in practice 80 to 90 per cent of these cases are also referred to the Committee for decision. This Committee consists of three persons: a physician, a layman (preferably a woman), and the Royal Medical Board Chief of the Bureau for Social Psychiatry. Their decision is based upon the written material presented to them.[40]

The record of abortions in Sweden showed 46 deaths for the five-year period from 1946 through 1951, during which 28,447 pregnancies

---

[37] Ekblad 1955:17.

[38] Olow 1947 recommended that no law should permit any woman of immoral behavior the right to have an abortion operation as a means of escape from her position. Rönne-Petersen 1951:340 stated that both legislation and practice in applying the abortion law should be much more restrictive. Ask-Upmark 1953:12 asserted that all social and medico-social indications should be prohibited.

It should be pointed out that part of the intention in extending the grounds for legal abortion was to encourage more women who were seeking abortion to apply at the advisory centers or at a doctor's office. In the cases in which there were insufficient grounds for legal abortion, the advisors would thus have an opportunity to have "a social and psychological influence" upon the woman (Gille 1948:40).

[39] Westman 1955:236.

[40] See Geijerstam in Planned Parenthood 1955 Abortion Conference, Calderone 1958.

were legally terminated. The fatality rate for abortion alone was 0.9 per thousand cases, and for induction of abortion in combination with sterilization, it was 3.5 per thousand.[41]

While the first reports seemed to indicate that half the cases of induced abortion had psychiatric after-effects, later more extensive investigations indicate that such effects are less widespread. In a sample of 479 women who had undergone a therapeutic abortion on psychiatric grounds, a follow-up study after a 2 to 3 year period showed that 75 per cent of them experienced no self-reproach, while 14 per cent felt mild self-reproach, and 11 per cent serious self-reproach. In only 1 per cent had the woman's working capacity been impaired, and in these cases there were other contributing factors. It was also shown that the psychically abnormal find it more difficult to stand the stress of a legal abortion, as might be expected.[42] According to Westman, who reported on a preliminary survey at the 1955 Planned Parenthood Conference in Tokyo, physical complications appeared to be rare.[43]

The problem of "recidivism" in applications for legal abortion has received attention in Sweden. Ekblad in his 1955 study reported that 38 per cent of a group of women therapeutically aborted but not sterilized were pregnant again within 2 to 4 years (the large majority of them unintentionally), despite renewed instruction in contraception. A part of these "recidivists" will be allowed to have another abortion, but in many of the cases it will be accompanied by a sterilization operation.[44] Over 25 per cent of all legal abortions in Sweden during 1946–1951 were associated with the radical measure of sterilization.[45] Since the fatality ratio in the double operation was nearly four times as great as it was when only an abortion was performed, this seems a fairly drastic measure to cut the future abortion figure.

The low birth rate in Sweden has been a cause for public concern since the 1930's,[46] and while net reproduction rates moved upward in 1941, the fact that they started a downward swing again in 1946 has given new weight to the problem.[47] There has been a natural apprehension that the legal abortion program was contributing to the lowering of the birth levels, rather than simply replacing the unauthorized operations. An effort has been made to answer this question by asking women who were granted a therapeutic abortion whether they had

---

[41] Westman 1955:237.
[42] Ekblad 1955:168-218.
[43] Westman 1955:237-283.
[44] Ekblad 1955:99-103, 225.
[45] Calculated from figures in Tietze 1955:239, Table 2.
[46] See Swedish Population Commission Report 1940, Part 1.
[47] Data from the 1951 Statistical Yearbook acc. to Kälvesten n.d.:22, 70, Table 8.

previously had an illegal one, by a follow-up of cases in which the abortion request was denied in order to see whether the pregnancy was carried through to term, and by a tabulation of unauthorized abortions requiring hospital care. So far, the results of these investigations do not show any clear-cut evidence of a "noteworthy" reduction in illegal abortion, and it has been claimed by some that the number has been actually increasing. The statement was made that the "termination of pregnancy has become a matter of every-day discussion," and that this has resulted in the population becoming increasingly "abortion minded."[48] One conjecture is that the legal abortion clientele is a group of women quite separate from those who would resort to illegal abortion.[49] If this were the case, it might well be that total abortions have risen.

The Swedish culture is so permissive toward sexual intercourse before marriage that approximately 80 per cent of the women and 90 per cent of the men have such experience.[50] Long engagements and late marriages are typical, the average age of first marriage for women being well over twenty-five. This situation brings about a considerable incidence of pre-marital pregnancy. The proportion of illegitimate births has been as high as 15 per cent of the total births in the 1920's, but it is now about 9 to 10 per cent.[51] It would be of interest to know the exact extent to which the Swedish authorities have used legal abortion in cases of pregnancies of unmarried females, but the figures do not seem to be readily available.[52] It is incorporated in the law that any girl who was under fifteen at the time she became pregnant is permitted abortion freely on "humanitarian" grounds. One series of young girls who had applied for abortion is described by Dr. Kule Palmstierna, chief gynecologist at the General Hospital of Gävle.[53] He reported that during the years 1950–1955, 83 girls, ages fourteen

[48] Westman 1955:236; Ekblad 1955:93.
[49] Ekblad 1955:93-98.
[50] Wikman 1937:17-162 presented wide material on the traditional courting practices in rural Sweden. The Swedish Population Commission Report 1940: 79-86, supplied clear evidence of prevailing liberal sex attitudes. Wangson et al. 1951:104, in the government report on sexual behavior of Swedish youth, provided figures on pre-marital experience. Kälvesten n.d.:23 stated, "sex relations among unmarried persons is and has always been fairly common and as a consequence the rate of births out of wedlock is high compared to other countries."
[51] Swedish Population Commission Report 1940:6-10; Kälvesten, n.d.:27, 72.
[52] In one sample of 479 women with legal abortions for psychiatric indications, 27 per cent were single, 12 per cent separated, widowed, or divorced, and 61 per cent married. See Ekblad 1955:33.
[53] Norrlands-Posten, May 21, 1955 (translation furnished by courtesy of Dr. Palmstierna).

to seventeen, came to the Bureau of Consultation for Sexual Problems and Abortions in order to ask for a legal abortion. Twenty-three of these requests were granted, and the records showed that 17 girls later reported spontaneous abortions. During the same years, 119 unmarried girls of the same ages were delivered at the maternity department of the hospital. If one tentatively combines these figures to make an over-all outcome ratio, it would show 75 per cent of the known pregnancies resulting in live births, 11 per cent in spontaneous abortions, and 14 per cent in legal abortions. These figures suggest that legal abortion is not used very extensively to prevent illegitimate births in Sweden, at least among young girls.

One of the interesting side lights on the abortion policy in Sweden is the role that the National League for Sex Education apparently has played in its development.[54] In 1934, this group adopted a program that included legalization of abortion and sterilization on eugenic, medical, and social grounds. The new abortion law was passed in 1938, and in 1940 the League set up the first institution for social case work for women wishing to terminate pregnancy. State and municipal authorities followed this example, and many such institutions now exist. Elise Ottesen-Jensen, president of the League, stated that "the intensive propaganda carried out by the organization has undoubtedly contributed to the sequence of practical social reforms carried through during the past decade." The impact of such efforts to mold public opinion cannot be measured, but women carrying the torch for a social cause can be a potent force.

ABORTION IN DENMARK

In Denmark, as in other northern European countries, there was an early movement toward reform in the abortion laws. Public concern was clear-cut by 1929, when a petition was submitted to the Danish parliament by a delegation of working women asking for abolition of the penalty for induced abortion.[55] A government commission was set up in 1932 to consider the problem, and in its 1936 report recommended that abortion be permitted on medical, socio-humanitarian, and eugenic grounds.[56]

Meanwhile, wide attention had been drawn to the 1935 trial of Dr. J. H. Leunbach, a Copenhagen physician, who openly did induced

---

[54] See the pamphlet that the League published in 1949 in celebration of its fifteenth anniversary, pp. 14-15, and Mrs. Ottesen-Jensen's address at the 1955 Planned Parenthood Conference in Tokyo, Proceedings, p. 314.

[55] Guyon 1936(4):61.

[56] Cille 1952:178.

abortions with a modified Heiser paste[57] injection upon request of the family physician. Only abortions for the purpose of saving the life of the mother were officially permitted then,[58] but Leunbach claimed that "many medical men refused poverty as an indication for abortion, but readily accepted wealth,"[59] and it appeared that the law had been ignored by many others.[60] Since Leunbach was, in fact, operating a clinic for working class women, it was claimed that he was attacked violently by the conservative press for having broken through a class privilege. His 1935 trial first resulted in acquittal, but later he was sentenced to three months in prison and five years' disqualification as a practicing doctor.[61] His defense pointed out that the three deaths in his 320 cases showed a lower rate than the government hospital record of two deaths in 200 induced abortion cases. But since his paste method was an unorthodox one, he was also accused of culpable neglect.

Following the lead of Sweden by a year, Denmark put into operation in 1939 a law providing for a broad interpretation of therapeutic abortion. The pure socio-economic reasons recommended by the abortion commission were not incorporated into the law, but the medical grounds were wider than those suggested. Thus, a socio-medical indication for interrupting pregnancy was permitted along with the purely medical, ethical, and eugenic reasons. The ethical indication covers pregnancy following certain sex crimes, and the eugenic covers "severe hereditary taint." Later, the terms of the law were further clarified following detailed recommendations of a Ministry of Justice Committee.[62]

Except for the cases with clear medical indications, a board of three members is responsible for passing on an applicant's request for a legal abortion in Denmark today. Two of these are physicians, one of whom must be a psychiatrist, and the third is a representative from the Mothers' Aid organization. Medical indications now being used include a consideration of psychiatric conditions either present or threatening, and of social circumstances if there is no other available

---

[57] Heiser, a chemist in Berlin, had developed a soft soap paste to be used as an abortifacient. Its basic ingredients were iodine and various oils. He is said to have used it in 11,000 cases without a resulting infection prior to his arrest and sentencing to three years in prison. While the method had the advantage that a general practitioner could use it as a home or office procedure, it produced acute cramps, severe bleeding, and was not always effective in bringing about the expulsion of the embryo. See Levy-Lenz 1931:181-182 and Leunbach in Sanger and Stone 1931:184-185.

[58] Gille 1952:178.

[59] Hodann 1937a:232.

[60] Jacobsen 1932:50-52; *Ztschr. f. polit. Psychol. u. Sexualök.* 1935:2:61.

[61] Hodann 1937b:203.

[62] Gille 1952:178; Clemmesen 1956.

solution to the social problem.[63] A report on over 500 cases of authorized abortion[64] revealed that over half of them fell under the psychiatric classification, 20 per cent were for purely medical reasons, 14 per cent were socio-medical, and 11 per cent were on eugenic grounds.

Legal abortions in Denmark have risen markedly since the new law has been in effect, and in some quarters concern has been expressed that its terms have been too liberally interpreted. Vera Skalts, director of the Mothers' Aid organization, has entered the controversy and defended the policy of her staff on recommendations.[65] At present the Mothers' Aid, after investigating the individual cases of the women who request abortions, recommends legal abortions for about two fifths of the applicants. Of the remainder, a check has shown that over 70 per cent complete their pregnancy.[66]

The broadened use of official abortions in Denmark has furnished the opportunity for extensive material in the Danish medical journals on the merits of various techniques of abortion and on treatment and incidence of post-abortal complications.[67] Low mortality figures and a low rate of complications is the typical picture in most of the medical reports.[68]

---

[63] Clemmesen 1956.

[64] Trolle 1950:78.

[65] Gille 1952:179; Hinrichsen 1952; Henningsen, Skalts, and Hoffmeyer, 1952.

[66] Danske Selskab 1957:27.

[67] Oram 1948a covered 38,122 total abortions treated in Danish hospitals during 1940-1946, with detailed material on Aarhus hospital sample. Oram 1948b described medical success of membrane puncture method of abortion. Oram 1949a reported on treatment of 1,823 induced abortion cases covering 1927-1948, no deaths, and three fourths of the cases fever free. Fabricius-Møller and Oram 1951 recommended conservative aftertreatment in illegal abortions, and membrane puncture method for inducing therapeutic abortions. Oram 1951 provided data on 436 legal abortions at Aarhus government hospital, 1928-1950. Fabricius-Møller and Oram 1952 provided further support of recommended method and suggested it as equally effective for ambulant patients. Schou and Østergaard 1954 reported on 200 cases with a new abortifacient, soap-creme.

When the gynecologic and obstetric services of such great metropolitan hospitals as Bellevue and New York Hospital report an average of 15 to 20 therapeutically induced abortions a year—see statements of Kleegman and McLane, Planned Parenthood 1955 Abortion Conference, Calderone 1958— it is evident that the Danish material represents experience with an impressive number of cases.

[68] Fabricius-Møller 1948:813 reported 1,800 cases without a fatality or noteworthy complication.

Oram 1949b:204 compared mortality during 6-year period in total abortion cases (0.17 per cent), with that in maternity cases (0.11 per cent).

Trolle 1950:786, in a series of 556 legally induced abortions, reported 10 per cent with minor and 1 per cent with severe complications, and no deaths.

Oram 1952 pointed out that although legal interruptions of pregnancy had increased during 1940-1950, fatalities decreased. Total mortality for 10-year period was 0.2 per cent, more than half of which was from illegal abortions.

With legal abortions increasing rapidly under the new law to about 5 per cent of all known pregnancies in 1956,[69] the problem of illegal abortions was still a matter of deep concern. The 67 convictions for illegal abortions in 1950,[70] 11 years after the inauguration of the liberalized provisions, reveal that the problem has been only partly solved. As in Sweden, it is thought by some that the permissive legislation has brought a sharp increase in illegal interruptions of pregnancy.[71] The discussion centers in the question of what proportion of all abortions is home treated, and hence not covered in the country-wide hospital statistics, and what proportion of the hospitalized "spontaneous" abortions is genuinely spontaneous.[72] Several writers have pointed out that caution must be used in basing conclusions on a time-series record of hospitalized abortions, since there may be an unknown shift in the attitude of women toward hospitalization for post-abortion care. Likewise, one must reckon with the lowered incidence of spontaneous abortion, if the proportion of induced abortions is sizable. The home-treated cases have been calculated at various figures, from 25 to 50 per cent of hospital cases, and the spontaneous figure has been estimated at from 6 to 10 per cent of all pregnancies. One study ended with a tentative figure of a 77 per cent increase in criminal abortions during the decade 1940-1950.[73] It may well be that the rate has fallen since then, with the increased emphasis on maternal help, contraceptive education, and psychiatric counseling, and with the use of sterilization for women who are unsuited to have further pregnancies.

The survey of Dr. Kirsten Auken on the sexual behavior of Danish women, published in 1953, seems to be the only Danish study with questions on abortion as part of a more general investigation. The material covers 1933-1947, but was gathered largely from 1940 on. Of the entire sample of 315 women, 187 (14 per cent of them single) reported 423 pregnancies, half of them undesired. A total of 13.5 per cent of all pregnancies resulted in abortion: 9.5 per cent spontaneous, 1.4 per cent legally induced, and 2.6 per cent self-induced. The high number of attempted abortions, 11.5 per cent, as against 2.6 per cent successful, provides a striking insight into the behavior of women with unwanted pregnancies.[74] It must be remembered that these data in part were gathered before the inauguration and full operation of the 1939 law.

[69] Clemmesen 1956.
[70] Denmark. Statistical Department 1952:24.
[71] Oram 1953.
[72] Østergaard 1947, 1948; Oram 1948c; Fenger and Lindhardt 1952; Gille 1952: 177; Oram 1953.
[73] Oram 1953.
[74] Auken 1953:248 ff.

An investigation into maternal deaths in Copenhagen, 1946-1947 (86 cases), showed that 54 per cent had occurred in early pregnancy, and that 61 per cent of these (excluding extra-uterine pregnancies) were associated with illegal abortion or abortion attempts, while another 20 per cent were suicides. The conclusion was that "deaths in early pregnancy make up a large proportion of the total deaths in pregnancy and the puerperium, and that their prevention is rather a social than a purely medical problem."[75]

The approach of these two Scandinavian countries to the problem of unwanted pregnancies is a forthright one, and while Sweden and Denmark are still far from a solution to the social and medical problems involved, it can be said with certainty that they are facing the issue in a realistic fashion.

ABORTION IN ICELAND, FINLAND, AND NORWAY

Iceland, although receiving very little public notice, has had a law allowing therapeutic abortion for social and medical indications for twenty-three years. This little outpost in the north Atlantic was, in fact, the very first of the northern European countries to cope with the problem of enacting an abortion law that would face the question of social and economic indications. Vilm Jónsson, at that time Chief Medical Officer in Iceland, in an account of the 1934 passage of the law by the Althing,[76] described the measure as a compromise between those who would have limited the law to strictest medical indications and those who claimed that social circumstances alone should sometimes justify such an operation.

The law was truly experimental, since it had no prototype in other countries at the time. The medical profession of Iceland supported the new legislation and according to Jónsson welcomed it as a clarification of the existing confusion in regard to when a doctor was justified in interrupting a pregnancy.

The law provided for legal abortions up to six months of pregnancy, with closer restrictions for pregnancies of over two months' duration. The indications listed covered danger to life or health of the mother, with the social considerations that were to be weighed stated in these words: "When estimating how far childbirth may be likely to damage the health of a pregnant woman . . . it may . . . be taken into consideration, whether the woman has already borne many children at short intervals and a short time has passed since her last confinement, also whether her domestic conditions are difficult, either on account of a

---

[75] Kærn 1950.
[76] This account of the abortion law of Iceland, including the direct quotations, is based on Jónsson 1937:220-224.

large flock of children, poverty or serious ill-health of other members of the family."

It appeared that the law, which for the first time in Iceland officially permitted what it called "feticide," actually resulted in a decline of such abortions during the period immediately following its enactment. In the first years of the law 75 per cent of the abortions were for purely medical reasons, while the remaining 25 per cent showed social as well as medical reasons, with poverty, unemployment, and large families specifically mentioned.

Jónsson in an interesting passage described his own change of beliefs on the subject of social indications. He wrote in 1937 that he had originally been in the camp of those who believed social indications alone were sufficient justification for inducing abortion of a pregnancy, but that

> . . . while working and considering the matter in every bearing, I came to the conclusion that estimates of social indications would be so difficult, at least under conditions like those of my country, that the alternative was, in fact, not between medical indication on one side and medical indication plus social indications on the other, but between medical indications and no restrictions at all, with the consequence that any woman could have her fetus destroyed whenever she desired. I do not think that any responsible person would consider this desirable or even practicable. This was the reason for our sticking to medical indication, but the compromise consisted in emphasizing that social indications may be taken into consideration when the medical indications are weighed.

In practice, social indications alone are thus never justification for abortion in Iceland, but "insufficient health indications may justify the measure if there are adequate social reasons as well."

Turning to Finland, we find that up to 1950 there were no provisions in the Finnish legal code for legal abortions, although the use of therapeutic abortions to save the mother's life was the accepted practice by physicians.

The typically rural pattern of culture in Finland over the past years had included approval of pre-marital sex relations for couples intending to marry, as in some other northern European countries.[77] As a concomitant, illegitimate births and births early in marriage were relatively frequent. One third of all marriages in Finland in 1947, for example, showed live births prior to eight months of marriage, with rural areas always ahead of urban figures.[78] In such a situation the

---

[77] Nieminen 1951:404.
[78] See Nieminen 1951:300. Illegitimacy figures are given on pp. 288-294.

single girl who has become pregnant is less likely to be subjected to the social pressures that would lead her to seek an illegal abortion. But the increasing industrialization of Finland has led to more women's finding employment in the urban areas and a shift from the older agrarian economy and culture. A recent four-year study based on absenteeism because of abortion showed the extent to which both married and single women, employed in a municipal establishment, were avoiding the problems of motherhood by obtaining abortions. The figures for total pregnancy loss (spontaneous plus induced abortions) were 83 per cent for the unmarried employees and 50 per cent for the married.[79] In another study, an analysis of the motives of the women involved in 200 cases of criminal abortion showed that almost half of them were related to social problems, and a fourth to ill health; the remainder were classified as medical, conventional, "erotic," eugenic, or ethical in origin.[80]

Concern with such problems led to the passage in 1950 of a law permitting legal abortion for medical, humanitarian, and eugenic reasons, with the hope that it would help to lower illegal terminations of pregnancy.[81] As in Iceland, no purely social indications were recognized in the law, unless one might consider as social the humanitarian classification, which permits a therapeutic abortion for the victim of rape if she is under sixteen.

A first report on abortions done in the Woman's Clinic of Helsinki University for an 18-month period showed a strong increase in therapeutic abortions under the encouragement of the new law.[82] The majority of cases had been referred for physical reasons, with tuberculosis heading the list. About one fifth were done because of mental or nervous conditions, and almost as many for conditions of "exhaustion and debility." Over 15 per cent of the women aborted were single, the remainder were married. While less than 1 per cent of these early Finnish therapeutic abortion cases had serious after-complications, 12 per cent of the total group showed some complications. From this report it appears that the typical method of therapeutic abortion in Finland involves the insertion of a plug (laminaria tent) into the cervical canal as the first stage, with instrumental evacuation following on the second day.[83] The plugs consist of pencils of seaweed, which

---

[79] Rouhunkoski and Olki 1953a:44. This study was based on 1,000 women of childbearing ages, and was derived from the records of the plant gynecologist.
[80] Timonen 1949.
[81] See *Jour. Amer. Med. Assoc.* 1953:574, and Rouhunkoski and Olki 1953b for an account of the Finnish legislation.
[82] Niemineva and Ylinen 1952:44-45.
[83] Niemineva and Ylinen 1952:45.

enlarge in the presence of moisture and gradually dilate the canal. This method of dilation has been in the past widely employed in Europe but has not been popular in this country.[84]

A follow-up study of over 1,000 women who had applied for legal abortion at the Social Consulting Bureau in Helsinki, but whose requests had been refused, showed that 60 per cent of them had completed their pregnancies, and 40 per cent had experienced either spontaneous or illegal abortions. The proportion delivered dropped to 37 per cent in the cases in which the wife was the chief supporter of the family.[85] This same study showed that the medical committee responsible for passing on the applications for legal abortions had rejected over three fourths of the requests that were investigated.

The last of the northern European countries to be covered is Norway, where there is at present no modern legislation in the field of legal abortion. The penal code of 1902 established prison sentences of up to two years for women committing illegal abortion and up to six years for professional abortionists. An official statement from the Department of Justice permits therapeutic abortions on only a strictly medical basis, but it is reported as being broadly interpreted.[86] It is of some interest to note that the agitation for a new, more liberal law has come in part from the Norwegian Medical Association, which as early as 1930 requested a radical revision of the abortion legislation. The various drafts of proposed laws from medical, government, and religious groups apparently resulted in a temporary deadlock on the matter, but new legislation now pending is likely to be somewhat more conservative than that proposed by the medical profession, but generally similar to practices in Sweden and Denmark.

Since 1951 the Maternal Health Clinic, a private social agency supported by municipal tax funds in Oslo, has had a special service for women applying for legal abortion. Counseling is directed toward the basic social as well as the medical problem involved. Psychiatric indications apparently furnish a large part of the medical reasons for abortion in Norway, and represent in the great majority of cases "worn-out housewives'" neurasthenia, a form of depressive exhaustion neurosis.

ABORTION IN ENGLAND

While abortion laws and practices in Great Britain appear to be similar in most respects to those in this country, there has been a

---

[84] See Taussig 1936:188.
[85] Niemineva and Olki 1953, acc. *Int. J. Sexol.* 7:249.
[86] See Dr. Bard Brekke's account at the Planned Parenthood 1955 Abortion Conference, Calderone 1958.

much more concerted movement in England toward their reform and liberalization. To date it has borne little fruit.

Accounts of the early history of the penalties against abortion in England[87] usually point out that induced abortion was originally a religious offense, and that prior to 1803 it was punishable only if done after the time of quickening, that is, after the movements of the embryo had been felt by the mother. This distinction, derived from early ecclesiastical doctrine on when the soul first entered the body of the unborn infant, was continued in the first two English statutory acts dealing with abortion, which were enacted in 1803 and 1828. If the child had quickened, destroying it was a capital offense; otherwise the penalty was imprisonment, transportation, or whipping. In 1837, during Queen Victoria's reign, this distinction was dropped,[88] as was the death penalty. In 1861 the law was extended to cover the case of a woman procuring her own abortion as well as the attempt to induce abortion by a second person, whether it was successful or not.

The present maximum penalty for the mother is life imprisonment, which, according to one English authority, Mr. Glanville Williams, is "one of the most ferocious in the world." He hastens to add that "In practice, however, she is not prosecuted at all."[89] In explanation of this total discrepancy Mr. Williams lists considerations that in some degree are also reflected in U.S. abortion practices, which we discussed in Chapter 8. They are: (1) the necessity of the woman's evidence against the professional abortionist; (2) the difficulty of convincing a jury that self-abortion is a genuine crime; (3) the importance of not deterring the woman, through threat of punishment, from seeking any needed medical aid following an illegal abortion; (4) a growing tendency to regard the crime of abortion as chiefly consisting of the possible injury done the mother by the unskilled abortionist rather than of the loss of the unborn child. Since there are approximately 50 prosecutions for abortion annually in all England, it is clear that few cases reach the courts.[90]

During the 1920's and 1930's the names of English social reformers such as Stella Browne, Dora Russell, Janet Chance, Joan Malleson, and Norman Haire were associated with a plea for greater concern

---

[7] Williams 1957:148 ff., provides a good survey. See also Ministry of Health 1939, Chapter 4, for full details of the development of the English law.

[8] Taylor 1954:58 points out the inconsistency between this new ruling and the British law that did not stay the execution of a pregnant woman until the fourth month of pregnancy.

[9] Williams 1957:153-154.

[0] Williams 1957:210 cited 52 prosecutions for abortion in 1955 as a representative figure and set beside it estimates of from 60,000 to 250,000 illegal abortions a year to point up the ineffectiveness of the law as it stands.

and sympathy for the plight of the pregnant woman, married or single, who was unwilling or felt physically unable to carry her pregnancy through to live birth.[91] In much of the writing there was also the demand for an immediate clarification and broadening of the English abortion law. Lack of adequate contraceptive knowledge was usually blamed for the unwanted pregnancies that led to induced abortions, and the pathetic letters from overburdened mothers pleading for contraceptive information were given wide publicity.[92] Some of the agitation was apparently political in tinge, and in part it was undoubtedly influenced by the Soviet example.

The English abortion law of 1861 made no special provision for therapeutic abortion to save the mother's life,[93] but the Infant Life (Preservation) Act, 1929, allowed for this contingency in the case of the viable fetus, defined as one of 28 weeks' gestation. This meant that abortion for therapeutic purposes was still not recognized if the embryo was less than 28 weeks old. The decision in the landmark case of *Rex v. Bourne* in 1938, by analogy with the 1929 law, extended the principal to include early therapeutic abortion, and also included the mother's mental health as an essential part of her life or of her longevity.[94] Each case, however, was to be considered on its own facts but the decision provided a significant precedent. In the Bourne case a fourteen-year-old girl had been raped by soldiers, and the resulting pregnancy was interrupted by Dr. Aleck Bourne, an obstetric surgeon and gynecologist, who then reported the operation to the authorities thus making a test case of it.

Continued agitation, chiefly by women's groups, led to two reports on abortion by official bodies, the Birkett report on medical aspects of abortion by a committee appointed by the British Medical Association in 1936, and the Report of the Inter-Departmental Committee on Abortion in 1937 under the joint auspices of the Ministry of Health and the Home Office. The latter is a notable pamphlet of over 150

---

[91] See Chance 1931:52-74; Hodann 1937a:213-215; Malleson in Ministry of Health 1939:154; Haire 1950, an account of Norman Haire's experiences with abortion as a young doctor in Sydney, Australia, pointing out the need for abortions to be done by more competent persons under better conditions; Brown 1952. This paper, entitled "The Right of Abortion," was first read at the 1929 Congress of the World League for Sexual Reform held in London. It was reprinted in the final issue of Norman Haire's *Journal of Sex Education* in 1952, following his death.

[92] See Chance 1931:54-57.

[93] Burns 1807:85, in an early British medical treatise on abortion, suggests by its text that therapeutic abortion was practiced, albeit illegally, "when the safety of the mother demands this interference."

[94] For a full exposition of the legal aspects of *Rex v. Bourne* see Williams 1957: 160-183.

pages in which the members of the Committee tried earnestly, as directed, "To enquire into the prevalence of abortion, . . . and to consider what steps can be taken by more effective enforcement of the law or otherwise to secure the reduction of maternal mortality and morbidity arising from this cause."[95]

While the conclusions of the Committee were considered "deeply disappointing, feeble, timid, and highly conservative" by some,[96] the report served the purpose of clarifying the problem by testimony from various points of view and brought the social implications of the subject into clearer focus. Their chief recommendations included: (1) better gathering of statistics on abortion, (2) tighter control of the sale of abortifacient drugs, (3) a somewhat wider dissemination of contraceptive advice by local authorities, (4) the clarification of the scope of therapeutic abortion, (5) measures to relieve the financial strain of childbirth, (6) a more enlightened attitude toward unmarried mothers, (7) wider facilities for pregnancy tests, and (8) adequate medical facilities for abortion care.[97] An extension of contraceptive education to those who wished to limit or space their families rather than only to those whose health would be adversely affected by pregnancy was recommended by two members of the Committee.[98] In a strong minority report, Mrs. Dorothy Thurtle drew attention to the low risks of induced abortion if properly employed, and stated unequivocally that she did not regard abortion induced in the period before the impregnated ovum has become a viable child as taking of life. She also favored the use of legal abortion (before the third month of pregnancy) for cases of rape, incest, and for eugenic reasons. In addition she proposed that any woman who has had four completed pregnancies should have the right to have further pregnancy terminated if she so desired.[99] While the Report of the Abortion Committee has probably had some effect during the eighteen years since it was published, no great changes have occurred. The lawmakers are apparently reluctant to put in statutory form any broadened or clarified legislation on abortion, although such bills have been introduced in Parliament several times, and there has been a continued agitation on the matter.[100]

---

[5] Ministry of Health 1939:vi.
[6] See Wood 1952:33.
[7] Ministry of Health 1939:117-126.
[8] Ministry of Health 1939:127-128.
[9] Ministry of Health 1939:146-151.
[00] See *Manchester Guardian*, October 22, 1955, for a report of a resolution of the Magistrates' Association advocating a change in abortion law pertaining to therapeutic abortion to save the mother's life, to prevent serious injury to her, or to avoid the risk of abnormal offspring.

ABORTION IN GERMANY

Social agitation for more liberal abortion laws in Germany dates back to before 1900. Early "feminists of the Left" were leaders in the movement to make abortion legal or at least to remove the punishment for the act.[101] The target for the attack was the much castigated "Paragraph No. 218," which carried the heart of the bitterly debated law in that it set the penalties for those involved in the illegal abortion. It appears that in the discussion of the question the women actually took over the lead from the church and the medical profession, whose more or less exclusive province such matters had been considered to be. Leading liberal lawyers of the day came to the feminists' support, and as early as 1911 a detailed draft of a proposed law was published that incorporated suggestions for abolishing the penalty for doctors who performed an abortion and for cutting the punishment to as little as a week in jail for others involved.[102]

Much of the discussion, especially that of the women, hinged on the old question of whether the early embryo was a part of the mother's body that she could do with as she saw fit, or whether it had become an animate being starting from the moment of conception. The problem was debated from a legal, moral, and biological point of view.[103] The fact that early canon law as well as civil law in the code established for the Holy Roman Empire by Charles V in 1532 had made distinctions between the inanimate and the animate embryo also gave a basis for the arguments. This code had set forth that the male abortionist of the living fetus should die of the sword, while the woman guilty of such an act should be drowned. The fate of the aborter of the not yet living fetus, it was added, should be decided by those "familiar with the law." This distinction of animation was canceled by Pope Gregory XIV in 1591, but was kept on in the lay law to a much later date, although gradually the principle had gained ground that in either case abortion was a crime, and that the fetus was alive from the time of conception.[104]

---

[101] Havelock Ellis in discussing the women active in the movement for abortion reform in Germany cites the work of Gisela von Streitberg as pioneering and adds the names of Helene Stöcker, Oda Olberg, Elisabeth Zanzinger and Camilla Jellinek. See Ellis 1913:607 and Hodann 1937a:214-215.

[102] See Heinitz 1911:127-130. The lawyers whose various proposals were presented were Professors Kahl, von Liszt, von Lilienthal, and Goldschmidt. Ellis 1913: 608 lists other lawyers such as Hans Gross and Siegfried Weinberg, who were for the more or less complete abolition of punishment for abortion.

[103] See, for example, Weinberg 1905; Menjago 1906; Zanzinger 1907; Papprit 1909; Zimmermann 1912; Werthauer 1921.

[104] See Heinitz 1911:22 and Rech 1950:4.

The much discussed Section 218 was originally established by the German Imperial Laws of 1871. It set a maximum punishment of five years' imprisonment for the woman who brought on an abortion and a minimum of six months under extenuating circumstances. The same penalty was prescribed for anyone aiding her, while a maximum ten-year sentence was set for the professional abortionist who accepted a fee. Therapeutic abortions were not legally provided for. The prolonged and bitter conflict that took place over the effort to change this law was, according to Dr. Taussig, unequaled.[105] He stated that the subject was the topic of "many ardent debates" in the medical societies, and it is evident that the liberal journals and newspapers of the period were full of proposals for revisions and of discussions supporting various points of view. The whole problem became a political issue, and the agitation reached the point where mass meetings were held; and books, novels, and plays were based upon the theme.[106]

Paralleling the agitation protesting the harshness of the law was the fight against criminal abortion itself. Proposals to reduce its reportedly high incidence[107] included occasional demands for stricter enforcement of the law or for compulsory reporting of all abortions, but more commonly suggested remedies were a wider knowledge of contraception, legal sterilization for the eugenically unfit, increased social aid for unmarried mothers, the establishment of broad grounds for official therapeutic abortion, alleviation of unemployment, and the improvement of housing facilities. The Soviet example with its record of low mortality for authorized abortions was often cited as an example to follow.[108]

The severity of the Imperial Law was modified in 1926, but not enough to satisfy those working for a major change. Minimum sentences were reduced to one day for the woman who obtained an

---

[105] Taussig 1936:423.
[106] See Hodann 1937a:229 and Dr. Abraham Stone's discussion in Appendix C of the Planned Parenthood 1955 Abortion Conference, Calderone 1958.
[107] Studies that aroused concern about the spreading practice of illegal abortions in Germany were Hamburger 1908, 1916; Marcuse 1913; Bumm 1916; Nürnberger 1917; and Hirsch 1918. See Tietze 1954:13,21 for a summarization of the statistical sources from which these and later German studies were drawn. Reports in *Sexual-Probleme* 1913, Volume 9, pages 407 and 705, indicate that surveys of doctors were in progress in Düsseldorf and Prussia to determine the causes of the continual increase of induced abortions.
[108] See the following authors for examples of discussions on these topics: Guttzeit 1911 (orig. 1905); Adner 1906; Bloch 1907; Wilhelm 1909; Hirsch 1910; Spier 1912; Vaerting 1917; Schaeffer 1918; Winter 1919:40; Kafemann 1921: 188; Timerding 1926; Riese 1929, 1930; Fürth 1929:53-83; Wolf 1930; Wolff 1931.

abortion, and to three months for the person inducing the abortion.[109]
That the law was being enforced was evident from the official criminal
statistics, which included a listing of convictions for the crime of abortion, but that the convictions were only a small fraction of the cases
that went unpunished was generally acknowledged. The majority of
those sentenced were women, and according to Klauber over 90 per
cent were from a low economic level.[110] The attitude of German doctors
toward the problem of regulating induced abortion during this period
is reflected in a survey conducted by the Hamburg Medical Association. Of the 1,100 physicians in the city, 800 returned the requested
questionnaires. All of them approved of induced abortion to save the
mother's life, and 95 per cent indicated that it should also be used to
protect her health. Almost the same number were in favor of an abortion in the case of a pregnancy resulting from rape, and 80 per cent
approved of social indications being taken into consideration in medically doubtful cases. Over half of those answering approved of the use
of pregnancy interruption when conceptions followed at too short intervals or if there were already four children in the family, while only
40 per cent recommended purely social indications.[111]

When Hitler and the National Socialist party came into power in
1933, the penalties against abortion were made more severe, and in
1943 they were extended to include the death penalty if the guilty
person "had continually impaired the vitality of the German people by
such deeds."[112] At the same time the Nazi regime inaugurated therapeutic indications for abortion, legally recognized in Germany for the
first time.[113] The newly recognized indications were limited to pre-
serving the life or health of the mother and to eugenic indications,
which were administered by the new "hereditary health" courts.

The medical writing of this period is full of praise for the lowering
of the incidence of illegal abortion, both through the stricter law and
also by aids to pregnant women, single and married. Jews and Marxists
were blamed for the exaggerated reports of the number of deaths from
septic abortions in the previous 15 years, which the Nazis claimed had

---

[109] Taussig 1936:424.
[110] See Klauber in Levy-Lenz 1926:151. Hagemann 1933:119, Volume I of the
German Dictionary of Criminology cites over 3,800 convictions for the year
1928 with an occupational breakdown that revealed their widespread nature.
[111] See *Sexus,* April, 1931:46.
[112] See Harmsen 1950:402 and Schönke 1951:504.
[113] That therapeutic abortions had been openly done in the past by doctors on
the basis of clear medical emergencies is evident from various sources. See,
for example, Stumpf in von Winckel 1907 (3):366.

been publicized for the purpose of forcing the legalization of abortion. The rapidly diminishing number of therapeutic abortion permits, less than one tenth of the number granted in the first years of the new law, was cited with pride. According to the published figures illegal abortion shrank to a minimum, for the ratio of total abortions to known pregnancies dropped to as low as 9.9 per 100 in 1940.[114]

With the end of the war, the Control Council Law replaced the German penal code, the death penalty was abolished, therapeutic abortions were retained, but otherwise the general provisions of the 1926 act were reinstated.

It is clear that there is still some agitation to abolish the penalties on illegal abortion in West Germany. It is of interest that the Allied Control Council at one point considered a proposal to establish the legality of abortion for social indications, such as non-marital pregnancies; however, this plan was later abandoned.[115] That current prosecutions are not insignificant can be seen from the West German official criminal statistics. In 1956, over 6,000 persons—72 per cent of them women—were listed as abortion offenders by the police. The 5,400 abortion crimes reported to the German police in that year represented a rate of 10 per 100,000 population.[116] The magnitude of this can best be appreciated if it is translated into figures for our own country. This level of enforcement here would mean that almost 17,000 abortion cases would be officially known to the police each year.[117]

Reports from the Eastern Zone of Germany indicate a more shifting policy in abortion law than in Western Germany. During the period of 1946-1947, Section 218 was still in force, but during the next few years broadened social indications for therapeutic abortion were introduced, and legal abortions reached a peak of 10 to 15 per 10,000 population. From 1951 on, indications for social reasons were again dropped, which led to a rapid decrease in both the requests for abortion and in the percentage of cases approved.[118] One study based on a survey of over 6,000 women from 65 localities in East Germany, between 1946 and 1954, showed a range of from 14 to 19 per cent of all pregnancies lost by induced abortion. The figures showed a steady decrease after

---

[114] For abortion articles of the Nazi period see: Eymer 1939; Dorsch 1939; Philipp 1940; Reichert 1942. See also Tietze 1954:22 for a summary table of registered abortions 1936-1940, a period when the reporting of all abortions was mandatory in Germany.

[115] Rech 1950:16, 17.

[116] Bundeskriminalamt 1957:35 ff.

[117] Compare this to the figure cited in Chapter 8, footnote 18.

[118] Mehlan 1956b.

1950, reflecting, according to the author, the shift in official policy, broadened maternity benefits, and improved economic conditions.[119]

ABORTION IN FRANCE

Severe penalties for the crime of inducing an abortion have a long history in France as in Germany. In the 8th century under Charlemagne it was punishable by death if the period of animation had arrived; this was established at 41 days from conception for the male embryo and at 81 for the female. At the time of Henry II in the 16th century, the death sentence was re-enacted, not primarily for humane reasons, but because the child had been deprived of baptism.[120] Again in the 20th century under the Vichy regime capital punishment was in force, this time against professional abortionists, and abortion was ranked with sabotage and treason.[121]

The text of Article 317 of the French Penal Code, which deals with abortion, was first established by the Napoleonic Code in 1810, and provided for imprisonment with hard labor both for the woman and for the person who procured the abortion for her.[122] In 1864 the law was modified to waive penalties for the woman and for the agent who procured the instruments if the attempt to bring about the abortion was unsuccessful.[123]

In 1920 the law was increased in severity, heavy penalties being added for the act of selling or of offering for sale abortifacient drugs or implements, even if these were not used or were ineffectual.[124] Three years later, however, further amendments reduced the fines and terms of imprisonment in the expectation of fewer acquittals,[125] and also took the cases out of the hands of juries. The punishment for the attempt to procure the abortion of a woman was also established at this point.[126]

In 1939 the French *Code de la Famille* was enacted, and it is still largely in force today. While in the main it followed earlier laws in its provisions on abortion, there were some important additions. For procuring or attempting to procure an abortion for a female believed to be pregnant, the penalty was, as before, one to five years in prison and

[119] Mehlan 1955:4.
[120] Desmeules 1954:24-25.
[121] Watson 1952:267.
[122] Code Pénal 1947:192.
[123] Taussig 1936:424.
[124] Code Pénal 1947:193.
[125] Watson 1952:265 wrote, "But abortion was so generally accepted as justified and the penalties considered so ridiculously harsh, that offenders were frequently acquitted. In an effort, therefore, to remedy this situation . . ."
[126] Code Pénal 1947:192.

a fine of from 30,000 to 600,000 francs; this penalty could be doubled for a habitual abortionist. (The term "habitual" was established by court decisions in 1940-1944 as two successive abortive actions.) The woman who had procured or attempted to procure an abortion, or had consented to make use of the means indicated for that purpose, was subject to six months to two years in prison and to a fine of from 6,000 to 120,000 francs. If a physician or other person employed in the field of medicine or health, such as a drug clerk, a nurse, or a medical student was involved, in addition to the penalty indicated he was debarred from his profession for a minimum of five years.[127]

Article 92 of the new Family Code put a tight control over pregnancy tests. To aid the enforcement of abortion laws, it made more difficult the use of the test by women who wished to obtain an early abortion. This section of the law required that pregnancy tests be executed on a medical prescription blank, which must be transcribed in turn on a numbered registry and countersigned by the mayor or police commissioner, and that the tests be done only by the laboratories authorized by the Ministry of Health. The inscriptions (including name, address, and means of identification) in the registry must be consecutive, without erasures or corrections, and must be entered before the diagnosis is made. Any infraction or fraud of these rules could be punished by three months to two years in prison plus a fine. A laboratory that broke the rules could be closed permanently.[128]

For the first time in France, the 1939 code also allowed for legal therapeutic abortions. The wording of the law was such that it fitted within the framework of the Catholic interpretation. It stated that a therapeutic intervention can be legally indicated, "When the necessity of saving the life of the mother, gravely threatened, demands either a surgical intervention or the use of a therapeutic medium liable to cause interruption of pregnancy. . . ." The attending doctor must then consult and obtain the agreement of two (later of three) other physicians, one of them chosen from an official list of experts.[129]

While the Roman Catholic Church is strongly opposed to induced abortion, including therapeutic abortion as ordinarily defined, it does permit the removal and death of the embryo in particular circumstances. The non-Catholic may be confused by this seeming inconsistency; to a Catholic or a theologian there is no confusion, but simply the operation of the principle of double effect. The principle of double effect depends in essence upon the question of intent. For example,

---

[127] *Ibid.*, 191-194.
[128] *Ibid.*, 195.
[129] *Ibid.*, 194-195.

surgery with the intent to save the life of the pregnant female is good and is permitted even though it involves the unintended death of the embryo. The important thing, from the theological viewpoint, is that the death of the embryo was not intended, but was merely the unfortunate by-product of the intention to save the pregnant female's life.

This principle of double effect is not shaken even in cases where the death of the embryo is known to be the inevitable consequence of medical treatment. Catholic theologians would sharply differentiate between a "direct abortion," wherein the intent was to cause the death of the embryo in order to save the mother's life, and an "indirect abortion," wherein the embryo died as a result of treatment intended to save the mother's life. "Direct abortion" is condemned as murder and is punishable by excommunication; "indirect abortion" is permissible even though the end results are the same.[130] Abortion under the principle of double effect can obviously be done only when the life of the pregnant female is seriously threatened. The Roman Catholic Church does not recognize social, psychiatric, and medical (short of danger of death) indications for abortion.

It does not appear that therapeutic abortion has been used very widely in French hospitals. A report from the Seine district, 1947-1950, showed one such operation to about 700 deliveries.[131] The ratio would certainly show a smaller proportion outside the urban centers. The traditional condemnation of therapeutic abortion is reflected in a statement cited with approval by Fédou 1946:90 that therapeutic abortions were the last gesture in the practice of medicine and surgery retained from barbarism.

With the collapse of France and the inauguration of the Pétain regime, the abortion laws were made extremely stringent during 1940 and 1941. By court decrees the code was extended so that even a nonpregnant woman or one who attempted abortion but was unsuccessful could be held guilty of the crime. Trials were held before a special state court whose judgments were final. Punishment included deportation and life sentences at hard labor, and even death. This final penalty was invoked in February 1942, under the consideration, as in Germany during the Nazi rule, that abortion was an act against the state. One female abortionist was executed.[132] Other severe penalties such as 20 years' hard labor, solitary confinement with hard labor for life, and

---

[130] See Ferreres 1955:161-163; Arregui 1927:141-144; Noldin 1905 (2):346-351; and Davis 1946 (2):166-182.

[131] Desmeules 1954:49.

[132] Madame Giraud, a laundress, who was found guilty of performing 26 abortions, was the sole victim of the death penalty. See Fédou 1946:118 and Watson 1952:286.

deportation with hard labor for life were passed in individual cases of women who had performed abortions on others.

Following the liberation of France in 1944 the death penalty was rescinded, the use of the special state court abolished, and there was a slight relaxation of other regulations. The general repression of abortion was still in effect, however.[133] In spite of such severely implemented laws, it is thought that abortion has been[134] and still is common in France. Various surveys have shown that the women using it are mostly married women who wish to space or to limit their families.[135] With contraception also largely illegal, it is inevitable that women will seek induced abortions if a small family appears to be a necessity.

The position of the Catholic Church on the subject of abortion, the dangerously low birth rate in France, and the depletion of manpower through war losses all combine to make for a strongly vocal official stand against the limitation of families either by contraception or abortion. Economic and political conditions have, however, apparently discouraged fertility. Since 1955 there has been some attempt to arouse public support for more liberal abortion laws, but this effort has not as yet affected the official stand for more restrictive laws and closer enforcement. High mortality figures for illegal abortion have often been cited in the past, from 10,000 to 60,000 deaths a year,[136] but recent reports point out that the use of antibiotics has very much modified these statistics. For 1954 the total deaths associated with pregnancy and delivery were 548 for all of France, and while another 1,723 deaths for women of childbearing ages were classified under "reasons not given or poorly defined," this differed only slightly from the deaths in the same classification for the male population within the same ages.[137]

Estimates of the number of illegal abortions occurring annually in France range from 400,000 to 1,000,000. Most of them, it is suggested, are done by midwives or by medical personnel connected with lying-in establishments.[138] Judges, juries, and popular opinion appear to be

---

[133] Watson 1952:269.
[134] Two early French books on the problems of abortion point this up. Tardieu 1868 presented figures for known criminal abortions for the Seine district and for all of France for 1851 to 1865. About three fourths of the accused were women, and the number of convictions for that period was 604. Larue 1866 in an essay presented an early plea for milder punishment of the unmarried mother and for a change in the law that would permit therapeutic abortion to save a mother's life.
    For later evidences see League of Nations 1930:282.
[135] See Fédou 1946:161; Sutter 1950:86; Watson 1952:274-276.
[136] Bouzat in Besson et al. 1956:296 estimated 10,000 to 20,000 a year, while Watson 1952:282-283 mentioned estimates of from 20,000 to 60,000 a year.
[137] For this report see Population 1956, Vol. 11, p. 220.
[138] Watson 1952:270, 281 and Desmeules 1954:45-46.

much less condemnatory than the official attitude or the laws. That in all classes of society those who excuse abortion are still more numerous than those who condemn it, is regretfully admitted by one author.[139] It seems clear that anti-abortion and anti-conception measures have not worked as hoped for. Many charged with abortion have been acquitted over the past years,[140] and there is no conclusive evidence that abortion has lessened. A special police detail of 12 men was set up in Paris in 1946 to work exclusively on the problem. There have been desperate suggestions for entrapping abortionists by using decoys and for making women register all pregnancies before the third month.[141] It seems clear that past and current government policies in France have failed to produce the results desired in the field of abortion control and population problems.

ABORTION IN LATIN AMERICA

The legal codes of Latin American nations have a common Catholic heritage, and more particularly are derived from the codes of their respective mother countries. Thus many of the statutes of South America are Spanish in origin, while those of Haiti and the Dominican Republic are essentially French. Italian influences are also reflected in various codes.[142] In addition, some of the nations obviously patterned their laws on those of their neighbors. There exists, in consequence, a degree of homogeneity which allows one to generalize about the abortion laws of Latin America.

The majority of codes differentiate sharply between abortions performed with the consent of the woman and those performed without her consent, the latter situation involving heavier penalties for those who procured or performed the abortion.[143] This concern over consent seems a product of the subservient status of women, formerly so marked in Latin America, and one can imagine that there were fairly numerous instances in which the father or brother forced an unmarried daughter or sister to have an abortion in order to preserve the family reputation.

Illegal abortion performed upon a consenting female ordinarily

---

[139] Fédou 1946:159.
[140] The French tradition of judicial leniency toward abortion as evidenced in acquittals, light sentences, suspended sentences, and fines as sole punishment is discussed in Watson 1952:171-172.
[141] Watson 1952:285.
[142] Jiménez de Asúa and Carsi Zacarés 1946 (1):Chapter 2.
[143] For example, Article 304 of the Penal Code of Guatemala calls for five years' imprisonment if the female's consent was lacking, but only one year if consent was given. Ibid., 1340-1341.

entails a minimal sentence of one year and a maximum of three to
four. However, there are some interesting exceptions: Uruguay provides a minimum of six months while Ecuador has a maximum of
five years.[144]

Persons in positions of professional responsibility, such as physicians,
nurses, and pharmacists, are singled out for additional penalties if they
are convicted of being connected with illegal abortion. The imprisonment and fine may be increased by from one sixth (as in Venezuela)
up to one half (as in Paraguay). In addition, the person may be disqualified from practicing his profession for varying lengths of time.
In Bolivia he is disqualified permanently.[145]

Self-induced abortion is nearly always clearly differentiated and
accorded lesser penalties in the legal codes of Latin America. Evidently
legislators gave serious thought to the problems of the woman with an
unwanted pregnancy, and as a result of such detailed consideration the
penalties stipulated vary rather widely from nation to nation. For
example, Article 197 of the Costa Rican Code calls for a minimum
sentence of six months' imprisonment,[146] whereas Article 441 of the
Cuban Code sets a minimum of three months if mitigating factors are
absent. Maximum also varies from one year (Cuba) to five years
(Puerto Rico, Article 267).

A study of what are deemed mitigating circumstances in these countries is most interesting. In keeping with the Latin concepts of family
and personal honor, illegal abortions obtained to preserve honor carry
decreased penalties. The penalty may be decreased by from one third
to two thirds in various nations, and in Colombia the guilty person may
receive a judicial pardon.[147] In Bolivia a woman of good repute who

---

[144] See *ibid.* (2) 776-777, (1) 1260-1261.
[145] See Article 516 of the Bolivian Code, Article 388 of the Colombian Code, Article
331 of the Mexican Federal Code, Article 352 of the Penal Code of Paraguay,
and Article 435 of the Venezuelan Code. These can be found in Jiménez de
Asúa and Carsi Zacarés 1946.
[146] Costa Rica, *Codigo Penal* 1941:45.
[147] For example, Article 330 of the Panamanian Code reads, when translated, "In
the case of an abortion induced to save the honor of the guilty person, of the
woman, her mother, her descendant, her adopted daughter or her sister, the
penalties indicated in the preceding articles will be diminished by from one
third to two thirds. . . . " Article 441 of the Cuban Code stipulates a sentence
of from three months to one year for a self-aborted female, but continues,
"If she commits the deed to hide her dishonor, or because of her poverty,
she will be deprived of her liberty from one month and one day to eight
months." The Colombian Code, Article 389, states, "If the abortion has been
caused to save one's honor or that of the mother, wife, descendant, adopted
daughter or sister, the penalty may be reduced by one half to two thirds, or
judicial pardon may be granted." The above quotations were translated from
the text in Jiménez de Asúa and Carsi Zacarés 1946(2).

obtains an abortion to save her reputation is subject to arrest but apparently is not imprisoned.[148] Illegal abortion of a pregnancy resulting from rape calls for lesser penalties in certain countries such as Uruguay and Cuba. Both nations also recognize economic factors as mitigating circumstances, and Cuba takes special cognizance of abortion in which the woman feared she would transmit a serious disease to the child if she were to carry it to term.[149]

While in parts of the United States and some other countries attempted abortion is penalized, at least two Latin American codes exempt attempted self-induced abortion from any legal sanctions. Article 197 of the Costa Rican Code provides no penalty for attempted self-induced abortion by an unmarried female providing it is her first pregnancy. Argentina apparently dismisses all attempted self-abortions as not punishable by law.[150]

Since most Latin American nations are strongly Roman Catholic, one might expect to find either no provision made for legal abortion or else the most stringent restrictions. However, thus far we have found only two nations, Bolivia and Colombia, that do not specifically recognize legal therapeutic abortion.[151] In Latin America the preservation of the mother's life is the major factor that carries weight in permitting legal abortion, but many codes recognize that serious damage to the woman's health is sufficient grounds for a therapeutic abortion. Other grounds are less commonly recognized: the codes of Brazil, Cuba, Ecuador, Argentina, and some Mexican states mention rape, insanity, and mental deficiency.[152] More purely socio-economic factors are, apparently, not deemed sufficient to justify abortion.

---

[148] Article 517 of the Bolivian Code gives a sentence of from one to two years to the female, "But if the woman is single or a widow, free from corruption and of good reputation previously, and if in the judgment of the judges the only and principal motivation for her action was the desire to cover up her moral lapse, she will be punished only by arrest from one to two years."

[149] See Article 328, Items 2 and 4 of the Code of Uruguay, and Articles 441 and 443 of Cuba.

[150] Mediano et al. 1946:221-224 comment on Article 85, which deals with abortion, and evidently feel that a simple attempt by the female is not punishable. They also quote Article 88, which stipulates the sentence for self-abortion, and which adds, "The attempt by the woman is not punishable."

[151] The lack of provision for therapeutic abortion in Colombia is mentioned by Carranca y Trujillo 1941:335. The absence in the case of Bolivia is understandable since the Bolivian Code in effect (as late as 1946 if not at present) was promulgated in 1834 and was based on the Spanish Code of 1822. See Jiménez de Asúa and Carsi Zacarés 1945 (1):8.

[152] Abortion for pregnancies resulting from rape and for pregnancies conceived by insane females was legalized as early as 1921 by Argentina. Hodann 1937a:231.

It is interesting to note that despite the European origins of the Latin American codes and the dominance of Roman Catholicism in most of the nations, the laws concerning abortion are at various points more liberal than those of the United States, France, and some other countries.

BIBLIOGRAPHY

Abramson, M. 1936. A Study of 2,113 cases given contraception at the Minnesota Birth Control League clinic. Journal-Lancet 56:446-449.

Adair, F. L. 1944. Introductory remarks. *In:* Taylor, H. C., ed. The abortion problem, pp. 58-59.

Adner, H. 1906. Die "Verbrechen" der unehelichen Mutter. Geschl. u. Gesellsch. 1:195-203.

Ärztekammer Schleswig-Holstein. 1956. Schwangerschaftsunterbrechung und Geburtenregelung. Report of Conference, Grenzakademie Sankelmark, Sept. 1-2, 1956.

Alexandrow, W. 1947. Untersuchungen über die Persönlichkeit der passiven Abtreiberin. Bern, Hans Huber.

Amen, J. H. 1944. Some obstacles to effective legal control of criminal abortions. Discussion. *In:* Taylor, H. C., ed. The abortion problem, pp. 134-147.

Aptekar, H. 1931. Anjea. Infanticide, abortion and contraception in savage society. New York, Godwin.

Aristotle. 1932. (Rackham, H., trans.) The politics. London, Heinemann, New York, Putnam.

Arregui, A. M. 1927. Summarium theologiae moralis, ad recentem codicem iuris canonici accommodatum. Bilbao, Spain, El Mensajero del Corazón de Jesús.

Ask-Upmark, E. 1953. Medicinska abortindikationer. Reprint: Svenska Läkartidn. 50:457. 16 p.

Auken, K. 1953. Undersøgelser over unge kvinders sexuelle adfærd. Copenhagen, Rosenkilde & Bagger.

Baldwin, B. T. 1928. The determination of sex maturation in boys by a laboratory method. J. Comp. Psychol. 8:39-43.

Barton, M. 1955. Fertility in women. *In:* Harrison, R. G., ed. Studies on fertility, pp. 99-104.

Batkis, G., and Gurwitsch, L. 1929. Einiges Material über die Sexualreform in der Union der sozialistischen Sowjetrepubliken. *In:* Sex. Ref. Congr., Proceedings of the second congress. Riese, H., and Leunbach, J. H., eds., pp. 37-63.

Baumgartner, L., and Erhardt, C. 1953. Some observations on the factors in the incidence of prematurity and fetal death. *In:* Engle, E. T., ed. Pregnancy wastage, pp. 146-171.

Becker, H., and Hill, R., eds. 1955. Family, marriage and parenthood. Boston, Heath.

Beebe, G. W. 1941. Differential fertility by color for coal miners in Logan County, West Virginia. Milbank Quart. 19:189-195.

1942. Contraception and fertility in the southern Appalachians. Medical aspects of human fertility series issued by the National Committee on Maternal Health. Baltimore, Williams & Wilkins.

Beebe, G. W., and Geisler, M. A. 1942. Control of conception in a selected rural sample. Human Biol. 14:1-20.

Berkusky, H. 1913. Der künstliche Abort bei den Naturvölkern. Sexual-Probl. 9:458-467, 556-567.

Bernard, J. 1956. Remarriage. A study of marriage. New York, Dryden.

Besson, A., et al., eds. 1956. La prévention des infractions contre la vie humaine et l'intégrité de la personne. 2 vols. Paris, Editions Cujas.

Bloch, I. 1907. Neomalthusianismus, sexueller Präventivverkehr, künstliche Sterilität und künstlicher Abort. Geschl. u. Gesellsch. 2:253-267.

Bouzat, P. 1956. Etude sociologique de l'avortement. In: Besson, A., et al., eds. La prévention des infractions contre la vie humaine et l'intégrité de la personne, Vol. 2, pp. 291-325.

Bowman, H. A. 1954. Marriage for moderns. New York, McGraw-Hill.

Brenman, M. 1943. Urban lower-class Negro girls. Psychiat. 6:307-347.

Brezina, E., and Reuterer, V. 1935. Über den Abortus in Österreich. Nach den Berichten der österreichischen Krankenanstalten in den Jahren 1929-1932. Arch. f. Hyg. u. Bakteriol. 114:320-336.

Bromley, D. D., and Britten, F. H. 1938. Youth and sex. A study of 1300 college students. New York, London, Harper.

Browne, F. W. S. 1952. The right of abortion. J. Sex Educ. 5:29-32.

Brunner, E. K. 1941. The outcome of 1556 conceptions. A medical and sociological study. Human Biol. 13:159-176.

Brunner, E. K., and Newton, L. 1939. Abortions in relation to viable births in 10,609 pregnancies. A study based on 4,500 clinic histories. Amer. J. Obstet. & Gynec. 38:82-90.

Bumm, E. 1916. Tagesfragen. Zur Frage des künstlichen Abortus. Mschr. f. Geburtsh. u. Gynäk. 43:385-395.

Bundesrepublik Deutschland. Bundeskriminalamt. 1957. Polizeiliche Kriminalstatistik 1956. Holle, R., ed. Wiesbaden, Author.

Bundesrepublik Deutschland. Statistisches Bundesamt. 1957. Die Abgeurteilten und Verurteilten 1954. Stuttgart, Kohlhammer.

Burch, T. K. 1955. Induced abortion in Japan under eugenic protection law of 1948. Eug. Quart. 2:140-151.

Burgess, E. W. 1944. Social and economic aspects of abortion. Discussion. In: Taylor, H. C., ed. The abortion problem, pp. 115-132.

Burns, J. 1807 (2nd ed.). Observations on abortion: containing an account of the manner in which it takes place, the causes which produce it, and the method of preventing or treating it. London, Longman, Hurst, Rees, & Orme.

Calderone, M. S., ed. 1958. Abortion in the U. S. A. Proceedings of the conference held under the auspices of the Planned Parenthood Federation of America, April and June 1955. New York, Harper. (This volume was in press as the present bibliography was being edited; therefore it has not been possible to cite contributing authors by individual pagination.)

Carmichael, L., ed. 1946. Manual of child psychology. New York, Wiley; London, Chapman & Hall.

Carranca y Trujillo, R. 1941 (2nd ed.). Derecho penál mexicano. Mexico City, José Porrua.

Carr-Saunders, A. M. 1922. The population problem. A study in human evolution. Oxford, Clarendon.

Cecil, R. L., ed. 1951. The specialties in general practice. Philadelphia, London, Saunders.

Chance, J. 1931. The cost of English morals. London, Noel Douglas.

Child, C. G. 1931 (orig. 1922). Sterility and conception. New York, London, Appleton.

Christensen, H. T. 1939. The time-interval between marriage of parents and the birth of their first child in Utah County, Utah. Amer. J. Sociol. 44:518-525.

——— 1950. Marriage analysis. Foundations for successful family life. New York, Ronald.

——— 1953. Studies in child spacing: I—Premarital pregnancy as measured by the spacing of the first birth from marriage. Amer. Sociol. Rev. 18:53-59.

Christensen, H. T., and Meissner, H. H. 1953. Studies in child spacing: III—Premarital pregnancy as a factor in divorce. Amer. Sociol. Rev. 18:641-644.

Clemmesen, C. 1956. State of legal abortion in Denmark. Amer. J. Psychiat. 112:662-663.

Code Pénal [France]. 1947. (Petits codes Dalloz, 44th ed.) Code pénal annoté d'après la doctrine et la jurisprudence avec renvois aux publications Dalloz. Paris, Dalloz.

Coghill, H. de J. 1941. Emotional maladjustments from unplanned parenthood. Va. Med. Monthly 68:682-687.

Collins, J. H. 1951. Abortions—a study based on 1,304 cases. Amer. J. Obstet. & Gynec. 62:548-558.

Coogan, T. F. 1946. Catholic fertility in Florida. Differential fertility among 4891 Florida Catholic families. Cath. Univ. of Amer., Stud. in Sociol., Vol. 20. Washington, D.C., Catholic University of America Press.

Costa Rica. Codigo penal. 1941. San José, National Printing Plant.

Croog, S. H. 1951. Aspects of the cultural background of premarital pregnancies in Denmark. Social Forces 30:215-219.

——— 1952. Premarital pregnancies in Scandinavia and Finland. Amer. J. Sociol. 57:358-365.

Danske Selskab. 1957. (Hagemann, E., trans.) The Danish mothers' aid centres. Review of their history and activities. Copenhagen, Author. Pamphlet.

Davis, A. 1950. 2665 cases of abortion. A clinical survey. Brit. Med. J. 2:123-130.

Davis, F. P. 1923 (2nd ed.). Impotency, sterility, and artificial impregnation. St. Louis, Mosby.

Davis, H. 1946 (5th ed.). Moral and pastoral theology. 4 vols. Vol. 2. Commandments of God. Precepts of the Church. New York, Sheed and Ward.

Davis, K. 1939. Illegitimacy and the social structure. Amer. J. Sociol. 45:215-233.

Davis, K. B. 1929. Factors in the sex life of twenty-two hundred women. New York, London, Harper.

Davis, M. E. 1952. Recent trends in the study of infertility. Ann. N. Y. Acad. Sci. 54:845-863.

Denmark. Statistical Department. 1952. Statistiske Meddelelser, Series 4, Vol. 149, no. 4. Crime statistics, 1950. Copenhagen, Author.

Dennis, W. 1946. The adolescent. In: Carmichael, L., ed. Manual of child psychology, pp. 633-666.

Desmeules, A. 1954. L'avortement et le contrôle des naissances. Aspect médico-social et légal. Lausanne, Payot.

Deutsch, H. 1945. The psychology of women. A psychoanalytic interpretation. 2 vols. Vol. 2, Motherhood. New York, Grune & Stratton.

Devereux, G. 1955. A study of abortion in primitive societies. A typological, distributional, and dynamic analysis of the prevention of birth in 400 pre-industrial societies. New York, Julian.

Dickinson, R. L. 1944. Discussion. In: Taylor, H. C., ed. The abortion problem, pp. 50-53.

Dickinson, R. L., and Beam, L. 1931. A thousand marriages. A medical study of sex adjustment. Baltimore, Williams & Wilkins.

——— 1934. The single woman. A medical study in sex education. Baltimore, Williams & Wilkins.

Diddle, A. W. 1944. The effect of travel on the incidence of abortion. Amer. J. Obstet. & Gynec. 48:354-360.

Dinkel, R. M. 1952. Occupation and fertility in the United States. Amer. Sociol. Rev. 17:178-183.

Dorsch, C. 1939. Erblichkeit, Rassenhygiene und Bevölkerungspolitik. Die Indikationen zur künstlichen Schwangerschaftsunterbrechung im Lichte der alten Regelung und der neuen Gesetzgebung. Münch. med. Wschr. 86: 1155-1161.

Drake, St. C., and Cayton, H. R. 1945. Black metropolis. A study of Negro life in a northern city. New York, Harcourt, Brace.

Drummond, I. 1953. The sex paradox. New York, Putnam.

Dück, J. 1954. Virginität und Ehe. In: Giese, H., and Willy, A., eds. Mensch. Geschlecht. Gesellschaft, pp. 191-200.

Duncan, J. M. 1871 (2nd ed.). Fecundity, fertility, sterility and allied topics. Edinburgh, Black.

Dunlop, J. C. 1914. The fertility of marriage in Scotland: a census study. J. Roy. Statis. Soc. 77:259-288.

Dunn, H. L. 1944. Frequency of abortion. Discussion. In: Taylor, H. C., ed. The abortion problem, pp. 1-14.

Eaton, J. W., and Mayer, A. J. 1953. The social biology of very high fertility among the Hutterites. The demography of a unique population. Human Biol. 25:206-264.

Ebbell, B., ed. and trans. 1937. The papyrus Ebers. The greatest Egyptian medical document. Copenhagen, Levin & Munksgaard, Ejnar Munksgaard. London, Humphrey Milford, Oxford University Press.

Ehrmann, W. 1956. Illegitimacy in Florida. Part II. Social and psychological aspects of illegitimacy. Eug. Quart. 3:223-227.

Ekblad, M. 1955. (Burton, D., trans.) Induced abortion on psychiatric grounds. A follow-up study of 479 women. Acta Psychiat. et Neurol. Scandinav., Supp. 99. Stockholm, Esselte.

Ellis, A. 1951. The folklore of sex. New York, Boni.

Ellis, H. 1913. Studies in the psychology of sex. 6 vols. Vol. 6, Sex in relation to society. Philadelphia, Davis.

Elster, A., and Lingemann, H., eds. 1933. Handwörterbuch der Kriminologie und der anderen strafrechtlichen Hilfswissenschaften. Berlin, Leipzig, Walter de Gruyter.

Engle, E. T., ed. 1953. Pregnancy wastage. Preceedings of a conference sponsored by the Committee on Human Reproduction, National Research Council in behalf of the Committee on Maternal Health, Inc. Springfield, Ill., Thomas.

Erhardt, C. L. 1952. Reporting of fetal deaths in New York City. Pub. Health Rept. 67:1161-1167.

Erhardt, C. L., and Jacobziner, H. 1956. Ectopic pregnancies and spontaneous abortions in New York City. Amer. J. Pub. Health 46:828-835.

Evans, M. 1938. Discussion. In: Van Hoosen, B., Report on maternal mortality and abortion. J. Assoc. Med. Women in India 26:47.

Eymer, H. 1939. Communication. J. Obstet. & Gynaec. 46:86-89.

Fabricius-Møller, J. 1948. Om abortbehandling. Ugeskr. f. Læger 110:813-814.

Fabricius-Møller, J., and Oram, V. 1951. Om tekniken ved legal og illegal svangerskabsafbrydelse. Ugeskr. f. Læger 113:664-669.

1952. Ambulant svangerskabsafbrydelse. Ugeskr. f. Læger 114:485-487.

Farris, E. J. 1956. Human ovulation and fertility. Philadelphia, Lippincott.

Fédou, G. 1946. L'avortement. De sa répression et de sa prévention dans le Code de la Famille et les lois postérieures. Villeurbanne, Marquès.

Fenger, M., and Lindhardt, M. 1952. Om antallet af aborter i Danmark 1940-1950. Ugeskr. f. Læger 114:617-621.

Ferreres, J. B. 1955 (4th ed., Mondría, A., ed.). Epítome de teología moral. Barcelona, Subirana.

Field, A. W. 1932. Protection of women and children in Soviet Russia. New York, Dutton.

Fishbein, M., and Burgess, E. W., eds. 1947. Successful marriage. Garden City, Doubleday.

Fisher, R. S. 1954. Criminal abortion. In: Rosen, H., ed. Therapeutic abortion, pp. 3-11.

Ford, C. S. 1945. A comparative study of human reproduction. New Haven, Yale University Press.

1952. Control of conception in cross-cultural perspective. Ann. N.Y. Acad. Sci. 54:763-768.

Frazier, E. F. 1932. The Negro family in Chicago. Chicago, University of Chicago Press.

1948 (orig. 1939). The Negro family in the United States. New York, Citadel.

1957. Black bourgeoisie. Glencoe, Ill., Free Press, Falcon's Wing Press.

Freedman, R., and Whelpton, P. K. 1950. Part X. Fertility planning and fertility rates by religious interest and denomination. *In:* Whelpton, P. K., and Kiser, C. V., eds. Social and psychological factors affecting fertility, Vol. 2, pp. 417-466.

1952. Part XV. Fertility planning and fertility rates by adherence to traditions. *In:* Whelpton, P. K., and Kiser, C. V., eds. Social and psychological factors affecting fertility, Vol. 3, pp. 675-704.

Fürth, H. 1929. Die Regelung der Nachkommenschaft als eugenisches Problem. Stuttgart, Julius Püttmann.

Fulton, J. F., ed. 1955. A textbook of physiology. Philadelphia, London, Saunders.

Galloway, C. E., and Paul, T. D. 1939. The treatment of early abortion. Amer. J. Obstet. & Gynec. 38:246-255.

Gens, A. 1930. The demand for abortion in Soviet Russia. *In:* Sex. Ref. Congr., Proceedings of the third congress. Haire, N., ed., pp. 143-154.

Giese, H., and Willy, A., eds. 1954. Mensch. Geschlecht. Gesellschaft. Das Geschlechtsleben unserer Zeit gemeinverständlich dargestellt. Paris, Guillaume Aldor.

Gille, H. 1948. Recent developments in Swedish population policy. Population Stud. 2:3-70, 129-184.

1949. The demographic history of the Northern European countries in the eighteenth century. Population Stud. 3:3-65.

1952. Family welfare measures in Denmark. Population Stud. 6:172-210.

Glass, D. V., and Grebenik, E. 1954. The trend and pattern of fertility in Great Britain. A report on the family census of 1946. Papers of the Royal Commission on Population. Vol. 6, Part I. London, Her Majesty's Stationery Office.

Glick, P. C. 1955. The life cycle of the family. Marr. & Fam. Liv. 17:3-9.

1957. American families. New York, Wiley.

Glueck, S., and Glueck, E. 1934. Five hundred delinquent women. New York, Knopf.

Gordon, E. S. 1955. Taking physical factors into account. *In:* Becker, H., and Hill, R., eds. Family, marriage and parenthood, pp. 305-340.

Grabill, W. H. 1955. Progress report on fertility monograph. *In:* Milbank Memorial Fund. Current research in human fertility, pp. 82-92.

Grotjahn, A. 1921. Geburten-Rückgang und Geburten-Regelung. Berlin, Oscar Coblentz.

Guaman Poma de Ayala, F. 1943. (Varallanos, J., ed.) El derecho Inca según Felipe Guaman Poma de Ayala. Lima, Peru, Varallanos.

Gunzert, R., ed. 1953. Statistisches Jahrbuch für Frankfurt am Main, 1952. Statistisches Amt und Wahlamt der Stadt Frankfurt am Main.

Guttmacher, A. F. 1947. Miscarriages and abortions. *In:* Fishbein, M., and Burgess, E. W., eds. Successful marriage, pp. 206-217.

1956. Factors affecting normal expectancy of conception. J. Amer. Med. Assoc. 161:855-860.

Guttmacher, M. S. 1954. The legal status of therapeutic abortions. *In:* Rosen, H., ed. Therapeutic abortion, pp. 175-186.

Guttzeit, J. 1911 (orig. 1905). Ein dunkler Punkt. Das "Verbrechen gegen das keimende Leben" oder die Fruchtabtreibung. Leipzig, Max Spohr (Ferd. Spohr).

Guyon, R. 1936. Etudes d'éthique sexuelle. 6 vols. Vol. 4, Politique rationnelle de sexualité. La reproduction humaine. Saint-Denis, Dardaillon & Dagniaux.

Hagemann, M. 1933. Beruf. *In:* Elster, A., and Lingemann, H., eds. Handwörterbuch der Kriminologie und der anderen strafrechtlichen Hilfswissenschaften, pp. 113-126.

Haire, N. 1947. Soviet Russia and abortion. Marr. Hyg. 1:8-10. 1950. Abortion in Australia. J. Sex Educ. 2:171-176.

Hall, G. S. 1904. Adolescence. Its psychology and its relations to physiology, anthropology, sociology, sex, crime, religion and education. 2 vols. New York, Appleton.

Hamburger, C. 1908. Über den Zusammenhang zwischen Konzeptionszustand und Kindersterblichkeit in grossstädtischen Arbeiterkreisen. Ztschr. f. soz. Med. 3:121-143.
    1916. Beitrag zu der Frage, ob Kinderzahl und Kindersterblichkeit zusammenhängen. Berlin. klin. Wschr. 53:1269-1271.

Hamilton, G. V. 1929. A research in marriage. New York, Boni.

Hamilton, V. C. 1940. Some sociologic and psychologic observations on abortion. Amer. J. Obstet. & Gynec. 39:919-928.

Harmsen, H. 1950. Notes on abortion and birth control in Germany. Population Stud. 3:402-405.

Haro, F. 1934. Concepción y anticoncepción. In: Noguera, E., and Huerta, L., eds. Genética, eugenesia y pedagogía sexual, Vol. 1, pp. 310-366.

Harris, J. A., and Gunstad, B. 1936. The relationship between number of pregnancies and number of births in man. In: Rosendahl, C. O., et al. J. Arthur Harris: botanist and biometrician, pp. 146-158.

Harrison, R. G., ed. 1955. Studies on fertility. Oxford, Blackwell.

Hart, H. 1922. Differential fecundity in Iowa. In: International Neo-Malthusian and Birth Control Conference, Report of the fifth conference. Pierpoint, R., ed., pp. 158-164.

Hartman, C. G. 1931. On the relative sterility of the adolescent organism. Science 74:226-227.

Heffernan, R. J., and Lynch, W. A. 1953. What is the status of therapeutic abortion in modern obstetrics? Amer. J. Obstet. & Gynec. 66:335-345.

Heinitz, A. 1911. Die Straftaten wider das keimende Leben. Leipzig, Spamer.

Hellman, L. M. 1951. Obstetrics. In: Cecil, R. L., ed. The specialties in general practice, pp. 355-415.

Henningsen, E. J., Skalts, V., and Hoffmeyer, H. 1952. Mødrehjælpen og abortus provocatus problemet siden svangerskabsloven af 1939. Ugeskr. f. Læger 114:502-510.

Henripin, J. 1954. La fécondité des ménages canadiens au début du XVIIIe siècle. Population 9:61-84.

Henry, L. 1951. Etude statistique de l'espacement des naissances. Population 6:425-444.
    1953. Fécondité des mariages. Nouvelle méthode de mesure. I.N.E.D. Travaux et Documents, Cahier no. 16. Paris, Presses Universitaires de France.

Hertig, A. T., and Livingstone, R. G. 1944. Spontaneous, threatened and habitual abortion: their pathogenesis and treatment. N. Eng. J. Med. 230:797-806.

Hertig, A. T., and Rock, J. 1949. A series of potentially abortive ova recovered from fertile women prior to the first missed menstrual period. Amer. J. Obstet. & Gynec. 58:968-993.

Hertig, A. T. and Sheldon, W. H. 1943. Minimal criteria required to prove prima facie case of traumatic abortion or miscarriage. An analysis of 1000 spontaneous abortions. Ann. Surgery 117:596-606.

Hertz, H., and Little, S. W. 1944. Unmarried Negro mothers in a southern urban community. Social Forces 23:73-79.

Hertzler, J. O. 1956. The crisis in world population. Lincoln, University of Nebraska Press.

Hinrichsen, S. 1952. Abortus provocatus in Copenhagen. Int. J. Sexol. 6:53.

Hirsch, M. 1910. Über Fruchtabtreibung. Sexual-Probl. 6:375-384.
    1911. Review: Weissenberg, 100 Fehlgeburten, ihre Ursachen und Folgen. Sexual-Probl. 7:220-221.
    1918. Part II. Zur Statistik des Aborts. Zentralbl. f. Gynäk. 42:758-769.

Hodann, M. 1937a. (Browne, S., trans.) History of modern morals. London, Heinemann.
1937b. A prosecution for abortion in Denmark. Marr. Hyg. 3:202-203.
Holmes, R. W., et al. 1929. Factors and causes of maternal mortality. J. Amer. Med. Assoc. 93:1440-1446.
Hudson, G., and Rucker, M. P. 1945. Spontaneous abortion. J. Amer. Med. Assoc. 129:542-544.
Human Fertility. 1941. A study of the abortion practice in New York. 6:184-187.
Hyman, H. T. 1946. An integrated practice of medicine. 5 vols. Philadelphia, London, Saunders.
Inghe, G. 1947. The abortion problem in Sweden. Human Fertil. 12:40-45.
International Neo-Malthusian and Birth Control Conference. 1922. Report of the fifth conference, London, July 1922. Pierpoint, R., ed. London, Heinemann.
International Planned Parenthood Federation. 1955. The fifth international conference on planned parenthood. Theme: Overpopulation and family planning. Report of the proceedings. Tokyo, Japan, 24-29 October, 1955. London, Author.
Jacobsen, J. 1932. Seksualreform. En social fremstilling af populær seksualoplysning. Copenhagen, Funkis.
Javert, C. T. 1957. Spontaneous and habitual abortion. New York, London, Blakiston, McGraw-Hill.
Jiménez de Asúa, L., and Carsi Zacarés, F. 1946. Codigos penales iberoamericanos. Estudio de legislación comparada. 2 vols. Caracas, Andrés Bello.
Johnson, W. O. 1931. Two years' résumé: abortion in Louisville City Hospital. Amer. J. Obstet. & Gynec. 22:778-782.
Johnwick, E. B. 1952. The control of gonorrhea. The problem. In: Public Health Service. Digest, Venereal Disease Control Seminar. Seattle, Washington, June 1952, pp. 14-16.
Jónsson, V. 1937. The Icelandic birth control and feticide act. J. Contracep. 2:219-224.
Journal of the American Medical Association. 1953. Foreign letters. Finland. Legal induction of abortion. 151:574.
Journal of Obstetrics and Gynaecology of the British Empire. 1939. The prohibition of abortion in the Soviet Socialist Republics. 46:89-90.
Journal of Venereal Disease Information. 1948. Statistics. 29:29.
Kærn, T. 1950. Dødeligheden i tilslutning til tidlig graviditet. Ugeskr. f. Læger 112:787-790.
Kälvesten, A. n. d. [1953?]. The social structure of Sweden. [Stockholm], Author. Mimeo. 75 p.
Kafemann, [?]. 1921. Gesetzliche Freigabe der freiwilligen künstlichen Frühgeburt. Geschl. u. Gesellsch. 10:112-129, 161-168, 185-198, 233-238.
Kammerer, P. G. 1918. The unmarried mother. Boston, Little, Brown.
Kinsey, A. C., Pomeroy, W. B., and Martin, C. E. 1948. Sexual behavior in the human male. Philadelphia, London, Saunders.
Kinsey, A. C., Pomeroy, W. B., Martin, C. E., and Gebbard, P. H. 1953. Sexual behavior in the human female. Philadelphia, London, Saunders.
Kiser, C. V. 1935. Fertility of Harlem Negroes. Milbank Quart. 13:273-285.
1939. Voluntary and involuntary aspects of childlessness. Milbank Quart. 17:50-68.
1942. Group differences in urban fertility. A study derived from the National Health Survey. Baltimore, William & Wilkins.
1956. Review: Third public opinion survey on birth control in Japan. Population Problems Research Council. Amer. J. Sociol. 62:348.
Kiser, C. V., and Whelpton, P. K. 1944. Social and psychological factors affecting fertility. Part II. Variations in the size of completed families of 6,551 native-white couples in Indianapolis. Milbank Quart. 22:72-105.
1950. Part IX. Fertility planning and fertility rates by socio-economic status.

In: Whelpton, P. K., and Kiser, C. V., eds. Social and psychological factors affecting fertility, Vol. 2, pp. 359-415.

Kitagawa, E. M. 1953. Differential fertility in Chicago, 1920-40. Amer. J. Sociol. 58:481-492.

Klauber, L. 1926. Die Abtreibung. *In:* Levy-Lenz, L., ed. Sexual-Katastrophen, pp. 107-170.

Kleegman, S. J. 1954. Planned parenthood: its influence on public health and family welfare. *In:* Rosen, H., ed. Therapeutic abortion, pp. 254-265.

Koguchi, Y. 1955. The prevalence of induced abortion in present-day Japan. *In:* International Planned Parenthood Federation. The fifth international conference . . . , pp. 231-234.

Koos, E. L. 1953. Marriage. New York, Holt.

Kopp, M. E. 1933. Birth control in practice. Analysis of ten thousand case histories of the Birth Control Clinical Research Bureau. New York, McBride.

Koya, Y. 1954. A study of induced abortion in Japan and its significance. Milbank Quart. 32:282-293.

———. **1957.** Family planning among Japanese on public relief. Eug. Quart. 4:17-23.

Koya, Y., et al. 1955. A survey of health and demographic aspects of reported female sterilizations in four health centers of Shizuoko Prefecture, Japan. Milbank Quart. 33:368-392.

Kuczynski, R. R. 1938. Childless marriages. Sociol. Rev. 30:120-144, 213-235, 346-364.

Kummer, J. M. 1953. Psychiatric contraindications to pregnancy, with reference to therapeutic abortion and sterilization. Calif. Med. 79:31-35.

Landis, J. T., et al. 1950. The effects of first pregnancy upon the sexual adjustment of 212 couples. Amer. Sociol. Rev. 15:766-772.

Larue, E. de V. 1866. Essai sur l'avortement considéré au point de vue du droit criminel, de la médecine légale et de la responsabilité médicale lorsqu'il est provoqué par le médecin pour le salut de la mère. Paris, Adrien Delahaye.

League of Nations. 1930. Monthly epidemiological report of the health section of the Secretariat. R. E. 140. Maternal mortality, pp. 279-306.

Leunbach, J. H. 1931. A new abortus provocatus method. *In:* Sanger, M., and Stone, H. H., eds. The practice of contraception, pp. 183-189.

Levy, D. 1955. A follow-up study of unmarried mothers. Social Casework 36:27-33.

Levy-Lenz, L. 1931. A new non-operative method for the interruption of pregnancy. *In:* Sanger, M., and Stone, H. M., eds. The practice of contraception, pp. 180-183.

Levy-Lenz, L., ed. 1926. Sexual-Katastrophen. Bilder aus dem modernen Geschlechts-und Eheleben. Leipzig, Payne.

Lewis-Faning, E. 1949. Report on an enquiry into family limitation and its influence on human fertility during the past fifty years. Papers of the Royal Commission on Population. Vol. 1. London, His Majesty's Stationery Office.

Lips, J. 1947. Naskapi law. Trans. Amer. Phil. Soc. 37: Part IV.

Lorimer, F., et al. 1954. Culture and human fertility. A study of the relation of cultural conditions to fertility in non-industrial and transitional societies. Paris, Zurich, UNESCO.

Mac-Lean y Estenós, R. 1942. Sociología peruana. Lima, Peru, Gil.

Malleson, J. 1939. A suggestion for lessening the incidence of criminal abortion. *In:* Ministry of Health. Report of the inter-departmental committee on abortion, pp. 152-155.

Manchester Guardian, October 22, 1955.

Mandy, A. J. 1954. Reflections of a gynecologist. *In:* Rosen, H., ed. Therapeutic abortion, pp. 284-296.

Marcuse, M. 1913. Zur Frage der Verbreitung und Methodik der willkürlichen

Geburtenbeschränkung in Berliner Proletarierkreisen. Sexual-Probl. 9:752-780.

Mayer, A., and Klapprodt, C. 1955. Fertility differentials in Detroit: 1920-1950. Population Stud. 9:148-158.

Mazer, C., and Israel, S. L. 1951 (3rd ed.). Diagnosis and treatment of menstrual disorders and sterility. New York, Hoeber.

Meaker, S. R. 1934. Human Sterility. Baltimore, Williams & Wilkins.

Mediano, J. M., et al., eds. 1946. Leyes penales comentadas . . . de la República Argentina Buenos Aires, Losada.

Mehlan, K. H. 1955. Abortstatistik und Geburtenhäufigkeit in der Deutschen Demokratischen Republik. Das Dt. Gesundheitsw. 10: 1648-1659.

1956a. Spätfolgen nach legalem Abort. Das Dt. Gesundheitsw. 11:876-880.

1956b. Die Schwangerschaftsunterbrechungen in der Deutschen Demokratischen Republik in den Jahren 1946/1950. In: Ärztekammer Schleswig-Holstein. Schwangerschaftsunterbrechung und Geburtenregelung, pp. 22-27.

Menjago, H. 1906. Verbrechen gegen die Leibesfrucht. Geschl. u. Gesellsch. 1:558-566.

Menken, H. P., and Lansman, H. H. 1940. The results in treatment of 600 incomplete abortions. Amer. J. Obstet. & Gynec. 40:1011-1017.

Metraux, A. 1946. Ethnography of the Chaco. In: Steward, J., ed. Handbook of South American Indians, Vol. 1, pp. 197-370.

Metropolitan Life Insurance Company. Statistical Bulletin, October 1956. The birth rate: Recent trends and outlook. 37:1-3.

Milbank Memorial Fund. 1955. Current research in human fertility. Papers presented at the 1954 annual conference of the Milbank Memorial Fund. New York, Author.

Millar, W. M. 1934. Human abortion. Human Biol. 6:271-307.

Ministry of Health. Home Office. 1939. Report of the inter-departmental committee on abortion. London, His Majesty's Stationery Office.

Mondat, V. 1844 (trans. from the 5th French ed.). On sterility in the male and female, its causes and treatment. New York, Redfield.

Montagu, M. F. A. 1946. Adolescent sterility. A study in the comparative physiology of the infecundity of the adolescent organism in mammals and man. Springfield, Ill., Thomas.

Moore, J. G., and Randall, J. H. 1952. Trends in therapeutic abortion. A review of 137 cases. Amer. J. Obstet. & Gynec. 63:28-40.

Moses, B. L. 1936. Contraception as a therapeutic measure. Baltimore, Williams & Wilkins.

Muramatsu, M. 1955. Recent trends in induced abortion and sterilization in Japan. In: International Planned Parenthood Federation. The fifth international conference . . . , p. 230.

Murdock, G. P. 1949. Social structure. New York, Macmillan.

Naiditch, [?], et al. 1935. Ginek. i. Akusherstvo 6:71, acc. J. Contracep. 1936. The after-effects of abortion. 1:167-168.

Nakatsu, Y. 1955. Survey of induced abortion in Japan. In: International Planned Parenthood Federation. The fifth international conference . . . , pp. 234-235.

National League for Sex Education. 1949. The National League for Sex Education. Stockholm, Author. Pamphlet.

Nelson, N. A., and Crain, G. L. 1938. Syphilis, gonorrhea and the public health. New York, Macmillan.

New York City, Department of Health, Bureau of Records and Statistics. n.d. [1954]. No title. Mimeo. 19 p.

n.d. [1955.] No title. Mimeo. 8 p.

New York Herald Tribune, October 25, 1956.

New York Times, November 23, 1955.

Newberger, C. 1946. An analysis of the obstetric activities in hospitals of Cook County during 1944. Amer. J. Obstet. & Gynec. 51:372-386.

Nieminen, A. 1951. Taistelu sukupuolimoraalista. Porvoo, Helsinki, Werner Söderström Osakeyhtiö.

Niemineva, K., and Olki, M. 1953. Eripainos Aikakauskirjasta, Dec. 11, acc. Int. J. Sexol. 1954. Observations on women who were refused requested abortion. 7:249-250.

Niemineva, K., and Ylinen, O. 1952. The new law concerning therapeutic abortion in Finland. Int. J. Sexol. 6:43-46.

Noguera, E., and Huerta, L., eds. 1934. Genética, eugenesia y pedagogía sexual. 2 vols. Madrid, Javier Morata.

Noldin, H. 1905. Summa theologiae moralis. 3 vols. Vol. 2. De praeceptis et ecclesiae. Innsbruck, Rauch.

Nordlinger, G., and Murray, L. 1943. The contraceptive service of the George Washington University School of Medicine. A study of 2000 cases. Human Fertil. 8:56-58.

Norrlands-Posten, May 21, 1955.

Notestein, F. W., and Kiser, C. V. 1935. Factors affecting variations in human fertility. Social Forces 14:32-41.

Nürnberger, L. 1917. Die Stellung des Abortus in der Bevölkerungsfrage. Mschr. f. Geburtsh. u. Gynäk. 45:23-39.

Okasaki, A. 1952. Le problème et la politique démographiques au Japon. Population 7:207-226.

Olow, J. 1947. Några erfarenheter om den svenska abortlagen. Menneske og Miljø 4:155-161.

Olson, H. J., et al. 1943. The problem of abortion. Amer. J. Obstet. & Gynec. 45:672-678.

Oram, V. 1948a. Om abortbehandling. Ugeskr. f. Læger 110:724-728.
    1948b. Bidrag til teknikken ved svangerskabsafbrydelse. Ugeskr. f. Læger 110:731-734.
    1948c. Om antallet af kriminelle aborter. Ugeskr. f. Læger 110:734-738.
    1949a. Abortbehandling. Reprint: Nordisk Med. 41:1027. 11 p.
    1949b. Abortdødeligheden i Danmark 1940-46. Ugeskr. f. Læger 111:201-204.
    1951. Om risikoen ved legal svangerskabsafbrydelse. Ugeskr. f. Læger 113:73-78.
    1952. Dødsårsag og dødelighed ved legal svangerskabsafbrydelse i årene 1940-50 i Danmark. Ugeskr. f. Læger 114:482-485.
    1953. De kriminelle aborters antal. Fortsatte undersøgelser. Ugeskr. f. Læger 115:1367-1369.

Østergaard, E. 1947. Aborthyppighed og abortprofylaxe. Ugeskr. f. Læger 109:883-887.
    1948. Om spontane og kriminelle aborter. Ugeskr. f. Læger 110:812-813.
    1949. The treatment of abortions, with special reference to the value of sulfonamide in febrile cases. Reprint: Acta Obstet. & Gynec. 28. 15 p.

Ottesen-Jensen, E. 1955. The National League for Sex Education, Sweden. In: International Planned Parenthood Federation. The fifth international conference . . . , pp. 313-314.

Panchaud, A. 1951. Code pénal suisse annoté. Lausanne, Payot.

Pappritz, A. 1909. Die Vernichtung des keimenden Lebens. Sexual-Probl. 5:491-498.

Parish, T. N. 1935. One thousand cases of abortion. J. Obstet. & Gynaec. Brit. Emp. 42:1107-1121.

Parry, L. A. 1932. Criminal abortion. London, J. Bale & Danielssohn.

Pasche-Oserski, N. 1929. Sexualstrafrecht in der Sowjetunion. In: Sex. Ref. Congr., Proceedings of the second congress. Riese, H., and Leunbach, J. H., eds., pp. 228-239.

Pearl, R. 1937. Fertility and contraception in New York and Chicago. J. Amer. Med. Assoc. 108:1385-1390.

1939. The natural history of population. London, Oxford University Press.

Peckham, C. H. 1936. Abortion. A statistical analysis of 2287 cases. Surg., Gynec. & Obstet. 63:109-115.

Peller, S. 1931. Abortus und Geburtenrückgang. Med. Klinik 27: 847-849.

Pemberton, L. 1955 (orig. 1948). The stork didn't bring you. New York, Nelson.

Philipp, E. 1940. Der heutige Stand der Bekämpfung der Fehlgeburt. Zentralbl. f. Gynäk. 64:225-255.

Pirkner, E. H. 1927. Praktische Erfahrungen über Präventivverkehr. Ztschr. f. Sexualwiss. 14:17-20.

Ploscowe, M. 1955. The truth about divorce. New York, Hawthorn.

Pommerenke, W. T. 1955. Abortion in Japan. Obstet. & Gynec. Survey 10:145-175.

Popenoe, P. 1946. Modern marriage. New York, Macmillan.

Population. 1956. La limitation des naissances en France. 11:209-345.

Population Bulletin. 1956. "Children in spite of ourselves." France struggles with a dilemma. 12:109-126.

Powdermaker, H. 1933. Life in Lesu. The study of a Melanesian society in New Ireland. New York, Norton.

Pritchard, J. B., ed. 1950. Ancient Near Eastern texts relating to the Old Testament. Princeton, N. J., Princeton University Press.

Public Health Service. 1952. Digest, Venereal Disease Control Seminar, Region X, Seattle, Washington, June 24-25, 1952. Washington, D. C., Author.

Pugh, W. S. 1935. The dangers of abortion. Pop. Med. 1:649-652.

Rech, H. 1950. Kampf dem §218. Lauf b/Nürnberg, Zitzmann. Pamphlet.

Reichert, F. 1942. Über die Häufigkeit der Fehlgeburten. Archiv f. Gynäk. 173:266-273.

Riese, H. 1929. Schwangerschaftsunterbrechung im Lichte medicin. Zeitfragen. In: Sex. Ref. Congr., Proceedings of the second congress. Riese, H., and Leunbach, J. H., eds., pp. 289-293.

1930. Die soziale Indikation zur Unterbrechung der Schwangerschaft. In: Sex. Ref. Congr., Proceedings of the third congress. Haire, N., ed., pp. 219-232.

Rock, J., and Loth, D. 1949. Voluntary parenthood. New York, Random House.

Rönne-Petersen, E. 1951. Provrörsmänniskan. Stockholm, Biopsykologi.

Rohden, F. v. 1956. Die Entwicklung der legalen Schwangerschaftsunterbrechung im Bundesgebiet im ersten Nachkriegsjahrzehnt. In: Ärztekammer Schleswig-Holstein. Schwangerschaftsunterbrechung und Geburtenregelung, pp. 7-21.

Rolph, C. H. 1955. Women of the streets. A sociological study of the common prostitute. London, Secker & Warburg.

Rongy, A. J. 1933. Abortion: legal or illegal? New York, Vanguard.

Rosen, H., ed. 1954. Therapeutic abortion. Medical, psychiatric, legal, anthropological and religious considerations. New York, Julian.

Rosendahl, C. O., et al. 1936. J. Arthur Harris: botanist and biometrician. Minneapolis, University of Minnesota Press.

Rouhunkoski, M., and Olki, M. 1953a. Sickness absenteeism due to criminal abortions. Int. J. Sexol. 7:44.

1953b. Therapeutic abortion in Finland. Int. J. Sexol. 7:81-82.

Rubin, I. C. 1931. Sterility secondary to induced abortion with special reference to the tubal factor. N. Y. State J. Med. 31:213-217.

Russell, K. P. 1951. Therapeutic abortion in a general hospital. Amer. J. Obstet. & Gynec. 62:434-438.

1952. Therapeutic abortions in California in 1950. West. J. Surg. Obstet. & Gynec. 60:497-502.

Sanger, M., and Stone, H. M., eds. **1931.** The practice of contraception. An international symposium and survey. Baltimore, Williams & Wilkins.
Schaeffer, R. 1918. Die Anmeldepflicht jeder Fehlgeburt. Dt. med. Wschr. 44:548.
Schlesinger, R. 1949. Changing attitudes in Soviet Russia. 2 vols. Vol. 1. The family in the U. S. S. R. London, Routledge & Kegan Paul.
Schönke, A. 1951. Strafgesetzbuch. Kommentar. Munich, Berlin, Beck.
Schou, P., and Østergaard, E. 1954. Abortus provocatus ved extraovulær injection af cremor saponis. *In:* Förhandlingar vid Nordisk Förenings för Obstetrik och Gynekologi Kongress i Göteborg, pp. 178-184.
Sexual Reform Congress. 1929. Proceedings of the second congress, Copenhagen, July 1928. Riese, H., and Leunbach, J. H. eds. Copenhagen, Levin & Munksgaard; Leipzig, Thieme.
  1930. Proceedings of the third congress, London, September 1929. Haire, N., ed. London, Kegan Paul, Trench, Trubner.
Sexual-Probleme. 1913. Untersuchung über Fehlgeburten. 9:407-408. Ministerial-Erlass an die Ärzte-Kammern Preussens betr. Fruchtabtreibung und Geburten-Rückgang. 9:705-706.
Sexus, Internationale Monatsschrift für Sexualwissenschaft u. Sexualreform. 1931. Wie verhalten sich die Aerzte zur Abtreibungsfrage? 1:46.
Sherwin, R. V. 1949. Sex and the statutory law. Part I and Part II. A comparative study and survey of the legal and legislative treatment of sex problems. New York, Oceana.
Siegler, S. L. 1944. Fertility in women. Philadelphia, London, Lippincott.
Simmons, F. A. 1951. Diagnosis and treatment of the infertile male. *In:* Monographs on surgery, pp. 267-307. New York, Nelson.
  1954. The diagnosis and treatment of the infertile female. Springfield, Ill., Thomas.
Simons, J. H. 1939. Statistical analysis of one thousand abortions. Amer. J. Obstet. & Gynec. 37:840-849.
Sjövall, T. 1953. Legal abortion and family counselling. Int. J. Sexol. 7:83-84.
Skidmore, R. A., and Cannon, A. S. 1951. Building your marriage. New York, Harper.
Sontheimer, M. 1955. Abortion in America today. Reprint: Woman's Home Companion, October 1955. New York, Planned Parenthood Federation of America. 3 p.
Soviet Union. Great medical encyclopedia. 1956 (2nd. ed., Bakulev, A. N., et al., eds.). Abortion, Vol. 1, cols. 21-47. Moscow, State Publishing House of Medical Literature.
Speert, H., and Guttmacher, A. F. 1956. Obstetric practice. New York, Landsberger.
Spier, I. 1912. Sozial-sexuelle Krisen. Geschl. u. Gesellsch. 7:439-449.
Steward, J. H., ed. **1946.** Handbook of South American Indians. 6 vols. Vol. 1. The marginal tribes. Smithsonian Institution, Bureau of American Ethnology. Bulletin 143. Washington, D.C., U.S.G.P.O.
Stewart, R. E. 1935. An analysis of 1,772 abortions and miscarriages with a consideration of treatment and prevention. Amer. J. Obstet. & Gynec. 29:872-875.
Stix, R. K. 1935. A study of pregnancy wastage. Milbank Quart. 13:347-365.
  1938. The medical aspects of variations in fertility. Amer. J. Obstet. & Gynec. 35:571-580.
  1940. Factors underlying individual and group differences in uncontrolled fertility. Milbank Quart. 18:239-256.
  1941. Contraceptive service in three areas. Part I. The clinics and their patients. Milbank Quart. 19:171-188.
Stix, R. K., and Notestein, F. W. 1940. Controlled fertility. An evaluation of clinic service. Baltimore, Williams & Wilkins.

Stix, R. K., and Wiehl, D. G. 1938. Abortion and the public health. Amer J. Pub. Health 29:621-628.

Stone, H. M., and Hart, H. 1932. Maternal health and contraception. A study of the social and medical data of 2,000 patients from the Maternal Health Center, Newark, N.J. Newark, Maternal Health Center. Pamphlet.

Storer, H. R., and Heard, F. F. 1868. Criminal abortion. Its nature, its evidence, and its law. Boston, Little, Brown.

Strandskov, H. H., and Einhorn, S. 1948. On the relation between age of mother and percentage of stillbirth in the total, the "white" and the "colored" U.S. populations. Amer. J. Phys. Anthrop. n. s. 6:187-198.

Studdiford, W. E. 1950. The common medical indications for therapeutic abortion. Bull. N. Y. Acad. Med. 26:721-735.

Stumpf, M. 1907. Die Schwangerschaft in ihrer Bedeutung für die gerichtliche Medizin. In: Winckel, F. von, ed. Handbuch der Geburtshülfe, Vol. III, Part 3, pp. 340-402.

Sullivan, K. 1956. Girls on parole. Boston, Houghton Mifflin.

Sutherland, I. 1949. Stillbirths. Their epidemiology and social significance. London, New York, Toronto, Oxford University Press.

Sutter, J. 1950. Résultats d'une enquête sur l'avortement dans la région Parisienne. Population 5:77-102.

    1955. Le movement dans le monde en faveur de la limitation des familles (1945-1954). Population 10:277-294.

Svanberg, N. 1949. Senkomplikationer vid legal abortprovokation. Nordisk Med. 42:1264-1268.

Sweden, Statistika Centralbryån, 1945. Folkräkningen den 31 December 1945. Vol. 7, no. 2.

Swedish Population Commission. 1940. (Hamilton, V. C., trans.) Report on the sex question. Baltimore, Williams & Wilkins.

Swyer, G. I. M. 1954. Reproduction and sex. London, Routledge & Kegan Paul.

Sydenstricker, E. 1932. A study of the fertility of native white women in a rural area of western New York. Milbank Quart. 10:17-32.

Taeuber, I. 1956. Fertility and research in Japan. Milbank Quart. 34:129-149.

Tappan, P. W. 1947. Delinquent girls in court. A study of the Wayward Minor Court of New York. New York, Columbia University Press.

Tardieu, A. 1868. Etude médico-légale sur l'avortement . . . Paris, Baillière.

Taussig, F. J. 1931. The abortion problem in Russia. Amer. J. Obstet. & Gynec. 22:134-139.

    1936. Abortion. Spontaneous and induced. Medical and social aspects. St. Louis, Mosby.

    1944. Effects of abortion on the general health and reproductive function of the individual. In: Taylor, H. C. ed. The abortion problem, pp. 39-48.

Taylor, G. R. 1954. Sex in history. New York, Vanguard.

Taylor, H. C., ed. 1944. The abortion problem. Proceedings of the conference held under the auspices of the National Committee on Maternal Health, Inc. Baltimore, Williams & Wilkins.

Terman, L. M. 1938. Psychological factors in marital happiness. New York, London, McGraw-Hill.

Thurtle, D. 1939. Minority report. In: Ministry of Health, Report of the inter-departmental committee on abortion, pp. 139-151.

Tietze, C. 1943. Differential reproduction in the United States. Paternity rates for occupational classes among the urban white population. Amer. J. Sociol. 49:242-247.

    1948. Abortion as a cause of death. Amer. J. Pub. Health 38:1434-1441.

    1049. Report on a series of illegal abortions induced by physicians. Human Biol. 21:60-64.

    1952. The clinical effectiveness of contraception. Reprint from: The third international conference on planned parenthood. Report of the proceedings. Bombay. 6 p.

1953. Introduction to the statistics of abortion. *In:* Engle, E. T., ed. Pregnancy wastage, pp. 135-145.

1954. Chapter III. Pregnancy wastage. *In:* United Nations. Foetal, infant and early childhood mortality, pp. 12-28.

1955. Maternal mortality associated with legal abortion. *In:* International Planned Parenthood Federation. The fifth international conference . . . , pp. 238-240.

1957. Reproductive span and rate of reproduction among Hutterite women. Fertil. & Steril. 8:89-97.

Tietze, C., et al. 1950a. Unintentional abortion in 1497 planned pregnancies. J. Amer. Med. Assoc. 142:1348-1350.

1950b. Time required for conception in 1727 planned pregnancies. Fertil. and Steril. 1:338-346.

Tietze, C., and Grabill, W. H. 1957. Differential fertility by duration of marriage. Eug. Quart. 4:3-7.

Tietze, C., and Lauriat, P. 1955. Age at marriage and educational attainment in the United States. Population Stud. 9:159-166.

Tietze, C., and Lewit, S. 1953. Patterns of family limitation in a rural Negro community. Amer. Sociol. Rev. 18:563-564.

Tietze, C., and Martin, C. E. 1957. Fœtal deaths, spontaneous and induced, in the urban white population of the United States. Population Stud. 11:170-176.

Time, October 19, 1936; July 28, 1941; March 6, 1944.

Timerding, H. E. 1926. Zum Problem der ledigen Frau. Ztschr. f. Sexualwiss. 13:210-224.

Timonen, S. 1949. Possibilities of preventing criminal abortion in the light of analysis of motive. Ann. Chir. et. Gynec. Fenniae 38: Supplem't 3, 484-494.

Trolle, D. 1950. Legal abortus provocatus. Ugeskr. f. Læger 112:779-787.

Truex, R. O. 1936. The size of family in three generations. Amer. Sociol. Rev. 1:581-591.

United Nations. 1949. Demographic yearbook, 1948. New York, Author.

United Nations. Department of social affairs, Population division 1954. Foetal, infant and early childhood mortality. Vol. 1. The statistics. Population studies, no. 13. New York, Author.

United Nations. Monthly Bulletin of Statistics. October 1957.

U. S. Bureau of the Census. 1945-1946. Judicial criminal statistics, 1944. Series J-13. Washington, D.C., U.S.G.P.O.

U. S. Bureau of the Census. Current Population Reports. Series P-20. June 30, 1948, no. 18. Fertility: April 1947.

March 28, 1956, no. 65. Fertility of the population: April 1954.

U.S. Bureau of the Census. 1953. U.S. census of population: 1950. Vol. 4, Special Reports, Part 3, Chapter B, Nonwhite population by race. Washington, D.C., U.S.G.P.O.

1955. U.S. census of population: 1950. Vol. 4, Special Reports, Part 5, Chapter C, Fertility. Washington, D.C., U.S.G.P.O.

1956. U.S. census of population: 1950. Vol. 4, Special Reports, Part 1, Chapter B, Occupational characteristics. Washington, D.C., U.S.G.P.O.

U.S. Department of Labor. Children's Bureau. 1934. Maternal mortality in fifteen states. Publication no. 223. Washington, D.C., U.S.G.P.O.

U.S. Vital Statistics. 1954. Vital Statistics of the United States 1950. 3 vols. Vol. 1, Analysis and summary tables with supplemental tables for Alaska, Hawaii, Puerto Rico, and Virgin Islands. U.S. Department of Health, Education and Welfare, National Office of Vital Statistics. Washington, D.C., U.S.G.P.O.

1957. Vital statistics of the United States 1955. 2 vols. Vol. 1, Introduction and summary tables. U.S. Department of Health, Education, and Welfare, National Office of Vital Statistics. Washington, D.C., U.S.G.P.O.

U.S. Vital Statistics—Special Reports. National Summaries. **1955.** Vol. 42, no. 11, pp. 247-265. Natality: Each state and territory, and specified possessions, 1953.

No. 12, pp. 269-278. Maternal mortality: Each state and territory, and specified possessions, 1953.

No. 13, pp. 281-294. Births by age of mother, race, and birth order: United States, 1953. U.S. Department of Health, Education, and Welfare, National Office of Vital Statistics. Washington, D.C. U.S.G.P.O.

1956. Vol. 42, no. 16, pp. 344-357. Fetal deaths: Each state and territory, and specified possessions, 1953.

Vol. 44, no. 6, pp. 104-133. Marriages: Detailed statistics for reporting areas, 1954.

No. 14, pp. 314-324. Maternal mortality: United States and each state, and Alaska, Hawaii, Puerto Rico, and the Virgin Islands (U.S.), 1954. U.S. Department of Health, Education, and Welfare, National Office of Vital Statistics. Washington, D.C., U.S.G.P.O.

U.S. Vital Statistics—Special Reports. Selected Studies. **1950.** Vol. 33, no. 5, pp. 70-106. Illegitimate birth statistics: United States, 1938-47. Federal Security Agency, National Office of Vital Statistics. Washington, D.C., U.S.G.P.O.

1956. Vol. 39, no. 7, pp. 303-429. Mortality from selected causes by marital status, United States, 1949-51. U.S. Department of Health, Education, and Welfare, National Office of Vital Statistics. Washington, D.C., U.S.G.P.O.

Vaerting, M. **1917.** Über den Einfluss des Krieges auf Präventivverkehr und Fruchtabtreibung und seine eugenischen Folgen. Ztschr. f. Sexualwiss. 4:137-144.

Van Hoosen, B. **1938.** Report on maternal mortality and abortion. J. Assoc. Med. Women in India 26:28-60.

Vernier, C. G. **1931.** American family laws. A comparative study of the family law of the forty-eight American states, Alaska, the District of Columbia, and Hawaii (to Jan. 1, 1931). 5 vols. Vol. 1. Introductory survey and marriage. Stanford University, Calif., Stanford University Press.

Vögel, [?]. **1928.** Wird die Fruchtbarkeit der Frau durch Aborte beeinträchtigt? Archiv f. Frauenkunde 14:189-198.

Wangson, O., et al. **1951.** Ungedomen möter samhället. Ungdomsvårdskommitténs slutbetänkande. Statens offentlige Utredningar: 41. Stockholm, Beckmans.

Watkins, R. E. **1933.** A five-year study of abortion. Amer. J. Obstet. & Gynec. 26:161-172.

1936. Abortion deaths. Adjunct report no. 1. West. J. Surg. Obstet. & Gynec. 44:338-342.

Watson, C. **1952.** Birth control and abortion in France since 1939. Population Stud. 5:261-286.

Webster, R. C., and Young, W. C. **1951.** Adolescent sterility in the male guinea pig. Fertil. and Steril. 2:175-181.

Weinberg, S. **1905.** Die Vernichtung des keimenden Lebens. Mutterschutz 1:312-319.

Werthauer, J. **1921.** Die Abtreibung. Geschl. u. Gesellsch. 10:228-232.

Westman, A. **1955.** The problem of abortion in Sweden. In: International Planned Parenthood Federation. The fifth international conference . . . , pp. 235-238.

Whelpton, P. K. **1944.** Frequency of abortion. Its effects on the birth rates and future population of America. *In:* Taylor, H. C., ed. The abortion problem, pp. 15-38.

1954a. Cohort fertility. Native white women in the United States. Princeton, N.J., Princeton University Press.

1954b. Future fertility of American women. Eug. Quart. 1:4-17.

1956. Too many people in the world? U.S. News and World Report, July 13, 80-91.

Whelpton, P. K., and **Kiser, C. V. 1943.** Social and psychological factors affecting fertility. Part I. Differential fertility among 41,498 native-white couples in Indianapolis. Milbank Quart. 21:221-280.

1950. Part VI. The planning of fertility. Part VIII. The comparative influence on fertility of contraception and impairments of fecundity. *In:* Whelpton, P. K., and Kiser, C. V., eds. Social and psychological factors affecting fertility, Vol. 2, pp. 209-257; 303-357.

Whelpton, P. K., and **Kiser, C. V.,** eds. **1950, 1952, 1954.** Social and psychological factors affecting fertility. 4 vols. Vol. 2, The intensive study. Purpose, scope, methods, and partial results. Vol. 3, Further reports on hypotheses in Indianapolis. Milbank Quart. 21:221-280.

other data from the Indianapolis study. New York, Milbank Memorial Fund.

Whitehead, J. 1848. On the causes and treatment of abortion and sterility. Philadelphia, Blanchard & Lea.

Whitehouse, B. 1929. Abortion. Its frequency and importance. Brit. Med. J. 2:1095-1099.

Wiehl, D. G. 1938. A summary of data on reported incidence of abortion. Milbank Quart. 16:80-88.

Wiehl, D. G., and **Berry, K. 1937.** Pregnancy wastage in New York City. Milbank Quart. 15:229-247.

Wikman, K. R. V. 1937. Die Einleitung der Ehe. Acta Academiae Aboensis. Humaniora XI.1. Åbo, Åbo Akademi.

Wilhelm, E. 1909. Die Abtreibung und das Recht des Arztes zur Vernichtung der Leibesfrucht. Sexual-Probl. 5:321-339, 426-443.

Williams, E. H., and **Thorner, R. M. 1956.** Illegitimacy in Florida. Part I. Reported illegitimate births in Florida, 1917-1953. Eug. Quart. 3:219-223.

Williams, G. 1957. The sanctity of life and the criminal law. New York, Knopf.

Wilson, D. C. 1954. The abortion problem in the general hospital. *In:* Rosen, H., ed. Therapeutic abortion, pp. 189-197.

Winckel, F. von, ed. **1903-1907.** Handbuch der Geburtshülfe. 3 vols. Wiesbaden, Bergmann.

Winter, G. 1919. Der künstliche Abort. Denkschrift für die praktischen Ärzte. Berlin, Schoetz.

Wisconsin Legislative Committee. 1914. Report and recommendations of the Wisconsin legislative committee to investigate the white slave traffic and kindred subjects. Madison, Wis., State of Wisconsin.

Witherspoon, J. T. 1933. An analysis of 200 cases of septic abortion treated conservatively. Amer. J. Obstet. & Gynec. 26:367-374.

Wolf, J. 1930. Mutter oder Embryo? Zum Kampf um den Abtreibungs-Paragraphen. Berlin, C. Heymann. Pamphlet.

Wolff, F. 1931. Im Namen des Volkes! (Fort mit dem §218). Sexus, Internatl. Mschr. f. Sexualwiss. u. Sexualref. 1:23-25.

Wolff, P. de, and **Meerdink, J. 1957.** (Zajicek, J., and Pressat, R., trans.) La fécondité des mariages à Amsterdam selon l'appartenance sociale et religieuse. Population 12:289-318.

Wood, R. 1952. Abortion 1929-1952. J. Sex Educ. 5:33-34.

Young, L. 1954. Out of wedlock. A study of the problems of the unmarried mother and her child. New York, Toronto, London, McGraw-Hill.

Zanzinger, E. 1907. Verbrechen gegen die Leibesfrucht. Beiträge zur Frage der Fruchtabtreibung. III. Paragraph 218. Geschl. u. Gesellsch. 2:206-228.

Zeitschrift für politische Psychologie und Sexualökonomie. 1935. Ein Abtreibungsprozess in Dänemark. 2:61-64.

Zimmermann, P. 1912. Das Verbrechen wider das keimende Leben. Geschl. u. Gesellsch. 7:450-463.

INDEX

All numbers refer to pages. Names of individuals are *italicized*. The letters T and F refer to material in Tables and Figures respectively.